MEDICALLY
REFRACTORY
REST
ANGINA

edited by
DOUGLASS ANDREW MORRISON

Veterans Affairs Medical Center and
University of Colorado Health Sciences Center
Denver, Colorado

PATRICK W. SERRUYS

Interuniversity Cardiological Institute
of The Netherlands and
Erasmus University
Rotterdam, The Netherlands

Marcel Dekker, Inc.   New York • Basel • Hong Kong

Library of Congress Cataloging-in-Publication Data

Medically refractory rest angina / edited by Douglass Andrew Morrison,
  Patrick W. Serruys.
       p.   cm.
   Includes bibliographical references and index.
   ISBN 0-8247-8630-0 (alk. paper)
   1. Angina pectoris.   I. Morrison, Douglass Andrew.
 II. Serruys, P. W.
      [DNLM: 1. Angina, Unstable--therapy.   WG 298 M489]
   RC685.A6M43   1992
   616.1'22-dc20
   DNLM/DLC
   for Library of Congress   91-46938
                                                              CIP

This book is printed on acid-free paper.

MARCEL DEKKER, INC.
270 Madison Avenue, New York, New York 10016

Current printing (last digit):
10 9 8 7 6 5 4 3 2 1

PRINTED IN THE UNITED STATES OF AMERICA

Foreword

Unlike other well-known syndromes in cardiovascular medicine—such as heart failure, sudden death, asymptomatic hypertension, and many others—unstable angina is a curious paradox. On the one hand, it is a serious condition of enormous proportions: in the United States approximately 750,000 patients with unstable angina are admitted to hospitals each year; countless others are treated at home. On the other, despite intensive study, unstable angina remains a wastebasket of diagnoses and there is considerable controversy regarding its management. Despite some efforts to provide more precise definitions and classifications, there is no consensus regarding precisely which clinical syndromes should be included under the general heading of unstable angina. Not surprisingly, the natural history of this condition appears to be influenced importantly by whether or not the patient's ischemia occurs at rest, whether it develops shortly after a myocardial infarction, whether it occurs despite intense treatment of myocardial ischemia, and whether it is accompanied by transient electrocardiographic changes. Insofar as the management of unstable angina is concerned, many cardiologists recommend medical therapy, that is, anti-ischemic measures, aspirin, and/or heparin, sometimes followed by cardiac catheterization, with a view to carrying out mechanical revascularization in those patients with lesions that appear particularly hazardous, but only after they "cool off." Others take a much more aggressive approach and move rapidly to catheterization and, in a large majority of patients, revascularization. There is widespread agreement that patients with unstable angina who are *refractory* to medical therapy should be revascularized whenever possible, but again there is no consensus regarding the relative roles of percutaneous transluminal coronary angioplasty as opposed to coronary bypass surgery.

This book makes a valuable contribution by attempting to bring order out of chaos. First, it provides a detailed, but eminently readable review of the varied clinical picture and natural history of unstable angina. Next, it provides an up-to-date exposition of the complex pathogenesis of this condition, as well as a detailed and thoughtful analysis of experiences with various treatment options.

iii

Finally, it proposes and ably defends a clinical trial in patients with medically refractory angina.

This excellent book is strongly recommended to the many physicians, invasive cardiologists, and surgeons who are called upon to care for patients with unstable angina, to trainees in cardiology, and to the rapidly increasing number of investigators interested in the design of cardiovascular clinical trials.

Eugene Braunwald, M.D.
Harvard Medical School and
Brigham and Women's Hospital
Boston, Massachusetts

Preface

This book arose from a dream. The dream was of a Veterans Affairs cooperative trial to compare percutaneous transluminal coronary angioplasty (PTCA) with coronary artery bypass graft (CABG) surgery in the care of patients with unstable angina. The Department of Veterans Affairs Cooperative Studies Program has approved and funded planning meetings for this study (VA Cooperative 385) and the participants for the meetings have been drawn from the contributors of this book. As such, the book has already helped the dream to become a reality.

Unstable angina is one of the most common and most difficult management problems in contemporary cardiology and internal medicine. The difficulty is compounded by problems in establishing concise, objective clinical definitions. Definitional issues plague not only the management of individual patients but also the design, conduct, and interpretation of clinical studies, which will permit us to provide better care in the future. Accordingly, the first task of the book has been to tackle definitional issues. Chapter 1 attempts to define "unstable angina"; Chapter 7 addresses "medically refractory"; Chapters 17–19 tackle "assisted" angioplasty and surgery; and Chapter 20 defines "high risk" and "prohibitive risk" for PTCA and CABG.

Another task of this book has been to bridge the gap between contemporary developments and their application to practical therapeutics. Chapters 3 and 4 summarize two recent pathophysiological insights, namely the unstable plaque and endothelial cell function, and their respective therapeutic implications.

The prospective, randomized trial is the most powerful tool available with which to assess therapeutic efficacy. Chapter 2 attempts to put the randomized trial in context by discussing where it fits among clinical studies and what some of its limitations are. With these factors in mind, much of the remainder of the book reviews the types of data, but prospective trial data in particular, which are available to support medical, surgical, or angioplasty options for unstable angina patients.

For academic physicians and health care planners, it is hoped that the book will help to more sharply focus management questions about unstable angina. For practicing cardiologists, internists, generalists, and surgeons, the book is intended to highlight controversies by placing them against the background of what is considered clear. For physicians and health care personnel in training, as well as aficionados of medical history, it is intended to emphasize that "not all the answers are in yet" and some of the ways in which "accepted treatment" changes.

We would like to thank all the contributors, our secretaries Trish Kent and Yvonne Lacock, and Elaine Grohman and all of the staff at Marcel Dekker, Inc.

This book is dedicated to the cardiologists, surgeons, and physicians in training, but mostly to the veteran patients who will make VA Cooperative 385 not only a reality but hopefully a contribution to the care of patients with unstable angina.

Douglass Andrew Morrison
Patrick W. Serruys

Contents

Foreword   Eugene Braunwald   *iii*

Preface   *v*

Contributors   *xi*

Part I: Introduction

1. Unstable Angina: Definition and Scope of the Problem   3
   Douglass Andrew Morrison

2. Unstable Angina: Design, Conduct, and Interpretation
   of Clinical Studies   33
   Douglass Andrew Morrison

Part II: Pathophysiology

3. The Unstable Plaque   41
   John A. Ambrose, Douglas H. Israel, and Sabino R. Torre

4. The Role of Endothelial Injury in Acute Coronary Events
   and Coronary Restenosis   59
   Lawrence D. Horwitz

5. Summary of Pathophysiology of Unstable Angina: Relevance
   to Therapeutic Options   69
   Douglass Andrew Morrison

Part III: Medical Therapy for Unstable Angina

6. Medical Therapy for Unstable Angina Supported by Controlled
   Studies   81
   H. Daniel Lewis, Jr.

7. What Constitutes Medically Refractory?   105
   Douglass Andrew Morrison

Part IV: Surgical Therapy for Unstable Angina

8. Veterans Administration Cooperative Study Comparing Medical
   and Surgical Therapy for Unstable Angina   121
   Stewart M. Scott, Robert J. Luchi, and Robert H. Deupree

9. National Cooperative Study of Unstable Angina   145
   Gary D. Plotnick

10. The Veterans Affairs Surgical Registry: Identification of the
    High-Risk Surgical Patient   157
    Frederick L. Grover

11. Surgery for Unstable Angina Pectoris   183
    Karl E. Hammermeister

Part V: Coronary Angioplasty for Unstable Angina

12. Percutaneous Transluminal Coronary Angioplasty in Patients
    with Unstable Angina: Historical Perspectives, Mayo Clinic
    Experience, and the BARI Study   215
    Malcolm R. Bell and David R. Holmes, Jr.

13. Coronary Angioplasty for Unstable Angina   237
    Pim J. de Feyter, Harry Suryapranata, and Patrick W. Serruys

14. Coronary Angioplasty in Patients with Unstable Angina
    and Depressed Left Ventricular Function   253
    Germano Di Sciascio and George Vetrovec

15. Coronary Angioplasty for Early Postinfarction Angina   269
    *Harry Suryapranata, Pim J. de Feyter, and Patrick
    W. Serruys*

16. Percutaneous Balloon Angioplasty of Saphenous Vein Bypass
Grafts: A Clinical and Morphological Review   293
Cass A. Pinkerton and Bruce F. Waller

Part VI: Bridge Techniques for Revascularization

17. Assisted Angioplasty: Adjuvant Techniques in Coronary
Angioplasty   317
Carl L. Tommaso and Robert A. Vogel

18. Pharmacological Support of Angioplasty in Unstable Angina   337
Paul T. Vaitkus and Warren Laskey

19. Bridging Techniques to Emergent Surgical Revascularization
After Failed Angioplasty   361
David William Nelson and Alden H. Harken

20. Summary of "High Risk" and "Prohibitive Risk" for Surgery
or Angioplasty in Unstable Angina   385
Douglass Andrew Morrison

Part VII: Summary and the Case for a Randomized Trial

21. The Internal Mammary Artery Experience: Can Nonrandomized
Observational Studies Substitute for the Randomized,
Controlled Clinical Trial?   405
William G. Henderson

22. New Methods of Catheterization Assessment: Will They
Change PTCA Practice in Unstable Angina Patients?   419
Douglass Andrew Morrison

23. Summary of Contemporary Care of the Unstable Angina
Patient and Proposal for a Prospective, Randomized Trial
of PTCA Versus CABG in Rest Angina   429
Douglass Andrew Morrison

Index   *453*

Contributors

John A. Ambrose, M.D., F.A.C.C. Director, Cardiac Catheterization Laboratory, and Professor of Medicine, Mount Sinai Medical Center, New York, New York

Malcolm R. Bell, M.B., B.S., F.R.A.C.P. Special Clinical Fellow, Division of Cardiovascular Diseases and Internal Medicine, and Assistant Professor of Medicine, Mayo Clinic and Mayo Foundation, Rochester, Minnesota

Pim J. de Feyter, M.D., F.E.S.C., F.A.C.C. Catheterization Laboratory, Thoraxcenter, University Hospital Rotterdam-Dijkzigt, and Erasmus University, Rotterdam, The Netherlands

Robert H. Deupree, Ph.D. Biostatistician, Veterans Affairs Medical Center, West Haven, Connecticut

Germano Di Sciascio, M.D., F.A.C.C. Associate Professor of Medicine (Cardiology), Department of Internal Medicine, Medical College of Virginia Hospitals, Virginia Commonwealth University, Richmond, Virginia

Frederick L. Grover, M.D. Chief, Department of Surgery, Veterans Affairs Medical Center, Denver, Colorado

Karl E. Hammermeister, M.D., F.A.C.C. Chief, Cardiology, Department of Veterans Affairs Medical Center, and Professor of Medicine, University of Colorado School of Medicine, Denver, Colorado

Alden H. Harken, M.D. Professor and Chairman, Department of Surgery, University of Colorado Health Sciences Center, Denver, Colorado

William G. Henderson, M.P.H., Ph.D. Chief, Cooperative Studies Program Coordinating Center, Veterans Affairs Hospital, Hines, Illinois

David R. Holmes, Jr., M.D., F.A.C.C. Professor of Medicine, Mayo Medical School, and Director, Adult Cardiac Catheterization Laboratory, Mayo Clinic, Rochester, Minnesota

Lawrence D. Horwitz, M.D., F.A.C.C. Professor of Medicine (Cardiology), Department of Medicine, University of Colorado Health Sciences Center, Denver, Colorado

Douglas H. Israel, M.D. Clinical Instructor in Medicine, Department of Medicine, Mount Sinai Medical Center, New York, New York

Warren Laskey, M.D., F.A.C.C. Director of Research, Cardiac Catheterization Laboratory, Department of Medicine, Hospital of the University of Pennsylvania and University of Pennsylvania School of Medicine, Philadelphia, Pennsylvania

H. Daniel Lewis, Jr., M.D. Chief, Cardiology Section, Veterans Affairs Medical Center, Kansas City, Missouri, and Professor of Medicine, University of Kansas School of Medicine, Kansas City, Kansas

Robert J. Luchi, M.D. Professor and Chief, Section of Geriatrics, Department of Medicine, Baylor College of Medicine and Veterans Affairs Medical Center, Houston, Texas

Douglass Andrew Morrison, M.D., F.A.C.C. Director, Cardiac Catheterization Laboratory, Veterans Affairs Medical Center, and Associate Professor (Cardiology), Department of Internal Medicine, University of Colorado Health Sciences Center, Denver, Colorado

David William Nelson, M.D. Chief Resident, Department of Surgery, University of California, Davis, Sacramento, California

Cass A. Pinkerton, M.D., F.A.C.C. Director, Interventional Cardiology, St. Vincent Hospital and Health Care Center, Indianapolis, Indiana

Gary D. Plotnick, M.D., F.A.C.C. Professor of Medicine, University of Maryland School of Medicine, and Associate Professor of Medicine, The Johns Hopkins University School of Medicine, Baltimore, Maryland

Stewart M. Scott, M.D. Consulting Professor of Surgery, Duke University Medical Center, and Chief, Surgical Service, Veterans Affairs Medical Center, Asheville, North Carolina

Patrick W. Serruys, M.D., Ph.D., F.E.S.C., F.A.C.C. Professor of Interventional Cardiology, Interuniversity Cardiological Institute of The Netherlands, and Thoraxcenter, Erasmus University, Rotterdam, The Netherlands

Harry Suryapranata, M.D., Ph.D., F.E.S.C. Catheterization Laboratory, Thoraxcenter, University Hospital Rotterdam-Dijkzigt, and Erasmus University, Rotterdam, The Netherlands

Carl L. Tommaso, M.D., F.A.C.C. Associate Professor of Medicine, Northwestern University Medical School, and Chief, Section of Cardiology, Veterans Administration Lakeside Medical Center, Chicago, Illinois

Sabino R. Torre, M.D. Fellow in Cardiology, Mount Sinai Medical Center, New York, New York

Paul T. Vaitkus, M.D. Fellow in Cardiology, Cardiology Section, Hospital of the University of Pennsylvania and University of Pennsylvania School of Medicine, Philadelphia, Pennsylvania

George Vetrovec, M.D., F.A.C.C. Professor of Medicine, Medical College of Virginia Hospitals, Virginia Commonwealth University, Richmond, Virginia

Robert A. Vogel, M.D., F.A.C.C. Head, Division of Cardiology, and Herbert Berger Professor of Medicine, Department of Medicine, University of Maryland Hospital, Baltimore, Maryland

Bruce F. Waller, M.D., F.A.C.C. Clinical Professor of Pathology and Medicine, Indiana University School of Medicine, Director, Cardiovascular Pathology Registry, St. Vincent Hospital, and Cardiologist, Nasser, Smith and Pinkerton Cardiology, Inc., The Indiana Heart Institute, Indianapolis, Indiana

MEDICALLY
REFRACTORY
REST
ANGINA

I
INTRODUCTION

1

Unstable Angina: Definition and Scope of the Problem

Douglass Andrew Morrison

Veterans Affairs Medical Center and
University of Colorado Health Sciences Center
Denver, Colorado

INTRODUCTION

It is axiomatic that to solve a problem, one must be able to adequately define the problem. The first thesis upon which this book has been developed is that unstable angina is a common and vexing clinical problem (1–12). The second thesis is that much of the difficulty in solving the problem derives from difficulties in developing precise clinical definitions. Definitional issues have hampered the design and interpretation of clinical studies aimed at solving the problem (1–28).

SUBJECTIVE SYMPTOMS

The entry point into the broad category (or, as Plotnick has described, "umbrella of syndromes") described as unstable angina is with patients' symptoms (12). Symptoms are of necessity subjective. Three broad categories of symptoms fall under this general umbrella (Tables 1–7) (13–250). One is angina, or chest discomfort, that occurs at rest. The first source of difficulty with this particular syndrome is certainty that the resting symptom is myocardial ischemic in origin. The second potential problem is that myocardial ischemia may manifest itself with other symptoms or "anginal equivalents" rather than chest pain. An example is dyspnea. The third and final problem with this particular subset of rest angina is that we now know many episodes of myocardial ischemia are

Table 1 Unstable Angina: Natural History Studies

First author	Ref	Symptom			Required				
		Rest angina	New onset	Progressive	ECG	Coronary anatomy	Post MI included	Med Rx	Med refractory
Vakil	33	+	−	−	+	−	−	−	−
Vakil	34	+	−	−	+	−	−	−	−
Krauss	35	+		−	−	−	−	−	−
Gazes	37	+	+	+	−	−	−	±	
Conti	38	+	±	±	+	+	+	+	±
Bertolasi	39	+	+	±	±	+	−	+	±
Duncan	40	±	±	±	−	−	−	−	−
Heng	41	+	±	±	−	−	−	±	−
Day	42	+	±	+	+	+	−	+	−
Mulcahy	43	±	±	±	+	−	−	−	−
Olson	44	+	−	−	−	−	−	±	−
Roberts	45	−	+	−	−	+	−	±	−
Schroeder	46	+	±	±	+	−	−	±	−
Schroeder	47	+	±	±	+	−	−	±	−
Lopes	48	+	±	±	+	−	−	±	−
Skjaeggestad	49	+	±	±	+	−	−	−	−
Gottlieb	25	±	±	±	+	−	−	+	±
Nedamanee	27	±	±	±	+	−	−	+	+
Wilcox	26	+	−	+	−	−	−	+	−
Scanlon	101	−		+	−	±	−	+	−
Wood	36	+	+	+	−	−	−	−	−
Resnik	104	+	+	+	−	−	−	±	−
Levy	106	+	+	+	−	−	−	−	−
Feil	109	+	+	−	±	−	−	+	−
Fischl	110	+	−	−	+	±	−	±	±
Fulton	146	+	+	+	−	−	−	−	−
Kannel	147	+			+	−	−	±	−
Scheidt	108	+	−	−	−	−	−	−	−

silent, or unaccompanied by symptoms. Preliminary data from a variety of sources suggest that this may have the same functional and pathophysiological consequences and perhaps prognostic significance as rest angina and/or angina equivalent (25–27).

A second category of subjective symptoms under the general umbrella of unstable angina is a change in pattern of angina. In this case a patient with typical exertional angina of a given frequency experiences either an increase in frequency or a significant diminution in the provocation required to elicit the symptom. This category is less likely to overlap with nonischemic syndromes than rest angina. The reason for this is that a patient with typical exertional angina is so highly likely to have significant coronary disease as an etiological factor. On the

Table 2 Unstable Angina: Pathophysiology

First author	Ref	Symptom			Required				
		Rest angina	New onset	Progressive	ECG	Coronary anatomy	Post MI included	Med Rx	Med refractory
Maseri	17	+	−	±	+	−	−	+	−
Sherman	18	+	−	+	−	+	−	+	±
Neill	19	±	+	+	±	+	−	+	±
Falk	20	+	−	−	−	−	−	+	− died
Horie	22	+	−	+	+	−	−	+	− died
Kruskal	23	+	−	−	±	−	−	±	−
Figueras	24	+	−	−	+	±	−	±	−
Beamish	31	+	+	+	−	−	−	−	−
Sampson	32	+	−	+	±	−	−	−	
Guazzi	58	+	−	−	+	−	−	?	−
Roughgarden	59	+	−	−	−	−	?		−
Moise	79	+	−	+	−	+	−	+	−
Ambrose	80	+	+	+	−	+	+	+	
Ambrose	82	+	−	+	−	+	−	?	−
Alison	83	+	+	+	−	+	+	+	−
Victor	84	−	+	−	−	+	−	?	−
Rehr	85	+	−	−	−	+	?	?	−
Freeman	86	+	−	+	−	+	−	+	−
Haft	87	+	+	+	?	+	?	?	−
Zack	88	+	−	+	−	+	−	?	−
deServi	89	+	−	−	+	+	−	−	−
Wilson	90	+	+	+	−	+	−	+	−
Levin	91	Postmortem			−	+		Postmortem	
Capone	92	+	+	−	−	+	−	?	−
deZwaan	93	±	+	+	±	+	+	+	−
Ambrose	94	+	+	+	−	+	−	±	−
Gotoh	96	+	−	−	+	+	−	+	+
Mandelkorn	97	+	−	−	−	+	−	?	−
Williams	98	+	−	+	−	+	−	+	−
Roberts	103	+	+	+	−	−	−	Postmortem	
Guthrie	105	+	+	+	−	−	−	Postmortem	
Maseri	64	+	−	−	+	+	−	+	−

other hand, the other two issues raised in regard to rest angina continue to be pertinent. That is, angina equivalent or dyspnea rather than chest pain is quite common and can change in pattern. Second, a change in pattern of silent ischemia is unlikely to be recognized by the patient or the physician unless sophisticated monitoring is used (25–27).

A third category of subjective symptoms is new onset of angina. This

Table 3 Unstable Angina: ECG References

First author	Ref	Rest angina	New onset	Progressive	ECG	Coronary anatomy	Post MI included	Med Rx	Med refractory
		Symptom				Required			
Plotnick	60	+	+	+	+	+	−	+	−
Plotnick	61	+	+	+	+	+	−	+	−
Papapietro	62	+	+	+	+	+	−	+	−
Yasue	63	+	−	−	+	+	−	?	−
deZwaan	66	+	+	+	+	+	+	?	−
Sclarovsky	67	+	+	+	+	−	−	+	−
Sclarovsky	68	+	+	+	+	+	−	?	−
Haines	69	+	+	+	−	−	−	+	−
Butman	70	−	+	+	−	−	−	+	−
Butman	71	−	+	+	−	+	−	+	−
Swahn	72	−	+	+	−	−	−	+	−
Johnson	73	+	+	+	−	−	−	+	−

Table 4 Unstable Angina: Medical Therapy

First author	Ref	Rest angina	New onset	Progressive	ECG	Coronary anatomy	Post MI included	Med Rx	Med refractory
		Symptom				Required			
Lewis	50	+	+	+	±	−	−	±	−
Cairns	117	+	+	+	+	−	−	+	−
Theroux	118	+	−	+	−	−	−	+	±
Parodi	129	+	−	−	+	−	−	+	−
Mehta	130	+	+	+	+	−	−	+	+
HINT	132	+	−	−	+	−	−	+	−
Theroux	133	+	−	+	+	−	+	+	±
Gottlieb	134	+	−	−	+	−	−	+	±
Muller	135	+	−	+	±	±	−	+	±
Gerstenblith	136	+	−	−	+	−	−	+	−
Mikolich	120	+	−	−	−	−	−	+	−
Kaplan	121	+	−	−	+	−	?	+	+
DePace	122	+	+	+	−	−	−	+	+
Roubin	123	+	−	−	−	+	−	+	+
Curfman	127	+	−	−	−	−	−	+	+
Telford	139	+	+	+	−	−	+	+	−
Ambrose	140	+			+	+	−	+	±
Gold	141	+			+	+	−	+	±
Shapiro	142	±	±		+	+	+	+	−
Rentrop	143	+			+	+	−	+	+
Vetrovec	144	+			+	+	−	+	±

Table 5 Unstable Angina: Surgery (CABG)

First author	Ref	Symptom				Required			
		Rest angina	New onset	Progressive	ECG	Coronary anatomy	Post MI included	Med Rx	Med refractory
Luchi	51	+	+	+	+	+	−	+	−
Russell	54–57	±	+	+	+	+	−		
Selden	159	±	−	−	+	+	−	+	−
Lambert	149	+	+	+	+	+	−	?	?
Segal	150	+		+	+	+	−	+	+
Favolaro	151	+	−	−	+	+	−	±	?
Douglas	152	+	+	+	−	+	?	+	+
Brown	158	+	+	+	+	+	−	+	−
Pugh	157	+	+	+	−	+	−	+	−
Bertolasi	39	+	−	+	±	+	−	+	−
Wiles	160	+	−	+	−	+	−	+	±
Hultgren	166	+	+	+	+	+	−	+	−
Langou	162	+	−	−	+	+	−	+	+
Olinger	163	+	+	+	+	+	−	+	−
Ahmed	164	+	−	+	−	+	−	+	+
Jones	165	+	+	+	+	+	−	+	−
Hultgren	166	+	+	+	−	−	−	+	−
Cobanoglu	167	+	+	+	−	+	+	+	−
Golding	168	+	+	+	+	+	−	?	?
Rankin	169	+	−	−	−	+	+	+	+
Goldman	170	+	−	+	−	+	+	+	+
Edwards	171	+	−	−	±	+	+	+	+
Cohn	172	+	+	+	+	+	−	+	+
Hatcher	173	+	+	+	−	+		+	−

category has the same problems as elicited for rest angina, that is: (a) confusion with new onset of nonischemic pain, (b) confusion arising from angina equivalent rather than angina, and (c) silent ischemia.

A fourth category that is highly relevant to the design of studies, interpretation of data, and clarification of an otherwise extremely confusing literature is the inclusion or exclusion of patients who have myocardial infarction and some form of ischemic instability in the early postinfarct period (Table 7) (208–244). A further subdivision is non-Q-wave versus Q-wave myocardial infarction.

In studies to date, there has been no consistent tendency to include or exclude any or all of these subjective subsets (Tables 1–7) (17–250). It is quite likely that over and above the three issues listed, nonischemic pain, angina equivalent, and silent ischemia, there is a substantial difference in prognosis and perhaps in pathophysiology between the patterns of rest angina and change in pattern of chronic stable angina. As we will subsequently review, patient selection has had

Table 6   Unstable Angina: Angioplasty (PTCA)

		Symptom				Required			
First author	Ref	Rest angina	New onset	Progressive	ECG	Coronary anatomy	Post MI included	Med Rx	Med refractory
Holmes	174	−	+	−	±	+	?	+	−
Detre	175	+	+	+	±	+	−	+	+
Mullin	178	+	+	+	±	+	−	+	+
Detre	177	+	+	+	±	+	−	+	+
Kent	179	+	+	+	±	+	−	+	+
Faxon	180	+	+	+	±	+	−	+	+
Shawl	182	+	+	+	+	+	−	+	−
Williams	183	+	+	+	+	+	−	+	+
Meyer	184	+	+	+	+	+	−	+	−
Meyer	185	+	+	+	+	+	−	+	+
deFeyter	186	+	−	−	+	+	−	+	±
Timmis	187	+	+	+	−	+	−	+	−
Tuczu	188	+			−	+			−
Faxon	189	+	+	+	−	+	−	+	−
Sharma	190	+	+	+	−	+	+	+	+
deFeyter	191	+	−	−	+	+	−	−	±
diMarco	192	+	+	+	+	+	−	+	+
Hartzler	194	?	?	?	?	+	?	+	?
Deligonul	195	+	+	+	−	+	−	+	+
Briesblatt	196	?	?	?	−	+	+	+	−
DiSciascio	197	+	?	?	−	+	+	+	−
Vandoermael	198	+	+	+	−	+		+	−
Cowley	199	+	?	?	−	+		+	−
Mabin	200	+	+	+	±	+	−	+	±

an enormous impact on the conclusions reached in studies of unstable angina
(Tables 1–7).

Representative Case I

A 67-year-old man was admitted for evaluation of new chest symptoms. He
described being awakened at night with substernal burning. This occasionally
occurred in the past several months with exertion, but was not reproducible. He
described fair exercise tolerance. The patient had been started on diltiazem, but
because his symptoms were atypical and rest ECG was normal, he was scheduled
for an exercise treadmill test.

On a standard Bruce protocol exercise, the patient experienced substernal
burning accompanied by 4–6 mm precordial ST elevation at 3 min of exercise.
The test was stopped; three sublingual nitroglycerine tablets were administered,
with relief of pain and ECG changes. The patient was admitted to the intensive

Table 7 Post Infarction Unstable Angina

First author	Ref	Symptom			Required				
		Rest angina	New onset	Progressive	ECG	Coronary anatomy	Post MI included	Med Rx	Med refractory
Bosch	208	+			+	+	+	+	±
Campolo	209	+		+	+	±	+	±	
Fioretti	210	+		+	±	±	+	±	
Bigger	211	±	+		−	−	+	±	−
Marmor	216	+			+	−	+	?	−
Fraker	217	+			+	−	+	?	−
Kronenberg	218	+			+	−	+	?	−
Stenson	219	+			+	−	+	?	−
Reid	220	±		+	+	−	+	−	−
Muller	221	±			+	−	+	±	−
McKay	222	−			−	+	+	?	−
Erlebacher	223	−			−	−	+	?	−
Schuster	224	+			+	±	+	±	−
Gibson	226	±			±	+	+	±	−
Gibson	228	±			−	−	+	+	±
Benhorin	229	±	±		−	−	+	±	±
Sellier	230	±	±		+	−	+	±	−
Tomkinson	235	+			+	+	+	±	−
Midwal	236	±	±		±	−	+	±	−
Williams	237		+		−	+	+	±	−
deFeyter	202	+			+	+	+	+	+
Hopkins	203	+			−	+	+	±	−
Gottlieb	204	±	±		+	+	+		
Suryapranata	206	±	±		−	+	+	+	±
Nunley	153	+	−	−	±	+	+	?	−
Williams	238	+			±	+	+	+	±
Rankin	169	+				+	+		
Baumgartner	238	+			±	+	+	+	±
Gertler	239	±			−	+	+	+	±
Singh	240	±			±	+	+	+	+
Brower	241	+		+	±	+	+	+	+
Breyer	242	+			+	+	+	+	±
Jones	155	+			±	+	+	+	+
Levine	154	+	−	−	±	+	+	+	+
Madigan	246	±			?	+	+	?	?
Bardet	244	+		+	+	+	+	+	+
Jones	245	±			−	+	+	+	+
Stuart	243	+			±	+	+	+	+
Brundage	247	+			±	+	+	+	+
Weintraub	248	+			±	+	+	+	+

care unit, where aspirin, intravenous heparin, low-flow oxygen, and intravenous nitroglycerin were added. He had no further chest pain on this regimen.

Coronary angiography revealed a discrete >95% stenosis in the proximal left anterior descending coronary artery after a large diagonal branch and before a large septal. This lesion was successfully dilated (PTCA) with a 4.0-mm, low-profile balloon. Three days after the dilatation, the patient exercised 7 min on a Bruce protocol with neither chest pain nor ECG changes of ischemia.

In retrospect, this patient clearly presented with unstable myocardial ischemia and "threatened" infarction of the anterior wall. Dilatation of the "culprit" lesion led to complete relief of his symptom complex.

For purposes of enrolling this patient in a study, where we might learn, for example, if he would be better served by PTCA or CABG, how does one classify such a patient? Prospectively, he was felt to have atypical chest pain. If one requires reversible ECG changes with resting pain, he would be excluded. Similarly, we did not make any effort to determine if he was "medically refractory." Although angioplasty to prevent infarction is an unproven hypothesis, we felt, given the stakes, it would have been clinically unjustifiable to forgo either PTCA or CABG. Given the issues of acute occlusion, restenosis, perioperative infarction, and surgical morbidity, we do not know whether PTCA was preferable to CABG in the long run for this patient.

PRESENCE OR ABSENCE OF ISCHEMIA

The most widely available means of insisting on the presence or absence of ischemia when interpreting resting pain or rest angina equivalent is the presence or absence of reversible electrocardiographic changes (Table 3) (24–28, 60–73). This leads to a variety of definitional and logistic problems in the study of unstable angina. First, the electrocardiogram is imperfect. Some areas of the heart, for example, the posterolateral wall, are represented with substantially lower sensitivity than, for example, the anterior wall of the heart. Second, it is not logistically possible to always have an electrocardiogram available, so the vast majority of symptomatic episodes occur in the absence of monitoring.

Despite these reservations, the majority of nonischemic episodes of chest pain can be eliminated for study purposes if one insists on the presence of reversible electrocardiographic changes. As we will see in our review of published studies of unstable angina, insistence on reversible electrocardiographic changes in patient selection has been quite variable (Tables 1–7).

Representative Case II

A 70-year-old man was admitted with crescendo angina. Eight months prior he had undergone two-vessel CABG to the left anterior descending artery and right coronary artery. He had done well without chest pain or dyspnea for 7 months.

One month prior to admission, he began to note resumption of exertional chest pressure, similar in character to the pain that had precipitated the CABG. In 1 month, he had noted that it took progressively less activity to elicit discomfort. He was admitted after a 20-min episode which occurred at rest and required four sublingual nitroglycerin tablets for relief. He was taking isordil, nifedipine, and aspirin. Oxygen and heparin were added, and the patient was scheduled for coronary angiography. Both vein grafts were widely patent. The other major change from his preoperative study was a new 70–90% proximal stenosis in a single obtuse marginal branch. The patient had two episodes of pain in the hospital. Neither was accompanied by changes on the 12-lead ECG, but intravenous nitroglycerin was started empirically, and the patient had symptomatic relief.

The decision was made to perform circumflex angioplasty (PTCA). During each balloon inflation, the patient's angina was reproduced, with gradual relief on deflation. Four days after successful angioplasty, the patient exercised for 5 min on a Bruce protocol, stopping with fatigue without chest pain or ECG changes.

Presumably due to the electrical silence of the circumflex distribution on a surface ECG, this patient had no objective substantiation that his crescendo symptoms were ischemic in origin. For a trial insisting on reversible ECG changes, this patient would have been excluded. Given the advantages of the "retrospectroscope," this patient almost certainly had crescendo angina secondary to isolated circumflex disease.

CORONARY ANATOMY/LEFT VENTRICULAR FUNCTION

Studies of unstable angina have been quite variable with regard to whether or not any or all subjects included in the study have had angiographic outline of their coronary anatomy (Tables 1–7) (74–98). On the one hand, we know that patients are no more likely to have unstable than stable angina, based on the number of coronary arteries involved. On the other hand, we know that both short- and long-term prognosis are directly related to the extent of anatomical coronary disease. Accordingly, studies that do not include this information are likely to give results that are difficult to interpret, with regard to both natural history and efficacy of therapy.

TREATMENT

As discussed by Braunwald in his recent editorial on the subject, previous studies of unstable angina have been highly variable with regard to treatment (Tables 1–7) (2–244). First, there are very few studies with patients on no therapy. Second, there is the historical matter that studies published before the 1970s are likely not to include such standard therapies today as intravenous nitroglycerin and/or calcium blockers. Similarly, bypass surgery has only been available since the late 1960s and angioplasty has only been available since the late 1970s. Accordingly, nearly all published studies include patients who have been treated with something, but there is a marked variability as to how much treatment. Clearly, this would have a major impact on studies purporting to demonstrate natural history. The additive effects of multiple therapies can profoundly influence the conclusions of studies designed to look at one specific form of therapy.

EXAMPLES OF CONCLUSIONS REGARDING UNSTABLE ANGINA THAT MAY REFLECT SELECTION BIASES OF "CLASSIC" STUDIES

Tables 1–7 are surveys of some of the most widely cited references in the literature of unstable angina. Table 1 includes a number of widely cited studies that deal with the natural history of unstable angina; Table 2 includes studies that deal with pathophysiology of unstable angina; Table 3 includes electrocardiographic references; and Tables 4, 5, and 6 deal respectively with medical therapy, surgical therapy, and angioplasty therapy for unstable angina. Table 7 specifically examines the subset of unstable angina occurring within 30 days of an acute myocardial infarction. The tables demonstrate which studies included patients from each of the three broad subjective symptom categories and which studies required resting electrocardiographic changes for inclusion and/or coronary arteriographic confirmation of disease prior to inclusion in the study. In addition, the tables describe whether the particular subset of patients with postinfarction unstable angina were included or excluded, and whether the subjects of the respective studies were on any medical therapy and/or deemed to be medically refractory (the definition of "medically refractory" will be discussed specifically in Chapter 7). From these few pieces of data we can make some inferences about the types of patients selected for the particular "classic" studies, and in turn, we can see how the selection process was likely to influence the conclusions drawn from these studies and the conclusions that practitioners now are likely to infer on even a casual perusal of the literature of unstable angina.

The inclusion of patients who do not manifest resting ECG changes in the category "unstable angina" is likely to provide a broader-based sample, but may very well do so by including patients whose symptoms are not myocardial in origin (46–48). This is even further emphasized if patients are not required to have coronary arteriographic confirmation. We know from a number of excellent arteriographic studies that if one takes all patients prospectively with rest angina, fully 10% will be found to have no coronary arteriographic abnormalities (61,83,101,157). Similarly, if one looks at the three broad symptom complexes, new onset of angina is likely to include a higher proportion of patients with either normal coronaries and/or single-vessel disease. Conversely, patients with progressive angina are more likely to have multivessel disease. Accordingly, a population that includes large numbers of patients with new onset of angina might be expected to demonstrate a natural history that is somewhat favorable compared to studies that include predominantly or exclusively patients with progressive angina (45). Nearly all the studies of natural history include patients who are on some form of therapy, and there is a clear historic bias. That is, early studies included only nitrates, because that is all that was available. More recent studies include patients who are more likely to be on calcium channel blockers, aspirin, and/or intravenous nitrates. The definition of medically refractory (see Chapter 7) is highly variable, and there is no uniformity with regard to attempting to include or exclude patients who are medically refractory in studies of natural history (146).

A number of pathophysiological alternatives have been used to explain the unstable angina syndrome, which have included progression of atherosclerosis, acute thrombosis, and coronary arterial spasm (13–28). The relative role of each of these possibilities can be sharply influenced, as one can see from a brief review of some of the most widely cited studies, depending on the selection process that went into obtaining patients for the study (Table 2). For example, to document progression of atherosclerosis over time, it is clearly necessary to have multiple coronary arteriograms (80,82,85,86). It is almost impossible to arrange a prospective angiographic study in patients who are not having symptoms over time. Therefore, there is a strong selection bias for patients with progressive symptoms in any study that includes serial angiography. Similarly, the frequency with which one sees a component of coronary arterial spasm is influenced by the presence of medical therapy (17,64,89): for example, the use of nitrates or calcium blockers, on the one hand, and/or the use of provocative agents, on the other. Postmortem studies may overestimate clot (20,91,92,103,105).

The inferences that one can make with regard to efficacy of any form of therapy are influenced by concomitant therapy. This point is relevant to all the widely cited studies in Tables 4–6, for there are almost no studies of any form of medical therapy, surgical therapy, or angioplasty therapy done in patients who are not on concomitant therapy. Even more confusing, the therapy is highly variable even within given widely cited studies.

In summary, these tables represent a sampling of some of the best work available in the English language on the entity of unstable angina. Clearly, this represents an enormous amount of work by numerous highly skilled clinicians and investigators. Nevertheless, our interpretation of much of this data and its relevance to our contemporary care of patients must take into account the highly variable selection process that went into each of these studies. The definitional issue will impact virtually every conclusion we attempt to reach about unstable angina, from natural history to pathophysiology to treatment.

IMPACT OF DEFINITIONAL AMBIGUITY IN THE DESIGN AND INTERPRETATION OF STUDIES

As will be discussed in a subsequent chapter, the major means by which new clinical therapies or new diagnostic techniques can be tested for (a) clinical effectiveness, (b) complications, and (c) cost is the controlled clinical trial. This method requires that a homogeneous population of patients are randomly assigned to the technique to be tested or its alternative and then the results in terms of the above three parameters can be compared. The most obvious problem for uncontrolled studies or studies not performed in a random fashion is that the intervention and control groups may not be homogeneous, so that any or all results may be attributable to patient selection rather than the intervention to be tested. This is an additional problem when it is not possible to compare the results of one controlled or even registry study with the results of an alternative study because patient selection is not comparable.

To consider this issue in the specific case of unstable angina, let us look at the three major prospective randomized trials in the therapy of unstable angina. The VA Cooperative Study of Aspirin (Table 4, Lewis), the National Cooperative Study of Medical Versus Surgical Therapy (Table 5, Russell), and the VA Cooperative Study of Medical Versus Surgical Therapy (Table 5, Luchi) are the three major prospective randomized trials in the management of patients with unstable angina. All three studies included specific exclusion of the diagnosis of myocardial infarction by enzymes and ECG criteria. For the VA Cooperative Study of Aspirin, the patient could not have had an infarction within 6 weeks; for both the others, patients could not have had an infarction within 3 months. Although all included a requirement for objective evidence of coronary artery disease, only the National Cooperative Study of Medical Versus Surgical Therapy and the VA Cooperative Study of Medical Versus Surgical Therapy required that all patients have cardiac catheterization. This is important not only in including only patients who had greater than 70% epicardial narrowing of at least one major epicardial branch and/or exclusion of patients with greater than 70% left main stenosis. In addition, it makes it possible to analyze specific subsets based on coronary anatomy. In a number of observational and prospective randomized trial types of studies, coronary anatomy has been associated as an important outcome variable in virtually every subset of coronary artery disease patients studied. The issue of comparability of patient populations becomes even more muddled when one turns to the specific definition of unstable angina. For example, only the VA Cooperative Study of Aspirin required resting chest pain; the other two studies included new onset or worsening of angina as potential categories. The requirement for electrocardiographic changes with rest paint was met by both National and VA Cooperative Studies of Medical Versus Surgical Therapy but not required in the VA Cooperative Study of Aspirin.

Table 8 Common Reasons for Exclusion from Studies of Unstable Angina

---

Age > 70 years
Recent myocardial infarction
Prior bypass surgery (CABG)
Medically refractory
Patient refusal
Follow-up impossible
Physician refusal
Significant comorbidity
    Diabetes
    COPD
    Hypertension

Similarly, exclusions among these and most studies are quite variable (Table 8). Relative to the previously mentioned issue of increasingly ill patients being subjected to revascularization procedures, it should be noted that two out of three of these studies excluded patients with left ventricular ejection fractions less than 30%, two of the three excluded patients aged over 70; all excluded patients with prior bypass surgery; and a variety of medical conditions were excluded primarily in terms of whether they were more likely than coronary artery disease to limit the patient's life expectancy.

These three studies are clearly the most excellent studies available of the care of unstable angina and each required a monumental effort of a large number of personnel. Nevertheless, there are significant differences in patient populations, making comparisons between studies difficult. At the same time, the results of these studies do not help us with the large number of patients who are in groups that would have been excluded from them.

SUMMARY: DEFINITIONS OF UNSTABLE ANGINA

A final point that deserves consideration is that different definitions might be appropriate for the same term under different circumstances. For example, a clinically useful definition might not be restrictive enough for a prospective clinical trial. Conversely, a retrospective case review might permit information that was only available to hindsight and thus not available for a prospective selection process.

Clinical Definition of Unstable Angina

New onset of angina, change in pattern of previously stable angina, and rest angina are the three broad symptom complexes. I think "angina equivalents" in each of these three categories should also be included where symptoms of dyspnea, pressure, nausea, or even vaguer symptoms might be allowed. Until more data are available, I would not include completely asymptomatic ECG changes (silent ischemia). Clearly, this reservation must be tempered with the realization that there is wide variety both in patients' abilities to describe symptoms and in doctors' abilities to elicit them.

For clinical purposes, any objective means of confirming the ischemic origin of symptoms is acceptable (reversible wall motion changes by angiography, echocardiography, or radionuclide vertriculography; perfusion imaging, etc., as well as reversible ECG changes). Similarly, a suggestive enough history in a patient with known coronary artery disease or strong exclusionary data for nonischemic alternatives may be adequate.

Retrospective Studies of Unstable Angina

Frequently, histories that seemed vague or atypical are substantially more lucid and typical when the light of the retrospectoscope is brought into play. In the study of patients with coronary disease, the most powerful retrospectoscopes are (a) ECG with pain, (b) ECG or wall motion or perfusion imaging during exercise, and (c) coronary arteriography. These kinds of data make it possible: to exclude patients whose symptoms, in retrospect, were not ischemic; to include patients who, in retrospect, were unstable; to compare comparable patient groups.

Prospective Studies of Unstable Angina

The power of the prospective, randomized trial is such that many have forgotten that it is an imperfect tool, that is, that there are shortcomings.

As stated previously, to insist on prospective objective confirmation of ischemia requires either expensive and potentially dangerous across-the-board interventions (e.g., every patient gets a thallium perfusion study or a balloon flotation catheter or coronary sinus cannulation or an echocardiogram) or the potential of excluding large numbers of patients who really belong in the population. Both these steps lead to increasing costs. The latter increases the risk that the study will commit a type II error (failure to detect a difference in a situation where it really exists). Concluding, for example, that surgery was no more effective than medical therapy (because of a type II error) in a population where it is really is beneficial is worse than no study at all! Similarly, insisting on coronary angiography will increase costs and lead to exclusions (patients who refuse to have it).

These kinds of contrasts are clear if one compares the Coronary Artery Surgery Study (CASS) to the Second International Study of Infarct Survival (ISIS-2) (250,251). The CASS study included only patients with angiographic coronary disease (250). ISIS probably included patients who had neither coronary disease nor an infarction (251). The homogeneity of the two tested groups is much more certain in CASS. Alternatively, the cost was much higher and, due to the numbers of patients randomized (780 versus 17,187), the statistical power much less in CASS than ISIS. Similarly, because of the proportions excluded, ISIS applies to a far larger proportion of clinical patients with infarction than does CASS to the clinical population potentially under consideration for surgery. The point of this comparison is not that one study is more valuable or more correct than the other. Rather, there is more than one way to conduct a study and tradeoffs are necessary, just as they are in clinical decision making.

SCOPE OF THE PROBLEM: DENVER VA MEDICAL CENTER

In one year, 1989, there were about 1800 admissions to the medical intensive care unit in our hospital. Of the intensive care unit admissions, 210 patients, approximately 20%, had the admitting diagnosis of unstable angina and 201 had the admitting diagnosis of "rule out" myocardial infarction. Many of the "rule outs" ruled out. Most of them then had a working diagnosis of unstable angina. Similarly, some patients admitted with other diagnoses, for example, stable angina, developed unstable symptoms and were transferred to the intensive care unit during their hospital stay. Accordingly, it can be seen that in our hospital unstable angina is a more frequent cause for intensive care unit admission than myocardial infarction.

In addition to being more common, unstable angina is frequently a more difficult problem than myocardial infarction. The majority of uncomplicated myocardial infarction patients have resolution of their pain syndrome and are then electively categorized as high or low risk pending the results of radionuclide ventriculography for left ventricular ejection fraction, low-level treadmill exercise testing, and/or 24-hr Holter monitoring. Based on these noninvasive evaluations, patients either go on to catheterization and interventional strategy (either bypass surgery or coronary angioplasty) or they are followed on medical therapy. For the most part, these patients are not a major clinical problem in terms of either evaluation or therapy. In contrast, patients with unstable angina frequently continue to have both ischemia and/or hemodynamic and electrical instability. As such, they continue to be diagnostic and therapeutic dilemmas. For example, in the same single year, 1989, unstable angina accounted for 92 of 115 bypass surgery operations performed in our hospital, 93 of 127 coronary angioplasties performed in our hospital, and 133 of 482 coronary arteriograms performed in our hospital. Finally, on a weekly basis, unstable angina is the subject of the most contentious discussions between internists, invasive and noninvasive cardiologists, and cardiac surgeons. In summary, it is a more common and more vexing clinical problem than myocardial infarction in our hospital.

SCOPE OF THE PROBLEM: U.S. VETERANS ADMINISTRATION MEDICAL CENTERS

Although serving a distinct segment of the U.S. population, the fact is the U.S. Veterans Administration (USVA) is the largest single provider of health care in this country. Accordingly, generalizations about this system have some relevance to health care delivery nationally. In addition, it is quite likely the USVA is the most thoroughly scrutinized health care delivery system in the United States. For example, it has been the VA policy since 1971 to keep statistics that are openly available on all cardiac surgeries performed within the system. We know from reports of the VA Surgical Registry that, for example, 8,569 of 10,440 patients undergoing bypass surgery between May 1987 and March 1989 within the 47 VA medical centers with cardiac surgery programs had registry reports filed (250). The indication for bypass surgery in this cohort of patients was rest angina in 4404 of 7904, or 56%.

There is currently no VA registry for coronary angioplasty, but we have attempted to survey catheterization laboratory directors in VA hospitals that have cardiac surgery programs (a requirement of angioplasty programs within the VA system). The response to our survey has been substantially less than 50%, but based on the data we have, it appears that approximately 50% of the angioplasties within the VA system are done to treat unstable angina.

Finally, the logistics/economics of the VA system are similar to the centrally planned and funded medical system of many European countries rather than the fee-for-service mode of most American hospitals. The necessity of trying to live within a preset budget rather than recompense for service delivered has had the effect of triaging only the sicker (medically refractory) patients to expensive intervention such as coronary artery bypass surgery (CABG) or percutaneous transluminal coronary angioplasty (PTCA). The result is that each year the proportion of patients coming to diagnostic catheterization for unstable symptoms is increasing and the proportion with stable symptoms or no symptoms is decreasing. The upshot: unstable angina was the leading reason for coronary angiography, bypass surgery, and angioplasty within the VA system in 1990.

SCOPE OF THE PROBLEM: U.S. PRIVATE HOSPITALS

Since early after its clinical inception in 1977, the percutaneous transluminal coronary angioplasty procedure has been closely followed in the United States by means of a National Health Institute Registry. Both early and late reports from the registry suggest that unstable angina is the indication for PTCA in approximately 60% of patients.

It is substantially more difficult to get a picture about what proportion of patients receiving coronary artery bypass surgery (CABG) do so for treatment of unstable angina. For example, unstable angina was a specific exclusion of the large scale NHLBI coronary artery surgery study (CASS). It is likely, based on the proportion of patients with normal coronary anatomy reported and the literature regarding silent ischemia, that more sizable proportions of patients with mild or minimal symptoms are being cathed in the private sector than in the VA system. Nevertheless, it can be stated that unstable angina constitutes a large proportion of patients undergoing coronary angiography and revascularization by either PTCA or CABG in the private sector as well.

REFERENCES

1. Bernard R, Corday, E, Eliasch H, et al. Report of the Joint International Society and Federation of Cardiology/World Health Organization Task Force on Standardization of Clinical Nomenclature: Nomenclature and criteria for diagnosis of ischemic heart disease. Circulation 1979; 59:607–8.
2. Braunwald E. Unstable angina; A classification. Circulation 1989; 80:410–4.
3. Conti CR, Hill JA, Mayfield WR. Unstable angina pectoris: Pathogenesis and management. Curr Prob Cardiol 1989; 14:553–623.
4. Farhi JI, Cohen M, Fuster V. Editorial: The broad spectrum of unstable angina pectoris and its implications for future controlled trials. Am J Cardiol 1986; 58:547–50.
5. Munger TM, Oh JK. Unstable angina. Mayo Clin Proc 1990; 65:384–406.
6. Fowler NO. Editorial: "Preinfarctional" angina: A need for an objective definition and for a controlled clinical trial of its management. Circulation 1971; 44:755–8.
7. Smitherman TC. Unstable angina pectoris: The first half century: Natural history, pathophysiology, treatment. Am J Med Sci 1986; 292:395–406.
8. Scanlon PJ. The intermediate coronary syndrome. Prog Cardiovasc Dis 1981; 23:351–64.
9. Cairns JA, Fantus IG, Klassen GA. Unstable angina pectoris. Am Heart J 1976; 92:373–86.
10. Patterson DLH. Unstable angina. Postgrad Med J 1988; 64:196–200.
11. Hecht HS, Rahimtoola SH. Unstable angina: A perspective. Chest 1982; 82:466–72.
12. Plotnick GD, ed. Unstable angina. Mt. Kisco, NY: Futura, 1985.
13. Maseri A. Pathogenetic classification of unstable angina as a guideline to individual patient management and prognosis. Am J Med 1986; 80: 45–55.
14. Forrester JS, Litvack F, Grundfest W, Hickey A. A perspective of coronary disease seen through the arteries of living man. Circulation 1987; 75:505–13.
15. Theroux P. A pathophysiologic basis for the clinical classification and management of unstable angina. Circulation 1987; 75 (suppl V): V–103–9.
16. Fuster V, Badimon L, Cohen M, Ambrose JA, Badimon JJ, Chesebro J. Insights into the pathogenesis of acute ischemic syndromes. Circulation 1988; 77:1213–20.
17. Maseri A, Severi S, L'Abbate A, et al. "Variant" angina: one aspect of a continuous spectrum of vasospastic myocardial ischemia. Am J Cardiol 1978; 42:1019–34.
18. Sherman CT, Litvack F, Grundfest W, et al. Coronary angioscopy in patients with unstable angina pectoris. N Engl J Med 1986; 315:913–9.

19. Neill WA, Wharton TP Jr, Fluri-Lundeen J, Cohen IS. Acute coronary insufficiency—Coronary occlusion after intermittent ischemic attacks. N Engl J Med 1980; 302:1157–62.
20. Falk E. Unstable angina with fatal outcome: Dynamic coronary thrombosis leading to infarction and/or sudden death. Circulation 1985; 71:699–708.
21. Fuster V, Chesebro JA. Editorial: Mechanisms of unstable angina. N Engl J Med 1982; 315:1023–5.
22. Horie T, Sekiguchi M, Hirosawa K. Relationship between myocardial infarction and pre-infarction angina. Am Heart J 1978; 95:81–8.
23. Kruskal JB, Commerford PJ, Franks JJ, Kirsch RE. Fibrin and fibrinogen related antigens in patients with stable and unstable coronary artery disease. N Engl J Med 1987; 317:1361–5.
24. Figueras J, Singh BN, Ganz W, Charuzi Y, Swan HJC. Mechanism of rest and nocturnal angina: Observations during continuous hemodynamic and electrocardiographic monitoring. Circulation 1979; 59:955–68.
25. Gottlieb SO, Weisfeldt ML, Ouyang P, Melits ED, Girstenblith G. Silent ischemia as a marker for early unfavorable outcomes in patients with unstable angina. N Engl J Med 1986; 314:1214–9.
26. Wilcox I, Freedman B, Kelly DT, Harris PJ. Clinical significance of silent ischemia in unstable angina pectoris. Am J Cardiol 1990; 65:1313–6.
27. Nademanee K, Intarachot V, Josephson MA, et al. Prognostic significance of silent myocardial ischemia in patients with unstable angina. J Am Coll Cardiol 1987; 10:1–9.
28. Oliva PB. Unstable rest angina with ST segment depression. Ann Intern Med 1984; 100:424–40.
29. Herrick JB. Clinical features of sudden obstruction of the coronary arteries. JAMA 1912; 59:2015–20.
30. Nichol ES, Fassett DW. An attempt to forestall acute coronary thrombosis. South Med J 1947; 40:631–7.
31. Beamish RE, Storrie VM. Impending myocardial infarction: Recognition and management. Circulation 1960; 21:1107–15.
32. Sampson JJ, Eliaser M Jr. The diagnosis of impending acute coronary artery occlusion. Am Heart J 1937; 13:675–86.
33. Vakil RJ. Intermediate coronary syndrome. Circulation 1961; 24:557–71.
34. Vakil RJ. Preinfarction syndrome—Management and follow-up. Am J Cardiol 1964; 14:55–63.
35. Krauss KR, Hutter AM, DeSanctis RW. Acute coronary insufficiency. Arch Intern Med 1972; 129:808–13.
36. Wood P. Acute and subacute coronary insufficiency. Br Med J 1961; 1:1779.
37. Gazes PC, Mobley EM Jr, Faris HM Jr, Duncan RC, Humphries GB. Preinfarctional (unstable) angina—A prospective study—Ten year follow up. Circulation 1973; 48:331–7.
38. Conti CR, Brawley RK, Griffith LSC, Pitt B, Humphries JO, Gott VL, Ross RS. Unstable angina pectoris: morbidity and mortality in 57 consecutive patients evaluated angiographically. Am J Cardiol 1973; 32:745–50.
39. Bertolasi CA, Tronge JE, Riccitelli MA, Villamayor RM, Zuffardi E. Natural

history of unstable angina with medical or surgical therapy. Chest 1975; 70: 596–605.

40. Duncan B, Fulton M, Morrison SL, Lutz W, Donald KW, Kerr F, Kirby BJ, Julian DG, Oliver MF. Prognosis of new and worsening angina pectoris. Br Med J 1976; 1:981–5.

41. Heng NK, Norris RM, Singh BN, Partridge JB. Prognosis in unstable angina. Br Heart J 1976; 38:921–5.

42. Day LJ, Thibault GE, Sowton E. Acute coronary insufficiency Review of 46 patients. Br Heart J 1977; 39:363–70.

43. Mulcahy R, Daly L, Graham I, Hickey N, O'Donoghue S, Owens A, Ruane P, Tobin G. Unstable angina: natural history and determinants of prognosis. Am J Cardiol 1981; 48:525–8.

44. Olson HG, Lyons KP, Aronow WS, Stinson PJ, Kuperas J, Waters HJ. The high risk angina patient. Circulation 1981; 64:674–84.

45. Roberts KB, Califf RM, Harrell FE, Lee KL, Pryor DB, Rosati RA. The prognosis for patients with new-onset angina who have undergone cardiac catheterization. Circulation 1983; 68:970–8.

46. Schroeder JS, Lamb IH, Harrison DC. Patients admitted to the coronary care unit for chest pain: High risk subgroup for subsequent cardiovascular death. Am J Cardiol 1977; 39:829–32.

47. Schroeder JS, Lamb IH, Hu M. Do patients in whom myocardial infarction has been ruled out have a better prognosis after hospitalization than those surviving infarction? N Engl J Med 1980; 303:1–5.

48. Lopes MG, Spivack AP, Harrison DC, Schroeder JS. Prognosis in coronary care unit noninfarction cases. JAMA 1974; 228:1558–62.

49. Skjaeggestad O. The natural history of intermediate coronary syndrome. Acta Med Scand 1973; 193:533–6.

50. Lewis, HD Jr., Davis JW, Archibald DG, Steinke WE, Smitherman TC, Doherty JE III, Schnaper HW, LeWinter MM, Linares E, Pouget JM, Sabharwal SC, Chesler E, DeMots H. Protective effects of aspirin against acute myocardial infarction and death in men with unstable angina. N Engl J Med 1983; 309:396–403.

51. Luchi RJ, Scott SM, Deupree RH, and the Principal Investigators and Their Associates of Veterans Administration Cooperative Study No. 28. Comparison of medical and surgical treatment for unstable angina pectoris. N Engl J Med 1987; 316:977–84.

52. Scott SM, Luchi RJ, Deupree RH, and the Veterans Administration Unstable Angina Cooperative Study Group. Veterans Administration cooperative study for treatment of patients with unstable angina. Circulation 1988; 78(Suppl I): I-113–21.

53. Parisi AF, Khuri S, Deupree RH, Sharma GVRK, Scott SM, Luchi RJ. Medical compared with surgical management of unstable angina 5 year mortality and morbidity in the Veterans Administration study. Circulation 1989; 80:1176–89.

54. Russell RO, Moraski RE, Kouchoukos N, et al. Unstable angina pectoris: National Cooperative Study Group to Compare Medical and Surgical Therapy. I. Report of protocol and patient population. Am J Cardiol 1976 37:896–902.

55. Russell RO, Moraski RE, Kouchoukos N, et al. Unstable angina pectoris: National Cooperative Study Group to Compare Surgical and Medical Therapy. II. In-hospital experience and initial follow-up results in patients with one, two, and three vessel disease. Am J Cardiol 1978; 42:839–48.

56. Russell RO, Moraski RE, Kouchoukos N, et al. Unstable angina pectoris: National Cooperative Study Group to Compare Surgical and Medical Therapy. III. Results in patients with S-T segment elevation during pain. Am J Cardiol 1980; 45:819–24.

57. Russell RO, Moraski RE, Kouchoukos N, et al. Unstable angina pectoris: National Cooperative Study Group to Compare Medical and Surgical Therapy. IV. Results in patients with left anterior descending artery disease. Am J Cardiol 1981; 48:517–24.

58. Guazzi M, Polese A, Fiorentini C, Magrini F, Olivari MT, Bartorelli C. Left and right heart haemodynamics during spontaneous angina pectoris. Br Heart J 1975; 37:401–13.

59. Roughgarden JW. Circulatory changes associated with spontaneous angina pectoris. Am J Med 1966; 41:947–61.

60. Plotnick GD, Conti CR. Transient S-T segment elevation in unstable angina: Prognostic significance. Am J Med 1979; 67:800–3.

61. Plotnick GD, Greene HL, Carliner NH, Becker LC, Fisher ML. Clinical indicators of left main coronary artery disease in unstable angina. Ann Intern Med 1979; 91:149–53.

62. Papapietro SE, Niess GS, Paine TD, Mantle JA, Rackley CE, Russell RO, Rogers WJ. Transient electrocardiographic changes in patients with unstable angina: relation to coronary arterial anatomy. Am J Cardiol 1980; 46:28–33.

63. Yasue S, Omote S, Masao N, Hyon H, Nishida S, Horie M. Comparison of coronary arteriographic findings during angina pectoris associated with S-T eleva-tion or sepression. Am J Cardiol 1981; 47:539–46.

64. Maseri A, L'Abbate A, Baroldi G, et al. "Variant" angina: One aspect of a continuous spectrum of vasospastic myocardial ischemia. Am J Cardiol 1978; 42:1019–33.

66. de Zwaan C, Bar FWHM, Wellens HJJ. Characteristic electrocardiographic pat-tern indicating a critical stenosis high in left anterior descending coronary artery in patients admitted because of impending myocardial infarction. Am Heart J 1982; 103:730–5.

67. Sclarovsky S, Davidson E, Lewin RF, Strasberg B, Arditti A, Agmon J. Unstable angina pectoris evolving to acute myocardial infarction: Significance of ECG changes during chest pain. Am Heart J 1986; 112:459–62.

68. Sclarovsky S, Davidson E, Strasberg B, Lewin R, Arditti A, Wurtzel M, Agmon J. Unstable angina: the significance of ST segment elevation or depression in patients without evidence of increased myocardial oxygen demand. Am Heart J 1986; 112:463–7.

69. Haines DE, Raabe DS, Gundel WD, Wackers FJ Th. Anatomic and prognostic significance of new T wave inversion in unstable angina. Am J Cardiol 1983; 52:14–8.

70. Butman SM, Olson HG, Gardin JM, Piters KM, Hullett M, Butman LK. Submaxi-

mal exercise testing after stabilization of unstable angina pectoris. J Am Coll Cardiol 1984; 4:667–73.

71. Butman SM, Olson HG, Butman LK. Early exercise testing after stabilization of unstable angina. Correlation with coronary angiographic findings and subsequent cardiac events. Am Heart J 1986; 111:11–8.

72. Swahn E, Areskog M, Berglund U, Walfridsson H, Wallentin L. Predictive importance of clinical findings and a predischarge exercise test in patients with suspected unstable coronary artery disease. Am J Cardiol 1987; 59:208–14.

73. Johnson SM, Mauritson DR, Winniford MD, Willerson JT, Firth BG, Cary JR, Hillis LD. Continuous electrocardiographic monitoring in patients with unstable angina pectoris: identification of high-risk subgroup with severe coronary disease, variant angina, and/or impaired early prognosis. Am Heart J 1982; 103:4–12.

74. Gregg DE, Patterson RE. Functional importance of the coronary collaterals. N Engl J Med 1980; 303:1404–6.

75. Rafflenbeul W, Smith LR, Rogers WJ, Mantle JA, Rackley CE, Russell RO. Quantitative coronary arteriography Coronary anatomy of patients with unstable angina pectoris reexamined 1 year after optimal medical therapy. Am J Cardiol 1979; 43:699–707.

76. Proudfit WL, Shirey EK, Sones FM Jr. Selective cine coronary arteriography: Correlation with clinical findings in 1,000 patients. Circulation 1966; 33:901–10.

77. Proudfit WL, Shirey EK, Sones FM Jr. Distribution of arterial lesions demonstrated by selective cinecoronary arteriography. Circulation 1967; 41:54–62.

78. Fuster V, Frye RL, Kennedy MA, Connolly DC, Mankin HT. The role of collateral circulation in the various coronary syndromes. Circulation 1979; 59: 1137–44.

79. Moise A, Theroux P, Taeymans Y, et al. Unstable angina in progression of coronary atherosclerosis. N Engl J Med 1983; 309:685–9.

80. Ambrose JA, Winters SL, Stern A, et al. Angiographic morphology and the pathogenesis of unstable angina pectoris. J Am Coll Cardiol 1985; 5:609–16.

81. Ambrose JA, Winters SL, Arora RR, et al. Coronary angiographic morphology in myocardial infarction: A link between the pathogenesis of unstable angina and myocardial infarction. J Am Coll Cardiol 1985; 6:1233–8.

82. Ambrose JA, Winters SL, Arora RR, et al. Angiographic evolution of coronary morphology in unstable angina. J Am Coll Cardiol 1986; 7:472–8.

83. Alison HW, Russell RO Jr, Mantle JA, et al. Coronary anatomy and arteriography in patients with unstable angina pectoris. Am J Cardiol 1978; 41:204–9.

84. Victor MF, Likoff MJ, Mintz GS, Likoff W. Unstable angina pectoris of new onset: A prospective clinical and arteriographic study of 75 patients. Am J Cardiol 1981; 47:228–32.

85. Rehr R, Disciascio G, Vetrovec G, Cowley M. Angiographic morphology of coronary artery stenoses in prolonged rest angina: Evidence of intracoronary thrombosis. J Am Coll Cardiol 1989; 14:1429–37.

86. Freeman MR, Williams AE, Chisholm RJ, Armstrong PW. Intracoronary thrombus and complex morphology in unstable angina. Circulation 1989; 80:17–23.

87. Haft JI, Goldstein JE, Niemiera ML. Coronary arteriographic lesion of unstable angina. Chest 1987; 92:609–12.

88. Zack PM, Ischinger T, Aker UT, Dincer B, Kennedy HL. The occurrence of angiographically detected intracoronary thrombus in patients with unstable angina pectoris. Am Heart J 1984; 108:1408–12.
89. deServi S, Specchia G, Ardeseno D, et al. Angiographic demonstration of different pathogenetic mechanisms in patients with spontaneous and exertional angina associated with ST segment depression. Am J Cardiol 1980; 45:1285–90.
90. Wilson RF, Holida MD, White CW. Quantitative angiographic morphology of coronary stenoses leading to myocardial infarction or unstable angina. Circulation 1986; 73:286–93.
91. Levin DC, Fallon JT. Significance of angiographic morphology of localized coronary stenoses: Histopathologic correlations. Circulation 1982; 66:316–20.
92. Capone G, Wolf NM, Meyer B, Meister SG. Frequency of intracoronary filling defects by angiography and angina pectoris at rest. Am J Cardiol 1985; 56:403–6.
93. deZwaan C, Bar FW, Janssen JHA, et al. Effects of thrombolytic therapy in unstable angina: Clinical and angiographic results. J Am Coll Cardiol 1988; 12:301–9.
94. Ambrose JA, Hjemdahl-Monsen CE, Borrico S, et al. Quantitative and qualitative effects of intracoronary streptokinase in unstable angina and non Q-wave infarction. J Am Coll Cardiol 1987; 9:1156–65.
95. Ambrose JA, Hjemdahl-Monsen CE. Arteriographic anatomy and mechanisms: Myocardial ischemia and unstable angina. J Am Coll Cardiol 1987; 6:1397–1402.
96. Gotoh K, Minamino T, Katoh O, et al. The role of intracoronary thrombus in unstable angina: Angiographic assessment of thrombolytic therapy during ongoing anginal attacks. Circulation 1988; 77:526–34.
97. Mandelkorn JB, Wolf NX, Singh S, et al. Intracoronary thrombus in non transmural myocardial infarction and unstable angina pectoris. Am J Cardiol 1983; 52:1–6.
98. Williams AE, Freeman MR, Chisholm RJ, Patt NL, Armstrong PW. Angiographic morphology in unstable angina pectoris. Am J Cardiol 1988; 62:1024–7.
99. Chahine RA. Unstable angina: The problem of definition. Br Med J 1975; 37: 1246–9.
100. Gunnar RM, Bourdillon DV, Dixon DW, et al. Guidelines for the early management of patients with acute myocardial infarction. ACC/AHA Task Force Report. J Am Coll Cardiol 1990; 16:249–92.
101. Scanlon PJ, Nemickas R, Moran JF. Accelerated angina pectoris: Clinical hemodynamic arteriographic and therapeutic experience in 85 patients. Circulation 1973; 47:19–26.
102. Wood B. Acute and subacute coronary insufficiency. Br Med J 1961; 1779–82.
103. Roberts WC, Virmani R. Quantification of coronary arterial narrowing in clinically unstable angina pectoris. Am J Med 1979; 67:792–9.
104. Resnik WH. The significance of prolonged anginal pain (preinfarction angina). Am Heart J 1962; 63:290–8.
105. Guthrie RB, Vlodaver Z, Nicoloff DM, Edwards JE. Pathology of stable and unstable angina pectoris. Circulation 1975; 51:1059–63.
106. Levy E. The natural history of changing patterns of angina pectoris. Ann Intern Med 1956; 44:1123–35.

107. Master AM, Jaffe HL, Field LE, Donoso E. Acute coronary insufficiency: Its differential diagnosis and treatment. Ann Intern Med 1956; 45:561–81.
108. Scheidt S, Wolk M, Killip T. Unstable angina pectoris: Natural history, hemo-dynamics, uncertainties of treatment and the ethics of clinical study. Am J Med 1976; 60:409–17.
109. Feil H. Preliminary pain in coronary thrombosis. Am J Med Sci 1937; 193:42–8.
110. Fischl SJ, Herman MV, Gorlin R. The intermediate coronary syndrome: Clinical, angiographic and therapeutic aspects. N Engl J Med 1973; 288:1193–8.
111. Graybiel A. The intermediate coronary syndrome. US Armed Forces Med J 1955; 6:1–21.
112. Ouyang P, Brinker JA, Mellits ED, Weisfeldt ML, Gerstenblith G. Variables predictive of successful medical therapy in patients with unstable angina. Selection by multivariate analysis from clinical, electrocardiographic and angiographic eval-uations. Circulation 1984; 70:367–76.
113. Plotnick GD. Approach to the management of unstable angina. Am Heart J 1979; 98:243–55.
114. Russell RO, Rackley CE, Kouchoukos NT. Editorial: Unstable angina pectoris: Do we know the best management? Am J Cardiol 1981; 48:590–1.
115. Brow BG, Dodge HT. Editorial: Unstable angina: Guidelines for therapy based on the last decade of clinical observations. Ann Intern Med 1982; 97:921–3.
116. Flaherty JT. Unstable angina: A rational approach to management. Am J Med 1984; 54:52–7.
117. Cairns JA, et al. Aspirin, sulfinpyrazone, or both in unstable angina. N Engl J Med 1985; 313:1369–75.
118. Theroux P, et al. Aspirin, heparin, or both to treat acute unstable angina. N Engl J Med 1988; 319:1105–11.
119. White CW, Chaitman B, Lassart A, et al. Abstract antiplatet agents are effective in reducing the immediate complications of PTCA. Results from the ticlopidine multicenter trial. Circulation 1987; 76 (Suppl IV):400.
120. Mikolich JR, Nicoloff NB, Robinson PH, Logue RB. Relief of refractory angina with continuous intravenous infusion of nitroglycerin. Chest 1980; 77:375–9.
121. Kaplan K, Davison R, Parker M, Przybylek J, Teagarden JR, Lesch M. Intra-venous nitroglycerin for the treatment of angina at rest unresponsive to standard nitrate therapy. Am J Cardiol 1983; 51:694–8.
122. DePace NL, Herling IM, Kotler MN, Hakki AH, Spielman SR, Segal BL. Intravenous nitroglycerin for rest angina. Ann Intern Med 1982; 142:1806–9.
123. Roubin GS, Harris PJ, Eckhardt I, Hensley W, Kelly DT. Intravenous nitro-glycerin in refractory unstable angina pectoris. Aust NZ J Med 1982; 12:598–602.
124. Squire A, Cantor R, Packer M. Abstract: Limitations of continuous intravenous nitroglycerin prophylaxis in patients with refractory angina at rest. Circulation 1982; 66 (Suppl II):120.
125. Dauwe F, et al. Abstract: Intravenous nitroglycerin-refractory unstable angina. Am J Cardiol 1979; 43:416.
126. Brodsky SJ, et al. Abstract: Intravenous nitroglycerin-infusion in unstable angina. Clin Res 608A.
127. Curfman GD, Heinsimer JA, Lozner EC, Fung HL. Intravenous nitroglycerin in

the treatment of spontaneous angina pectoris: A prospective randomized trial. Circulation 1983; 67:276–82.

128. McGregor M. Pathogenesis of angina pectoris and role of nitrates in relief of myocardial ischemia. Am J Med 1983; 56:21–7.

129. Parodi O, Maseri A, Simonetti I. Management of unstable angina at rest by verapamil. Br Heart J 1979; 41:167–74.

130. Mehta J, Pepine CJ, Day M, Guerrero JR, Conti CR. Short term efficacy of oral verapamil in rest angina. Am J Med 1981; 71:977–82.

131. Multicenter Diltiazem Postinfarction Trial Research Group. The effect of diltiazem and reinfarction after myocardial infarction. N Engl J Med 1988; 319:385–92.

132. Holland Interuniversity Nifedipine-metoprolol Trial Research Group (HINT). Early treatment of unstable angina in the coronary care unit: A randomized double-blind placebo controlled comparison of recurrent ischemia in patients treated with nifedipine and metoprolol or both. Br Heart J 1986; 56:400–13.

133. Theroux P, Taeymans Y, Morrissette D, et al. A randomized study comparing propanolol and diltiazem in the treatment of unstable angina. J Am Coll Cardiol 1985; 5:717–22.

134. Gottlieb SO, Weisfeldt ML, Ouyang P, et al. The effect of the addition of propanolol to therapy with nifedipine for unstable angina pectoris: A randomized double-blind placebo controlled trial. Circulation 1986; 73:331–7.

135. Muller JE, Turi ZG, Pearl ED, et al. Nifedipine in convential therapy for unstable angina pectoris: A randomized double-blind comparison. Circulation 1984; 69: 728–39.

136. Gerstenblith G, Ouyang P, Achuff SC, et al. Nifedipine in unstable angina. N Engl J Med 1982; 306:885–9.

137. Norris RM, Sammel NL, Clark ED, Smith WN, Williams B. Protective effect of propanolol on recurrent myocardial infarction. Lancet 1978: 907-9.

138. Yusuf S, Peto R, Bennett D, et al. Early intravenous atenolol treatment of suspected acute myocardial infarction. Lancet 1980:273–6.

139. Telford AM, Wilson C. Trial of heparin vs. atenolol in prevention of myocardial infarction in intermediate coronary syndrome. Lancet 1981:1225–8.

140. Ambrose JA, Alexopoulos D. Thrombolysis in unstable angina with a beneficial effect of thrombolytic therapy in myocardial infarction: The plight of patients with unstable angina. J Am Coll Cardiol 1989; 13:1666–70.

141. Gold HK, Johns JA, Leimbach RC, Yasuda T, Cohen D. Thrombolytic therapy for unstable angina pectoris: Rationale and results. J Am Coll Cardiol 1987; 10: 91b–95b.

142. Shapiro EP, Brinker JA, Gottlieb SO, Guzman PA, Bulkley BH. Intracoronary thrombolysis 3-13 days after acute myocardial infarction for postinfarction angina pectoris. Am J Cardiol 1985; 55:1453–8.

143. Rentrop P, Blanke H, Karsch KR, et al. Selective intracoronary thrombolysis in acute myocardial infarction and unstable angina pectoris. Circulation 1981; 63: 307–17.

144. Vetrovec GW, Leinbach RC, Gold HK, Cowley MJ. Intracoronary thrombolysis in syndromes of unstable ischemia: Angiographic and clinical results. Am Heart J 1982; 104:946–92.

145. Scheidt S, Wolk M, Killip T. Unstable angina pectoris: Natural history, hemo-

dynamics, uncertainties of treatment and the ethics of clinical study. Am J Med 1976; 60:409–17.

146. Fulton M, Lutz W, Donald KW, et al. Natural history of unstable angina. Lancet 1972; 1:860–5.

147. Kannel WB, Feinleib M. Natural history of angina pectoris in the Framingham study: Prognosis and survival. Am J Cardiol 1972; 29:154–63.

148. Firth BG, Hillis LD, Willerson JT. Unstable angina pectoris: Medical vs. surgical treatment. Herz 1890; 1:16–24.

149. Lambert CJ, Adam M, Geisler GF, et al. Emergency myocardial revascularization for impending infarctions and arrhythmias. J. Thorac Cardiovasc Surg 1971; 62:522–8.

150. Segal BL, Likoff W, Van den Broek H, Kimbiris D, Najmi M, Linhardt JW. Saphenous vein bypass surgery for impending myocardial infarction. JAMA 1973; 223:767–72.

151. Favaloro RG, Effler DB, Cheanvecha C, Quint RA, Sones FM, Jr. Acute coronary insufficiency (impending myocardial infarction). Am J Cardiol 1971; 28:598–607.

152. Douglas BC, Adelman AG, Huckell VF, et al. Unstable angina: A clinical, angiographic and surgical profile. Cardiovasc Med 1978; 167–76.

153. Nunley DL, Grunkemeier GL, Teply JF, et al. Coronary bypass operation following acute complicated myocardial infarction. J. Thorac Cardiovasc Surg 1983; 85:485–91.

154. Levine FH, Gold HK, Leinbach RC, et al. Safe early revascularization for continuing ischemia after acute myocardial infarction. Circulation 1979; 60 (Suppl I):5–8.

155. Jones RN, Pifarre R, Sullivan HJ, et al. Early myocardial revascularization for post-infarction angina. Ann Thorac Surg 1987; 44:159–63.

156. Kennedy JW, Kaiser GC, Fisher LD, et al. Clinical and angiographic predictors of operative mortality from the collaborative study in coronary artery surgery (CASS). Circulation 1981; 63:793–801.

157. Pugh B, Platt MR, Mills LJ, et al. Unstable angina pectoris: A randomized study of patients treated medically and surgically. Am J Cardiol 1978; 41:1291–8.

158. Brown CA, Hutter AM, Jr., DeSanctis RW, et al. Prospective study of medical and urgent surgical therapy in randomizable patients with unstable angina pectoris: Results of in-hospital and chronic mortality and morbidity. Am Heart J 1981; 102:959–64.

159. Selden R, Neill WA, Ritzmann LW, Okies JE, Anderson RP. Medical versus surgical therapy for acute coronary insufficiency. N Engl J Med 1975; 293:1329–33.

160. Wiles JC, Peduzzi PN, Hammond GL, Cohen LS, Langou RA. Preoperative predictors of operative mortality for coronary artery bypass grafting in patients with unstable angina pectoris. Am J Cardiol 1977; 39:939–43.

161. Hultgren HN, Pfeiffer JF, Angell WW, Lipton MJ, Bilisoly S. Unstable angina: Comparison of medical and surgical management. Am J Cardiol 1977; 39:734–40.

162. Langou RA, Geha AS, Hammond GL, Cohen LS. Surgical approach for patients with unstable angina pectoris: Role of the response to initial medical therapy and intraaortic balloon pumping and perioperative complications after aortocoronary bypass grafting. Am J Cardiol 1978; 42:629–32.

163. Olinger GN, Bonchek LI, Keelan MH, et al. Unstable angina: The case for operation. Am J Cardiol 1978; 42:634–40.

164. Ahmed M, Thompson R, Searbra-Gomes R, et al. Unstable angina: A clinical arteriographic correlation and long term results of early myocardial revascularization. J. Thorac Cardiovasc Surg 1980; 79:609–16.

165. Jones EL, Waites TF, Craver JM, et al. Unstable angina pectoris: Comparison with the National Cooperative Study. Ann Thorac Surg 1982; 34:427–34.

166. Hultgren HN, Shettigar UR, Miller DC. Medical versus surgical treatment of unstable angina. Am J Cardiol 1982; 50:663–70.

167. Cobanoglu A, Freimanis I, Grunkemeier G, et al. Enhanced late survival following coronary artery bypass graft operation for unstable versus chronic angina. Ann Thorac Surg 1984; 37:52–9.

168. Golding LAR, Loop FD, Sheldon WC, et al. Emergency revascularization for unstable angina. Circulation 1978; 58:1163–6.

169. Rankin JS, Newton JR, Jr., Califf RM, et al. Clinical characteristics and current management of medically refractory unstable angina. Ann Surg 1984; 200:457–64.

170. Goldman BS, Katz A, Christakis G, Weisel R. Determinants of risk for coronary artery bypass grafting in stable and unstable angina pectoris. Can J Surg 1985; 28:505–8.

171. Edwards FH, Bellamy R, Burge JR, et al. True emergency coronary artery bypass surgery. Ann Thorac Surg 1990; 49:603–11.

172. Cohn LH, Alpert J, Koster JK, Mee RBB, Collins JJ, Jr. Changing indications for the surgical treatment of unstable angina. Arch Surg 1978; 113:1312–6.

173. Hatcher CR, Jr., King SB III, Kaplan A. Surgical management of unstable angina. World J Surg 1978; 2:689–700.

174. Holmes DR, Jr., Holubkov R, Vliestra R, et al. Comparison of complications during percutaneous transluminal coronary angioplasty from 1977–1981, and 1985–1986: The National Heart, Lung and Blood Institute Percutaneous Transluminal Coronary Angioplasty Registry. J Am Coll Cardiol 1988; 12:1149–55.

175. Detre K, Myler RK, Kelsey, SF, VanRaden M, To M, Mitchell. Baseline characteristics of patients in the National Heart, Lung and Blood Institute Percutaneous Transluminal Coronary Angioplasty Registry. Am J Cardiol 1984; 54:7C–11C.

176. Firth BG, Hillis LD, Willerson JT. Unstable angina pectoris: Medical versus surgical treatment. Herz 1980; 5:16–24.

177. Detre K, Holubkov PH, Kelsey S, et al. Percutaneous transluminal coronary angioplasty in 1985–1986 and 1977–1981. N Engl J Med 1988; 318:265–70.

178. Mullin SM, Passamani ER, Mock MB. Historical background the National Heart, Lung and Blood Institute Registry for Percutaneous Transluminal Angioplasty. Am J Cardiol 1984; 53:3C–6C.

179. Kent KM, Bentivoglio LG, Block PC, et al. Percutaneous transluminal coronary angioplasty—Report from the Registry of the National Heart, Lung and Blood Institute. Am J Cardiol 1982; 49:2011–20.

180. Faxon DP, Kelsey SF, Ryan TJ, McCabe CH, Detre K. Determinants of successful percutaneous transluminal coronary angioplasty-report from the National Heart, Lung and Blood Institute Registry. Am Heart J 1984; 108:1019–23.

181. Mock MB, Smith HC, Mullaney, CJ. The second generation NHLBI Percutaneous Transluminal Coronary Angioplasty Registry: Have we established the role for PTCA in treating coronary disease? Circulation 1989; 80:700–2.

182. Shawl FA, Velasco CE, Goldbaum TS, Forman MB. The effect of coronary angioplasty on electrocardiographic changes in patients with unstable angina secondary to left anterior descending coronary artery disease. J Am Coll Cardiol 1990; 16:325–31.

183. Williams DO, Riley RS, Singh AK, Gewirth H, Most AS. Evaluation of the role of coronary angioplasty in patients with unstable angina pectoris. Am Heart J 1981; 102:1–9.

184. Meyer J, Schmitz H, Erbel R, et al. Treatment of unstable angina pectoris with percutaneous transluminal coronary angioplasty (PTCA). Catheterization Cardiovasc Diag-1981; 7:361–71.

185. Meyer J, Schmitz HJ, Kiesslicht, et al. Percutaneous transluminal coronary angioplasty in patients with stable and unstable angina pectoris: Analysis of early and late results. Am Heart J 1983; 106:973–80.

186. deFeyter PJ, Serruys PW, Suryapranata H, Beatt K, Van den Brand M. Coronary angioplasty early after diagnosis of unstable angina. Am Heart J 1987; 114:48–54.

187. Timmis AD, Griffin B, Crick CP, Sowton E. Early percutaneous transluminal coronary angioplasty in the management of unstable angina. Int J Cardiol 1987; 14:25–31.

188. Tuzcu EM, Simpendorfer C, Badwar K, et al. Determinants of primary success in elective percutaneous transluminal coronary angioplasty for significant narrowing of a single major coronary artery. Am J Cardiol 1988; 62:873–5.

189. Faxon DP, Detre KM, McCabe Ch, et al. Role of percutaneous transluminal coronary angioplasty in the treatment of unstable angina. Report from the National Heart, Lung and Blood Institute Percutaneous Transluminal Coronary Angioplasty and Coronary Artery Surgery Study Registries. Am J Cardiol 1983; 53:131C–135C.

190. Sharma B, Wyeth RP, Kolath GS, Gimenez HJ, Franciosa JA. Percutaneous transluminal coronary angioplasty of one vessel for refractory unstable angina pectoris (efficacy and single end multi-vessel disease). Br Heart J 1988; 59:280–6.

191. deFeyter PJ, Serruys PW, Arnold A, et al. Coronary angioplasty of the unstable angina related vessel in patients with multi-vessel disease. Eur Heart J 1986; 7:460–7.

192. DiMarco RF, McKeating JA, Pellegrin RV, et al. Contraindications for percutaneous transluminal coronary angioplasty in treatment of unstable angina pectoris. Texas Heart Inst J 1988; 15:152–4.

193. Holmes DR, Reeder GS, Vliestra RA. Role of percutaneous transluminal coronary angioplasty in multivessel disease. Am J Cardiol 1988; 61:9G–14G.

194. Hartzler GO, Rutherford BD, McConahay DR, et al. High risk percutaneous transluminal coronary angioplasty. Am J Cardiol 1988; 61:33G–37G.

195. Deligonul U, Vandormael MG, Kern MH, et al. Coronary angioplasty: A therapeutic option for symptomatic patients with 2 and 3 vessel coronary disease. J Am Coll Cardiol 1988; 11:1173–9.

196. Breisblatt WM, Barnes JV, Weiland F, Spaccavento LJ. Incomplete revascularization in multi-vessel percutaneous transluminal coronary angioplasty: The role for stress-thallium 201 imaging. J Am Coll Cardiol 1988; 11:1183–90.

197. Disciascio G, Cowley MJ, Vetrovec GW, Kelly KM, Lewis SA. Triple vessel

coronary angioplasty—Acute outcome and long term results. J Am Coll Cardiol 1988; 12:42–8.

198. Vandormael MG, Chaitman BR, Ischinger T, et al. Immediate and short term benefit of multi-lesion coronary angioplasty—Influence of degree of revascularization. J Am Coll Cardiol 1985; 6:983–91.

199. Cowley MJ, Vetrovec GW, Disciasco G, et al. Coronary angioplasty of multiple vessels—Short term outcome and long term results. Circulation 1985; 72:1314–20.

200. Mabin TA, Holmes DR, Smith HC, et al. Follow up clinical results in patients undergoing percutaneous transluminal coronary angioplasty. Circulation 1985; 71:754–60.

201. Thomas ES, Most AS, Williams DO. Coronary angioplasty for patients with multi-vessel coronary artery disease—Follow up clinical status. Am Heart J 1988; 115:8–13.

202. deFeyter PH, Serruys PW, Soward A, et al. Coronary angioplasty for early post-infarction/unstable angina. Circulation 1986; 74:1365–70.

203. Hopkins J, Savage M, Zalewski A, et al. Recurrent ischemia in the zone of prior myocardial infarction: Results of coronary angioplasty of the infarct related artery. Am Heart J 1988; 115:14–9.

204. Gottlieb SO, Walford GD, Ouyang P, et al. Initial and late results of coronary angioplasty for early postinfarction unstable angina. Cath Cardiovasc Diag 1987; 13:93–9.

205. Safian RD, Snyder LD, Snyder BA, et al. Usefulness of percutaneous transluminal coronary angioplasty for unstable angina pectoris after non Q-wave acute myocardial infarction. Am J Cardiol 1987; 59:263–6.

206. Suryapranata H, Beatt K, deFeyter PJ, et al. Percutaneous transluminal coronary angioplasty for angina pectoris after a non Q-wave myocardial infarction. Am J Cardiol 1988; 61:240–3.

207. Sabbah HN, Brymer JF, Gheoghiadez M, Stein PD, Kahja A. Left ventricular function after successful percutaneous transluminal angioplasty for post-infarction angina pectoris. Am J Cardiol 1988; 62:358–62.

208. Bosch X, Theroux P, Waters DD, Pellettier GB, Roy D. Early post infarction ischemia: Clinical angiographic and prognostic significance. Circulation 1987; 75:988–95.

209. Campolo L, DeBiase AM, Cataldo MG, et al. Indications for surgical treatment in post infarction angina. Eur Heart J 1986; 7(Suppl):103–9.

210. Fioretti P, Brower RW, Balakumaran R. Early post infarction angina; incidents and prognostic relevance. Eur Heart J 1986; 7(Supp C):73–7.

211. Bigger JT Jr. Angina pectoris early after myocardial infarction: Clinical experience of a multi-center post infarction program. Eur Heart J 1986; 7(Supp C):37–41.

212. Borer JS. Editorial: Unstable angina: A lethal gun with an invisible trigger. N Engl J Med 1980; 302:1200–2.

213. Mounsey P. Prodromal symptoms in myocardial infarction. Br Heart J 1951; 13:215–26.

214. Solomon HA, Edwards AL, Killip T. Prodromata in acute myocardial infarction. Circulation 1969; 40:463–71.

215. Hochberg HM. Characteristics and significance of prodromes of coronary care in patients. Chest 1971; 59:10–4.
216. Marmor A, Sobel BE, Roberts R. Factors prestaging early recurrent myocardial infarction (extension). Am J Cardiol 1981; 48:603–10.
217. Fraker TD, Wagner GS, Rosati RA. Extension of myocardial infarction: Incidence and prognosis. Circulation 1979; 60:1126–9.
218. Kronenberg MW, Hodges M, Akiyama T, et al. ST segment variations after acute myocardial infarction. Circulation 1976; 54:756–61.
219. Stenson RE, Flamm MD, Zaret BL, McGowan RL. Am Heart J 1975; 89:449–54.
220. Reid PR, Taylor DR, Kelly DT, et al. Myocardial infarct extension detected by proc ial ST mapping. N Engl J Med 1974; 290:123–8.
221. Muller JE, Rude RE, Braunwald E, et al. Myocardial infarct extension; occurrence at common risk factors in the multicenter investigation of the limitation of infarct size. Ann Intern Med 1988; 108:1–6.
222. McKay RG, Pfeffer MA, Pasternak RC, et al. Left ventricular remodeling after myocardial infarction; a corollary to infarction expansion. Circulation 1986; 74:693–702.
223. Erlebacher JA, Weiss JL, Weisfeldt ML, Bulkley BA. Early dilatation of the infarcted segment in acute transmural myocardial infarction. Role of infarct expansion in acute left ventricular enlargement. J Am Coll Cardiol 1984; 4:201–8.
224. Schuster EH, Bulkley BH. Early post infarction angina; ischemia at a distance and ischemia in the infarct zone. N Engl J Med 1981; 305:1101–5.
225. deFeyter PJ, van den Brand M, Serruys PW, Wyns W. Early angiography after myocardial infarction: What have we learned? Am Heart J 1985; 194–9.
226. Gibson RS, Beller GA, Gheorghiade M, et al. The prevalence and clinical significance of residual myocardial ischemia two weeks after non-complicated non Q-wave infarction; a prospective natural history study. Circulation 1986; 73:1186–98.
227. DeWood MA, Stifter WF, Simpson CS, et al. Coronary angiographic findings soon after non Q-wave myocardial infarction. N Engl J Med 1986; 315:417–23.
228. Gibson RS, Boden WE, Theroux P, et al. Diltiazem in re-infarction patients with non Q-wave myocardial infarction. N Engl J Med 1986; 315:423–9.
229. Benhorin J, Andrews ML, Carleen ED, et al. Occurrence characteristics and prognostic significance of early post acute myocardial infarction; angina pectoris. Am J Cardiol 1988; 62:679–85.
230. Sellier P, Plat F, Corona P, et al. Prognostic significance of angina pectoris recurring soon after myocardial infarction. Eur Heart J 1988; 9:447–553.
231. Falk E. Unstable angina fatal outcome; dynamic coronary thrombosis leading to infarction and/or sudden death. Circulation 1985; 71:699–708.
232. Theroux P, Waters DD, Halphen C, et al. Prognostic value of exercise testing soon after myocardial infarction. N Engl J Med 1979; 301:341–5.
233. Sobel BE, Bresnahan GF, Shell WE, Yoder RD. Estimation of infarct size in man and its relation to prognosis. Circulation 1972; 46:640–8.
234. DeServi S, Vaccari L, Graziano G, et al. Clinical and angiographic data in early post infarction angina. Eur Heart J 1986; 7(Suppl C): 69–72.
235. Tomkinson GC, Kern KB, Lancaster LD, Gay RG, Goldman S. Cardiac catheterization for patients with post infarction angina. Clin Cardiol 1987; 10:399–403.

236. Midwal J, Ambrose J, Pickard A, Abedin Z, Herman MV. Angina pectoris before and after myocardial infarction. Angiographic correlations. Chest 1982; 81:681–6.

237. Williams DB, Ivey TD, Bailey WW, Ivey SS, Redeout JT, Stewart D. Post infarction angina: Results of early revascularization. J Am Coll Cardiol 1983; 2:859.

238. Baumgartner WA, Borkon AM, Zibulewsky J, Watkins L, Gardner TJ, Bulkey BH, Achuff SC, Baughman KL, Traill TA, Gott VL, Reitz RA. Operative intervention for postinfarction angina. Ann Thorac Surg 1984; 38:265.

239. Gertler JP, Elefteriades JA, Kopf GS, Hashim SW, Hammond GL, Geha AS. Predictors of outcome in early revascularization after acute myocardial infarction. Am J Surg 1985; 149:441.

240. Singh AK, Rivera R, Cooper GN, Karlson KE. Early myocardial revascularization for post infarction angina: Results and long term follow-up. J Am Coll Cardiol 1985; 6:1121.

241. Brower RW, Fioretti P, Simoons ML, Haalebos M, Ruff ENR, Hugenholtz PG. Surgical vs. non-surgical management of patients soon after myocardial infarction. Br Heart J 1985; 54:460.

242. Breyer RH, Engelman RM, Rousou JA, Lemeshow S. Post infarction angina: An expanding subset of patients undergoing bypass surgery. J Thorac Cardiovasc Surg 1985; 90:532.

243. Stuart RS, Baumgartner WA, Soule L, Borkion AM, Gardner TJ, Gott VL, Watkins SL, Reitz BA. Predictors of perioperative mortality in patients with unstable postinfarction angina. Circulation 1988; 78(Supp I):I163–I165.

244. Bardet J, Rigand M, Kahn JC, et al. Treatment of post myocardial infarction angina by intraaotic balloon pumping and emergency revascularization. J Thorac Cardiosvasc Surg 1977; 74:299–305.

245. Jones EL, Waites TF, Craver JM, et al. Coronary bypass for relief of persistent pain following acute myocardial infarction. Ann Thorac Surg 1981; 32:33–43.

246. Madigan NP, Rutherford BD, Barnhorst DA, Danielson GK. Early saphenous vein grafting after endocardial infarction. Circulation 1977; 56 (Suppl 2):II-1–3.

247. Brandage BH, Ullyot DJ, Winokur S, Chatterjee K, Ports TA, Turley K. The role of aortic balloon pumping in postinfarction angina. Circulation 1980; 62(Suppl I):I-119–I123.

248. Weintraub RM, Aroesty JM, Paulin S, et al. Medically refractory unstable angina pectoris. Long term follow-up of patients undergoing intraaortic balloon counter-pulsation and operation. Am J Cardiol 1979; 43:877–82.

249. Grover F, Hammermeister KE, Burchfiel C, and the cardiac surgeons of the Department of Veterans Affairs: Initial report of the Veterans Administration preoperative risk assessment study for cardiac surgery. Ann Thorac Surg 1990; 50:12–28.

250. The principal investigators of CASS and their associates. The National Heart, Lung and Blood Institute Coronary Artery Surgery Study (CASS). Circulation 1983; 63 (Suppl I): I-1–I-81.

251. Second International Study of Infarct Survival Collaborative Group. Randomized trial of intravenous streptokinase, oral aspirin, both, or neither among 17,187 cases of suspected acute myocardial infarction: ISIS-2. Lancet 1988:349–60.

2

Unstable Angina: Design, Conduct, and Interpretation of Clinical Studies

Douglass Andrew Morrison

Veterans Affairs Medical Center and
University of Colorado Health Sciences Center
Denver, Colorado

HOW MUCH INFORMATION IS "ENOUGH"?

Each day, all of us are called upon to make decisions. In the care of the patient with unstable angina, one must decide on a course of medical therapy, when medical therapy has failed, whether to proceed to cardiac catheterization, and whether either an angioplasty or bypass strategy is preferable to continued medical therapy. Each of these, and many other decisions, must be made based on information that is incomplete. Whenever possible, we try to increase our information base upon which to make decisions. For example, we add to our patient history, obtain electrocardiograms during symptomatic periods, or make serial cardiac enzyme determinations. Obviously, there are limits to this type of individual information that can be obtained.

Far more limited is our information base about how patients will fare with a particular type of therapy. Our information base for these kinds of decisions consists of personal experience, case reports, retrospective series, prospective consecutive case series, controlled series, and prospective, randomized trials.

Each of these types of clinical study involve some degree of patient risk, doctor or investigator inconvenience, and cost. As a simple (and cynical) rule of thumb, the more clinically useful studies nearly always involve greater degrees of risk, inconvenience and cost!

WHAT KINDS OF CLINICAL INFORMATION BASE ARE AVAILABLE?

Single case reports are only useful in suggesting ideas. Many of the "classic" studies of unstable angina are retrospective case series. In other words, a hypothesis was not formulated first and data collected to test that hypothesis. Rather, case material was assembled and an hypothesis teased out of the data. Patient selection biases and data selection (what parameters to look at) biases can obviously enter such studies easily. This kind of observational data is most useful for formulating questions that can be more rigorously tested prospectively. Examples of important studies of this type from the tables in Chapter 1 include the natural history studies of Vakil, Krauss et al., Gazes et al., Conti et al., and Bertolasi et al. (1–5).

A prospective observational approach represents the next level of complexity. Especially if a hypothesis to be tested is formulated before the data gathering begins, this represents a significant step toward reducing bias. Additional validity may be gained by insisting on inclusion of consecutive cases (meeting some entry criteria). The alternative, indiscriminate exclusion, allows for major selection bias.

The multicenter registry extends the database of a single center (Refs. 16–18 from NHLBI PTCA registry versus Refs. 19–21 from Erasmus University and Ref. 24). Whether such data is prospective depends on when the hypothesis was formulated.

Another major step toward clinically useful decision-making data is the concept of control cases. Some of the retrospective series, such as Vakil's compared consecutive cases given a therapy (like Coumadin) with cases denied the therapy. If there is no provision for random assignment, there is almost certainly some selection bias in the choice between therapy case and control case (see Chapter 21 on the types of selection bias that have gone into the choice between internal mammary artery and saphenous veins as bypass graft conduits). Nonetheless, control cases at least provide some attempt to separate out the effects of concomitant therapy.

Historical controls, for example, comparing two different periods in the NHLBI PTCA Registry have some value (16–18). An alternative, with even greater selection bias, is to compare registries of different therapies, such as the CASS experience with bypass surgery versus the NHLBI Registry of angioplasty (22).

The most powerful type of clinical study to assess the merits of diagnostic or therapeutic approaches is the prospective, randomized clinical trial (6–15). The prospective and randomized nature of such studies assures that the control and treated groups are comparable. In turn, this means that any observed differences accrue from the intervention rather than as an artifact of selection bias, observation bias, or concomitant therapy. Among the best examples of this type of study applied to unstable angina are the VA Cooperative Aspirin Study (6), the VA Cooperative Medical Versus Surgical Trial (7–9), and the National Cooperative Medical Versus Surgical Trial (10–13).

POTENTIAL PROBLEMS IN THE DESIGN AND CONDUCT OF EACH TYPE OF CLINICAL STUDY

All the selection bias problems alluded to above lead to results that are not representative of the studied situation. It is important to emphasize that even though the controlled trial allows us to correctly compare the effect of therapy versus control in a given population, if control versus therapy homogeneity has been achieved by eliminating 90% of the available patients, the study results will apply only to ~10% of patients! As far-fetched as this may sound, large studies, like CASS, have typically excluded ≥90% of screened patients! (23)

A related issue to selection bias is sample size. A variety of commercially available computer programs allow one to manipulate the numbers to demonstrate the importance of sample size. It is intuitively clear that the smaller the difference to be detected between therapeutic and control groups, the larger the numbers of patients who must be randomized to detect this difference. Clearly, one must be sure when reviewing clinical data that failure to detect a difference does not represent inadequate sample size rather than truly no difference.

In uncontrolled or nonrandomly assigned control studies, a difference detected may represent changes in natural history or changes in therapy over time rather than a difference specific to the therapy.

Even the best-controlled, prospective randomized studies may be accused of generating results that are unique to the study setting and not generalizable. For example, a number of surgeons have criticized VA Cooperative surgical data as being unique to VA patients or surgeons (7–9). Because every study is performed in some unique setting, to some extent this criticism is unavoidable. Nevertheless, it is reasonable to assume that multicenter studies might be more representative than single-center studies.

In the real world, cost is always an issue. Larger, more representative studies with adequate sample sizes and randomized controls clearly cost much more in dollars and man-hours than retrospective observational data (especially with computers).

PROBLEMS IN INTERPRETATION OF CLINICAL STUDIES

When a trial, like the VA Cooperative Aspirin Study, detects a difference between control and treatment groups in mortality, the implication is clear (6). Alternatively, the "softer" the end-points, the less clear a "difference" really matters clinically. For example, of the six ongoing trials of PTCA versus CABG, only the NIH BARI was designed to have a chance to detect mortality or infarction differences. The other five will detect (or not detect) differences in some measure of relief of angina. It is predictable that these results will be of limited value in clinical decision making.

Sample size issues were alluded to under consideration of design and conduct. They reappear when one considers study interpretation because most studies do not recruit patients nearly as well as they anticipated. Alternatively, far more patients must be excluded than the designers anticipated.

A major problem in interpreting therapeutic studies accrues from concomitant therapy and/or crossovers. In unstable angina, nearly all patients are on some medical therapy whether they receive CABG or PTCA. Similarly the most vexing clinical decisions involve patients who already have had at least one CABG and/or PTCA. Intention to treat provides only a tool, but not a complete solution, to this difficult problem.

SUMMARY AND SUGGESTIONS FOR THE DESIGN, CONDUCT, AND INTERPRETATION OF A THERAPEUTIC STUDY OF UNSTABLE ANGINA

1. The study should be prospective with hypotheses formulated prior to data gathering.
2. Multicenter studies will provide more representative results and larger sample size.
3. A registry for all screened patients will permit evaluation of the selection biases that went into selecting the study and control populations.
4. Randomization is a key to comparable control and therapeutic groups.
5. An adequate clinical database will allow one to determine if statement #4 is true, namely, that the control and therapeutic groups are comparable.

REFERENCES

1. Vakil RJ. Preinfarction syndrome—Management and follow-up. Am J Cardiol 1964; 14: 55–63.
2. Krauss KR, Hutter AM, DeSanctis RW. Acute coronary insufficiency. Arch Intern Med 1972; 129: 808–13.
3. Gazes PC, Mobley EM Jr., Faris HM Jr., Duncan RC, Humphries GB. Preinfarctional (unstable) angina—A prospective study—Ten year follow up. Circulation 1973; 48: 331–7.
4. Conti CR, Brawley RK, Griffith LSC, Pitt B, Humphries JO, Gott VL, Ross RS. Unstable angina pectoris: Morbidity and Mortality in 57 consecutive patients evaluated angiographically. Am J Cardiol 1973; 32: 745–50.
5. Bertolasi CA, Tronge JE, Riccitelli MA, Villamayor RM, Zuffardi E. Natural history of unstable angina with medical or surgical therapy. Chest 1976; 70: 596-605.

6. Lewis, HD Jr., Davis JW, Archibald DG, Steinke WE, Smitherman TC, Doherty JE III, Schnaper HW, LeWinter MM, Linares E, Pouget JM, Sabharwal SC, Chesler E, DeMots H. Protective effects of aspirin against acute myocardial infarction and death in men with unstable angina. N Engl J Med 1983; 309: 396–403.

7. Luchi RJ, Scott SM, Deupree RH, and the Principal Investigators and their Associates of Veterans Administration Cooperative Study No 28. Comparison of medical and surgical treatment for unstable angina pectoris. N Engl J Med 1987; 316: 977–84.

8. Scott SM, Luchi RJ, Deupree RH, and the Veterans Administration Unstable Angina Cooperative Study Group: Veterans Administration Cooperative Study for Treatment of Patients with Unstable Angina. Circulation 1988; 78 (Supple I): I-113–I-121.

9. Parisi AF, Khuri S, Deupree RH, Sharma GVRK, Scott SM, Luchi RJ. Medical compared with surgical management of unstable angina: 5 Year mortality and morbidity in the Veterans Administration study. Circulation 1989; 80: 1176–89.

10. Russell RO, Moraski RE, Kouchoukos N, et al. Unstable angina pectoris: National Cooperative Study Group to Compare Medical and Surgical Therapy. I. Report of protocol and patient population. Am J Cardiol 1976 37: 896–902.

11. Russell RO, Moraski RE, Kouchoukos N, et al: Unstable angina pectoris: National Cooperative Study Group to Compare Surgical and Medical Therapy. II. In-hospital experience and initial follow-up results in patients with one, two, and three vessel disease. Am J. Cardiol 1978; 42: 939–48.

12. Russell RO, Moraski RE, Kouchoukos N, et al. Unstable angina pectoris: National Cooperative Study Group to Compare Surgical and Medical Therapy. III. Results in patients with S-T segment elevation during pain. Am J Cardiol 1980; 45: 819–24.

13. Russell RO, Moraski RE, Kouchoukos N, et al. Unstable angina pectoris: National Cooperative Study Group to Compare Medical and Surgical Therapy. IV. Results in patients with left anterior descending artery disease. Am J Cardiol 1981; 48: 517–24.

14. Cairns JA, et al. Aspirin, sulfinpyrazone, or both in unstable angina. N Engl J Med 1985; 313: 1369–75.

15. Theroux P, et al. Aspirin, heparin, or both to treat acute unstable angina. N Engl J Med 1988; 319: 1105–11.

16. Holmes DR, Jr., Holubkov R, Vliestra R, et al. Comparison of complications during percutaneous transluminal coronary angioplasty from 1977–1981, and 1985–1986: The National Heart, Lung and Blood Institute Percutaneous Transluminal Coronary Angioplasty Registry. J Am Coll Cardiol 1988; 12: 1149–55.

17. Detre K, Myler RK, Kelsey SF, VanRaden M, To M, Mitchell. Baseline characteristics of patients in the National Heart, Lung and Blood Institute Percutaneous Transluminal Coronary Angioplasty Registry. Am J Cardiol 1984; 54: 7C–11C.

18. Detre K, Holubkov PH, Kelsey S, et al. Percutaneous transluminal coronary angioplasty in 1985–1986 and 1977–1981. N Engl J Med 1988; 318: 265–70.

19. deFeyter PH, Serruys PW, Soward A, et al. Coronary angioplasty for early post-infarction/unstable angina. Circulation 1986; 74: 1365–70.

20. Safian RD, Snyder LD, Snyder BA, et al. Usefulness of percutaneous tranluminal coronary angioplasty for unstable angina pectoris after non Q-wave acute myocardial infarction. Am J Cardiol 1987; 59: 263–6.

21. deFeyter PJ, van den Brand M, Serruys PW, Wyns W. Early angiography after myocardial infarction: What have we learned? Am Heart J 1985; 194–9.

22. Faxon DP, Detre KM, McCabe Ch, et al. Role of percutaneous transluminal coronary angioplasty in the treatment of unstable angina. Report from the National Heart, Lung and Blood Institute Percutaneous Transluminal Coronary Angioplasty and Coronary Artery Surgery Study Registries. Am J Cardiol 1983; 53: 131C–135C.

23. The National Heart, Lung and Blood Institute Coronary Artery Surgery Study (CASS). Circulation 1981; 89: 513–24.

24. Grover F, Hammermeister KE, Burchfiel C, and the cardiac surgeons of the Department of Veterans Affairs. Initial report of the Veterans Administration preoperative risk assessment study for cardiac surgery. Ann Thorac Surg 1990; 50: 12–28.

II
PATHOPHYSIOLOGY

3

The Unstable Plaque

John A. Ambrose, Douglas H. Israel, and Sabino R. Torre

Mount Sinai Medical Center
New York, New York

INTRODUCTION

The acute coronary syndromes of unstable angina, non-Q-wave myocardial infarction, Q-wave myocardial infarction, and ischemic sudden death have fascinated cardiologists and generated controversy for nearly a century. Historically, the syndrome now known as unstable angina and referred to in the past as acute coronary insufficiency, preinfarction angina, or the intermediate coronary syndrome has been explained by a variety of pathogenetic mechanisms. Early studies proposed that rest angina occurred due to an imbalance between myocardial oxygen supply and demand, as in angina related to effort. In the 1970s, the concept of vasospasm was suggested to be important not only in the pathogenesis of classic Prinzemetal's angina, with ST segment elevation at rest, but also in the case of chest pain at rest with ST-segment depression or T-wave changes. More recently, there has been a large body of data derived from pathological, angiographic, and angioscopic studies suggesting that the acute coronary syndromes share a common pathogenesis related to spontaneous atherosclerotic plaque disruption with superimposed thrombosis. The syndromes of unstable angina, non-Q-wave infarction, and Q-wave infarction thus appear as a continuum, with the exact clinical scenario dependent on a number of factors, including the degree and acuteness of obstruction, the thrombotic burden, the sufficiency of endogenous thrombolytic systems, and the adequacy of collateral support. Newer evidence also suggests that recurrent minor plaque disruptions with deposition, organization, and incorporation of nonocclusive mural thrombus may be an important mechanism of subacute progression of the stable atherosclerotic plaque.

PATHOLOGICAL STUDIES

Very early pathological studies suggested coronary thrombosis as the cause of acute myocardial infarction (1–3), and in the 1940s and early 1950s, anticoagulation was routinely recommended in the postmyocardial infarction patient. In the 1970s, however, the pathophysiological relevance of thrombus as the proximate cause of myocardial infarction was challenged. In some studies, coronary thrombi were present in only about 50% of patients with myocardial infarction (4,5), and it was suggested that coronary thrombosis, when present, could be a secondary phenomenon. In addition, kinetic studies by Erhardt et al. (6), using iodine-135 labeled fibrinogen given intravenously to patients during acute myocardial infarction, appeared to indicate that the thrombi formed after the onset of infarction, supporting the notion that they were the consequence, rather than the cause, of infarction.

In spite of these data, however, the majority of pathological studies conducted during this period showed a high incidence of occlusive coronary thrombi (range 86–100%) (6–9) in arteries subtending an area of acute transmural myocardial infarction. Frequently, these thrombi were anchored to the site of an acute intimal disruptions, such as an ulcer or fissure (2,6,8). More recent pathological data, derived form patients dying following acute myocardial infarction or ischemic sudden death, have confirmed that there is a marked prevalence of major plaque disruptions, including ulcers, fissures, and frank atheromatous rupture complicated by varying degrees of thrombosis. In patients with ischemic sudden death, Davies and Thomas found coronary thrombi complicating a disrupted plaque in 74% of patients. Even in those in whom thrombi were not detected, there was an injured plaque in 80% of cases (10,11). Falk (12) performed postmortem examinations of the heart and coronary arteries in selected patients with a prodromal history of unstable angina culminating in acute coronary thrombosis and sudden death. He demonstrated that 81% of the thrombi had a layered appearance, with thrombotic material of varying ages, suggesting that they were formed by repeated deposition and organization of mural thrombi with progressive luminal narrowing occurring over an extended period of time.

It is possible that such episodic cycles of plaque disruption, mural thrombosis, and organization may be a major mechanism of plaque progression even when the patient's symptoms are stable, and that unstable symptoms occur only when there is acute progression to critical luminal narrowing. In many cases, however, the lesion responsible for the development of unstable angina or acute myocardial infarction arises through the mechanism of plaque disruption and thrombosis from a previously insignificant stenosis (13,14). In such cases, one may speculate that the inciting plaque injury may be very severe, creating a very thrombogenic milieu, and the resulting changes in plaque geometry with superimposed thrombus creates luminal obstruction. In the study by Falk (12), laminated thrombi were associated with intermittent distal microembolization in 73% of the cases, resulting in occlusion of small intramyocardial arteries and microinfarcts.

The angiographic features of such complex lesions were first described by Levin and Fallon (15). These investigators established histopathological and angiographic correlations by comparing postmortem coronary angiographic morphology and histological sections in 73 coronary lesions from patients dying following myocardial infarction, or after coronary artery bypass surgery. Histologically "complicated" stenoses exhibiting plaque rupture, plaque hemorrhage, superimposed partially occlusive thrombus, and/or recanalized thrombus had a distinctive angiographic appearance characterized by eccentric irregular and ragged borders with intraluminal lucency (Fig. 1). They further concluded that "complicated" lesions are associated with a higher risk of developing an acute myocardial infarction or sudden death than uncomplicated lesions. The relationship between cineangiography and postmortem histology was recently reexamined by Onodera et al. (16). In patients with acute myocardial infarction who died after intracoronary thrombolysis, postmortem angiographic findings of ragged and irregular stenosis borders with translucency and filling defects corresponded to histological findings of plaque rupture with thrombosis and hemorrhage in 80% of cases.

ANGIOGRAPHIC STUDIES

Complex Lesions

Unstable angina is often defined as ischemic cardiac pain at rest or with minimal effort. It may occur either de novo or as an abrupt acceleration of previously stable angina. Unstable and stable angina do not differ in the number of vessels with significant disease, the percent stenosis of the diseased vessels, or the degree of left ventricular dysfunction (17). However, sequential angiographic studies in patients with angina studied before and after the development of unstable symptoms have shown that the onset of unstable angina is associated with a marked progression of coronary stenosis in about 75% of cases (18,19), and that these new lesions demonstrate specific morphological features. Thus, whereas quantitative analysis of the coronary arteriogram cannot distinguish between stable and unstable angina, qualitative analysis of coronary morphology may often reliably differentiate the two syndromes. Coronary morphology refers to a qualitative assessment of the stenosis, with emphasis on the presence or absence of intracoronary filling defects, symmetry of the lesion, and whether the borders are regular or irregular. Morphology is best determined in orthogonal projections avoiding foreshortening of the lesion or overlap of vessels.

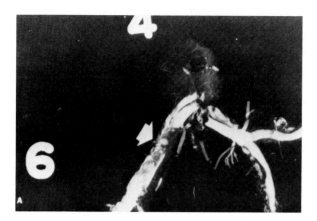

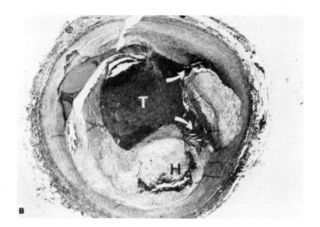

Figure 1 (A) Postmortem angiogram of a complex stenosis of the proximal left anterior descending artery (arrow). The borders of the lesion are markedly irregular and there are numerous intraluminal lucencies in the area of and distal to the narrowing. (B) The corresponding histological section shows a complicated atherosclerotic plaque with plaque rupture (arrows), intraplaque hemorrhage (H), and an intraluminal thrombus (T) that occludes the lumen almost totally. Hematoxylineosin stain; original magnification × 30. (Reprinted, with permission of D. C. Levin, J. T. Fallon, and the American Heart Association, from Ref. 15.)

In our studies, we found that coronary lesion morphology determined at angiography was predictive of unstable angina (19,20). The angiograms of more than 100 patients with either stable or unstable angina were assessed qualitatively at the time of angiography without knowledge of the patient's clinical status. Coronary lesions were categorized according to their angiographic morphology based on observations made by Levin and Fallon (15), as described above. Each significant coronary obstruction (>50% diameter stenosis) was categorized into one of the following morphological groups (Fig. 2): concentric (symmetrical narrowing); type I eccentric (asymmetrical with smooth borders and/or a broad neck); type II eccentric (asymmetrical with a narrow neck, or irregular borders,

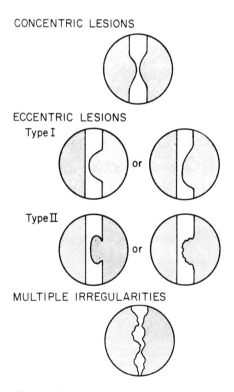

CONCENTRIC LESIONS

ECCENTRIC LESIONS
Type I   or

Type II   or

MULTIPLE IRREGULARITIES

Figure 2 Original classification scheme of coronary artery morphological findings. Concentric lesions were symmetrical and usually smooth. Type I eccentric lesions were asymmetrical and smooth. Most type I lesions were like those depicted on the right. Type II eccentric lesions either were smooth with a narrow neck (left side) or had irregular borders (right side). Multiple irregularities included vessels with serial lesions or severe diffuse disease. (Reprinted with permission of J. A. Ambrose and the American College of Cardiology, from Ref. 25.)

or both); and multiple irregular coronary narrowings in series. Type II eccentric lesions (Fig. 2) were significantly more frequent in patients with unstable angina, whereas concentric and type I eccentric lesions were seen more frequently in patients with stable angina. Type II eccentric lesions were present in 71% of ischemia-related vessels in patients with unstable angina but in only 16% of vessels associated with stable angina (19,20).

Our qualitative observations were later confirmed by other authors who described unstable lesions with similar angiographic morphology as complex plaques, intracoronary thrombi, or "type T" lesions (21–24). In patients who present with recent non-Q-wave or Q-wave myocardial infarction and a patent infarct-related artery, angiography discloses a similarly high incidence of eccentric irregular stenoses, whether or not thrombolytic agents have been administered (25,25a). Because the ischemia- or infarct-related artery in unstable angina or acute myocardial infarction may be a concentric or symmetrical stenosis with very irregular borders, as opposed to an eccentric lesion, we currently prefer the term complex or complicated stenosis, rather than type II eccentric lesion, to describe the culprit angiographic lesion in the acute coronary syndromes. An updated classification scheme of simple and complex coronary stenoses with the most common lesion geometries encountered is illustrated in Fig. 3, and exam-

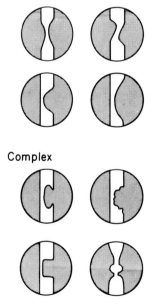

Complex

Figure 3 Updated classification scheme of coronary artery morphological findings. Simple lesions may be eccentric but do not have sharp overhanging edges or irregular borders, as found in complex lesions.

ples of complex plaques are illustrated in Fig. 4. In addition, the unstable angina-producing lesion may appear concentric with smooth borders, morphological characteristics often associated with stable coronary lesions. This can occur for a number of reasons. In some cases, angiography may have been performed long enough after the onset of unstable symptoms for the lesion to have undergone remodeling. In other cases, the plaque complexity or the presence of intracoronary thrombus may not be evident because of the relative insensitivity of angiography for detecting such features. Finally, instability of symptoms may occur without the presence of a complex lesion owing to transient increases in myocardial oxygen demand, coronary vasospasm, or the development of anemia.

In an attempt to make the assessment of coronary lesion morphology more objective, Kalbfleisch et al. (26) recently quantitated the irregularity of coronary lesions using a complex computer algorithm and verified a strong correlation between irregular borders and the presence of unstable symptoms. Unfortunately, this technique may not be better than qualitative analysis in the prediction of unstable symptoms since the sensitivity and specificity are similar to what we reported in our study (19,20). In addition, such methods do not account for the presence of intralesional lucency or filling defects suggestive of thrombus—an important aspect of the qualitative analysis of lesion morphology discussed in the next section.

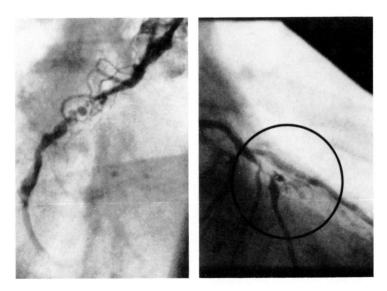

Figure 4 Selected angiographic images from two patients with a complex lesion. (Right) A discrete eccentric plaque with sharp overhanging edges in the left anterior descending artery. (Left) A complex plaque of the type with multiple irregularities in the right coronary artery.

Thrombi

Angiographic studies have conclusively proved the importance of coronary occlusion by thrombosis in the pathogenesis of acute myocardial infarction. Of patients studied within an hour of the onset of symptoms, up to 90% will have an occluded coronary artery (27), often with evidence of acute thrombosis, such as a funnel-shaped occlusion, or luminal dye staining. When angiography is performed later, such as at 12–24 hr after the onset of symptoms, the incidence of total coronary occlusion is as low as 50% (27,28). This high rate of spontaneous recanalization occurs secondary to the activation of the powerful endogenous fibrinolytic system. Moreover, spontaneous lysis likely caused much of the confusion generated by the pathological studies that found variable rates of coronary thrombi in patients dying following acute myocardial infarction (4,5).

The incidence of intracoronary thrombi detected angiographically in patients with unstable angina varies widely and has been quoted between 1 and 85%. Vetrovec et al. (29) reported a 6% incidence of intracoronary thrombi in patients who had unstable angina within 30 days prior to angiography, while Zack et al. (30) reported a 12% incidence of intracoronary thrombi within 90 days after the onset of unstable angina symptoms. However, a much greater incidence of intracoronary thrombi is detected when patients are studied soon after the onset of unstable symptoms. For example, Capone et al. (31) reported a 52% incidence of intracoronary thrombi in patients with unstable angina who underwent angiography within 24 hr from the onset of symptoms, and Gotoh et al. (32) reported a 57% incidence of intracoronary thrombi in patients with unstable angina catheterized during an episode of angina at rest. The variable angiographic detection of thrombus relates to several factors, including the administration of intravenous heparin prior to catheterization and the timing of angiography in relation to the onset of unstable angina or the last episode of ischemia at rest. Thus it is not surprising that in a later study, Vetrovec et al. (33) reported intracoronary thrombi in 85% of patients within 5 days of the onset of unstable angina symptoms.

Another important confounding factor in defining the true incidence of intracoronary thrombi in unstable angina is the lack of a standardized angiographic definition of intracoronary thrombus in an artery that is not completely occluded. Because a patient ischemia-relation artery is the most common finding in unstable angina, this would apply to 85–90% of patients with the syndrome (19,20). It has been our practice to define an intracoronary thrombus in a nontotally occluded artery as one or more filling defects located proximal or distal to a stenotic lesion and surrounded by contrast material on at least three sides (Fig. 5). A filling defect located within the borders of a lesion is classified as a complex lesion. Despite these reservations, the distinction between a complex lesion and an intracoronary thrombus is not absolute. As shown by pathological

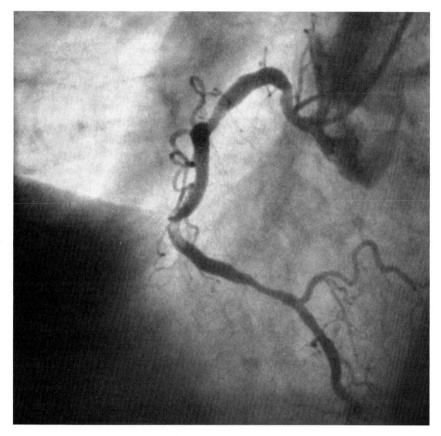

Figure 5 An intracoronary filling defect in the right coronary artery in a patient with chest pain following a Q-wave myocardial infarction. In the LAO projection (not shown), the filling defect is seen to be distal to a mildly stenotic lesion.

(15) and angioscopic (34–36) studies, most complex plaques contain mural thrombus, although these thrombi may be angiographically unapparent or indefinite.

It is likely that when filling defects are clearly identified angiographically, a large volume of thrombus has propagated into the lumen. Alternatively, in some cases, altered hemorrheology proximal or distal to a severe stenosis may favor the development of thrombi. Further evidence for the frequent coexistence of thrombus with complex lesions derives from an angiographic study by Nakagawa et al. (37). Patients with acute myocardial infarction received intracoronary urokinase and were restudied angiographically after 1 month of intense anticoagulation with heparin followed by oral warfarin. Of the arteries initially recanalized by urokinase, all had less luminal narrowing at 1 month, presumably due to endogenous thrombolysis in the setting of systemic anticoagulation. With such resolution of thrombus, complex features of the underlying plaque were revealed, including endoluminal and intraluminal lucencies, outpouchings, and sharp overhanging edges. These are similar to the morphological features noted in our studies (19,20,25).

Coronary Morphology and Prognosis

As indicated, the analysis of coronary lesion morphology is of proven value in distinguishing between stable and unstable coronary lesions (19,20). Recent data suggest that morphological criteria may also be predictive of the risk of adverse coronary events. Using angiographic data compiled in the registry of the Coronary Artery Surgery Study, Ellis et al. conducted a case-control study comparing the angiographic morphology of the left anterior descending coronary artery in patients who subsequently sustained an anterior myocardial infarction versus those who remained free of anterior infarction during a 3-year follow-up period (38). In a multivariate analysis, lesion "roughness," defined as irregular luminal borders or borders with a sawtooth component, and lesion length were the strongest predictors of future myocardial infarction. Although lesion ulceration and filling defects also predicted increased risk, the predictive value was weaker because of the low incidence of these features in the clinically stable population under study. Additionally, these features usually were noted in association with rough lesions. Unfortunately, patients were not restudied angiographically following infarction to confirm that the site of coronary occlusion was the lesion found on the earlier angiogram.

Freeman et al. (39) prospectively studied 78 patients with new onset of unstable angina. Patients were randomly assigned to coronary arteriography within 24 hr of hospitalization or angiography within the first week of hospitalization. If patients experienced further episodes of chest pain at rest despite medical therapy, they crossed over to late urgent angiography. Coronary stenoses were analyzed for complex morphology (defined as irregular borders and or overhanging edges) or thrombus (defined as filling defects or intraluminal dye staining). By the definition used, thrombus was detected in 43% of the early angiography group, 75% of the late urgent group, but in only 21% of the late elective group. Complex morphology was described to occur in about 40% of each group of patients. The presence of an intracoronary thrombus (defined as an intraluminal filling defect) most strongly predicted the risk of an adverse outcome, including death, infarction, or the need for revascularization. In addition to establishing the prognostic significance of intracoronary thrombus in unstable angina, this study underscores its dynamic nature and the importance of the timing of angiography in relation to the last episode of rest pain for the detection of such thrombi.

ANGIOSCOPY AND INTRAVASCULAR ULTRASOUND

Coronary angioscopy offers an alternative for directly inspecting the intima and identifying intravascular pathology. This technique has proved valuable in establishing clinical, anatomical, and pathophysiological correlations in the acute coronary syndromes. It has also demonstrated the relative insensitivity of angiographic analysis in identifying specific morphological features such as intimal disruptions and mural thrombus (Fig. 6). In a study by Sherman et al. (34), angioscopy was performed by inserting the instrument through the coronary arteriotomy during coronary artery bypass grafting surgery and passing it retrograde to visualize the lesion. Of their patients with angina at rest, all had angioscopic evidence of coronary thrombus, and patients with angina in a crescendo pattern had endothelial ulcerations and other plaque disruptions. None of the patients with stable anginal symptoms were found to have a complex plaque or intracoronary thrombus. Preliminary results by Ramee et al. (35) corroborated the finding that angiography is insensitive in detecting morphological features of complex plaques made obvious by angioscopy. During cardiac catheterization using an angioscope passed over an angioplasty guide wire, Mizuno et al. in another preliminary report (36) studied one group of patients with unstable angina within 20 hr of the last episode of chest pain and another group with myocardial infarction within 8 hr of the onset of symptoms. Over 90% of both groups had thrombi visible angioscopically. Interestingly, 73% of patients with unstable angina had "white" thrombi comprised almost exclusively of platelets, while all patients with myocardial infarction had mixed platelet-fibrin thrombi appearing white and red. This may be one explanation for the relatively minor angiographic impact of fibrinolytic agents on coronary lesions in patients with unstable angina, since platelet thrombi would be resistant to such agents (40).

While angioscopy has been able to provide fine detail of endoluminal surfaces, intravascular ultrasound, another new catheter-based technology, shows great promise in assessing the morphology of the vascular wall. In vitro studies have shown that intravascular ultrasound can detect the geometry of intimal disruptions after balloon angioplasty (41). Another in vitro study has demonstrated an ability to accurately measure intimal thickness and distinguish between fatty, fibromuscular, and calcified atheromata (42). However, from preliminary study, it appears that it may be difficult to distinguish between soft plaques and intracoronary thrombi (P.D. Yock, personnel communication), and the role of intravascular ultrasound in the evaluation of the patient with an acute coronary syndrome or in guiding coronary interventions remains to be defined.

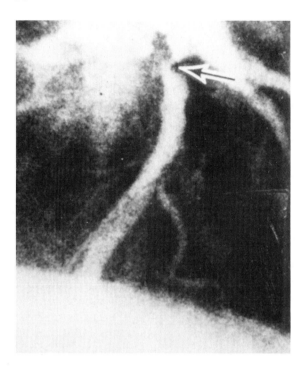

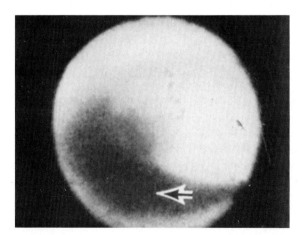

Figure 6 Angiographic and angioscopic images from a patient with unstable angina. Although there is no evidence of intracoronary thrombus on the angiogram, it may be clearly seen angioscopically. (Reprinted with permission from Ref. 34.)

UNIFYING HYPOTHESIS OF THE EVOLUTION OF STABLE AND UNSTABLE CORONARY DISEASE

Early Lesions

The earliest lesion of atherosclerosis, the raised fatty streak, is ubiquitous in the aorta of infants and children (43,44). By age 20, these lesions, consisting of lipid-laden macrophages, are nearly always present in the coronary circulation as well (43,44). Presumably such lesions arise in response to hemorrheological stresses, because they are invariably located at bend points and bifurcations in the coronary tree (45). In some individuals, lipid begins to accumulate in smooth muscle cells and pool in the extracellular matrix in the second decade of life.

Over the next decade, some of these lesions develop a fibrous cap of smooth muscle cells and collagen. Intermittently, platelets may deposit on the surface of these caps, due to minor defects in endothelial integrity, and this may lead to a rapid increase in the thickness of the cap and the beginning of luminal encroachment (45). Such progression of fatty streaks does not occur in all individuals and has been shown in autopsy studies to be related to geographic and ethnic influences and the presence of other risk factors for vascular disease (46).

Progression

The pathophysiology of early progression of the fibroatheroma is incompletely understood. It is likely that a gradual progression occurs in some lesions. This might occur as the result of mild, but chronic endothelial injury precipitated by hemodynamic stresses and vascular risk factors. Such endothelial injury is nondenuding but leads to functional alterations that favor monocyte accumulation and unregulated lipid uptake, thereby increasing the bulk of the lesion (47). Monocytes also release factors promoting smooth muscle cell chemotaxis and hyperplasia and connective tissue synthesis (48). Monocytes may also oxidatively modify lipoproteins or release other oxidation products toxic to the endothelium, thus perpetuating the cycle of chronic endothelial injury. In these early stages, gross endothelial integrity is maintained, as demonstrated angioscopically in the atheroma of patients with stable angina. Angiographically, lesions of this type are either concentric or eccentric, but have smooth borders.

It is also likely that early progression of the atheroma may occur rapidly in some cases, due to episodic deposition and organization of mural thrombi, triggered by focal minor losses in endothelial continuity. This mechanism could lead to a type of "subacute" progression of the plaque with incremental lumenal encroachment and progression of stable anginal symptoms. Evidence for this mechanism of progression is found in the experimental primate model (47) and in human autopsy studies (49,50).

Transition to the Unstable State

The development of an acute coronary syndrome is most frequently associated with a major plaque disruption leading to thrombosis because of the exposure of collagen, lipid, and tissue factor. Major plaque disruptions most frequently occur in the fibrous cap overlying an eccentric collection of macrophages and extracellular lipid. Such plaques may be prone to fissuring because of mismatches in the deformability and tensile strength of the fibrous cap in comparison to the underlying lipid pool, when exposed to hemodynamic stress (51). The fibrous cap may also be susceptible to erosion from within because of the release of proteolytic enzymes from macrophages undergoing autolysis.

Plaque disruption and thrombosis is the common pathophysiological link among the acute coronary syndromes of unstable angina, non-Q-wave and Q-wave myocardial infarction (52). The presenting clinical syndrome is determined by the severity and acuteness of vascular obstruction, which depends in part on the degree of vascular injury and the subsequent thrombotic response. Other important factors in determining whether the patient will progress to myocardial necrosis include the stability of the thrombus, (i.e., its ability to overcome endogenous inhibitors of thrombosis) and the degree of collateral support.

In unstable angina, plaque disruption is followed by increasing luminal obstruction, but it may be relatively less severe than that which occurs in myocardial infarction. Mural thrombi comprised mostly of platelets compound luminal obstruction, and the lesions that develop have the angiographic characteristics described above. Episodes of chest pain at rest may occur due to dynamic changes in the thrombus, as suggested by biochemical evidence (53,54), but may also occur due to vasoconstriction or transient increases in myocardial oxygen demand. Non-Q-wave myocardial infarction represents an intermediate stage in the spectrum of the acute coronary syndromes. The infarct-related artery is occluded with collaterals in 25% of patients (55), but the majority of such patients have a patent artery at angiography with angiographic lesion morphology very similar to that seen in patients with unstable angina (25a). The occurrence of ST-segment elevation and early peaking creatinine kinase washout in many patients with non-Q-wave infarction suggests that coronary thrombosis with total occlusion, but early spontaneous lysis, causes the syndrome (56). With Q-wave myocardial infarction, it is likely that the inciting plaque disruption is very severe, resulting in an occlusive, well-anchored fibrin-platelet thrombus, which may ultimately undergo spontaneous thrombolysis, but persists long enough for transmural myocardial necrosis to occur. As the underlying plaque is often less than critical in the degree of narrowing, collaterals are not able to open acutely to limit the degree of myocardial damage.

REFERENCES

1. Herrick JB. Clinical features of sudden obstruction of the coronary arteries. JAMA 1912; 59:2015.
2. Benson RL. The present status of coronary disease. Arch Pathol 1926; 2:879–916.
3. Blumgart HL, Schlesinger MI, Davis D. Studies on the relation of the clinical manifestations of angina pectoris, coronary thrombus and myocardial infarction to the pathological findings. Am Heart J 1940; 19:1–91.
4. Spain DM, Brandess VA. The relationship of coronary thrombosis to coronary atherosclerosis and ischemic heart disease (a necropsy study over 25 years). Am J Med.
5. Roberts WC, Buja LM. The frequency and significance of coronary arterial thrombi and other observations in fatal acute myocardial infarction. Am J Med 1972; 52:425.
6. Erhardt LR, Lundman T, Mellstedt H. Incorporation of 125 I-labelled fibrinogen into coronary arterial thrombi in acute myocardial infarction in man. Lancet 1973; 1:387–90.
7. Chandler B, Chapman I, Erhardt LR, Roberts WC, Schwartz CJ, Sinapius D, Spain DM, Sherry S, Ness PM, Simon TL. Coronary Thrombosis in myocardial infarction. Report of a workshop on the role of coronary thrombosis in the pathogenesis of acute myocardial infarction. Am J Cardiol 1974; 34:823–33.
8. Chapman I. Relationships of recent coronary artery occlusion and acute myocardial infarction. J Mt Sinai Hosp 1968; 35:149–54.
9. Friedman M, Van den Bovenkamp GJ. Role of thrombus in plaque formation in the human diseased coronary artery. Br J Exp Pathol 1966; 47:550–9.
10. Davies MJ, Thomas A. Thrombosis and acute coronary artery lesions in sudden cardiac ischemic death. N Engl J Med 1984; 310:1137–40.
11. Davies MJ, Thomas A. Plaque fissuring—The cause of acute myocardial infarction, sudden ischemic death, and crescendo angina. Br Heart J 1985; 53:363–73.
12. Falk E. Unstable angina with fatal outcome: Dynamic coronary thrombosis leading to infarction or sudden death. Circulation 1985; 71:699–708.
13. Ambrose JA, Tannenbaum M, Alexopoulos D, et al. Angiographic progression of coronary artery disease and the development of myocardial infarction. J Am Coll Cardiol 1988; 12:56–62.
14. Little WC, Constantinescui M, Appelgate RT. Can coronary angiography predict the site of a subsequent myocardial infarction in patients with mild to moderate coronary artery disease. Circulation 1988; 78:457–66.
15. Levin DC, Fallon JT. Significance of the angiographic morphology of localized coronary stenoses: histopathologic correlations. Circulation 1982; 66:316–20.
16. Onodera T, Fujiwara H, Tanaka M, Wu D-J, Matsuda M, Takemura G, Ishida M, Kawamura A, Kawai C. Cineangiographic and pathological features of the infarct-related vessel in successful and unsuccessful thrombolysis. Br Heart J 1989; 61:385–9.
17. Alison HW, Russell RO, Mantle JA, Kouchoukos NT, Moeaski RE, Rackley CE.

Coronary anatomy and arteriography in patients with unstable angina pectoris. Am J Cardiol 1978; 41:204–9.

18. Moise A, Theroux P, Taeymans Y, et al. Unstable angina and progression of coronary atherosclerosis. N Engl J Med 1983; 309:685–9.

19. Ambrose JA, Winters SL, Stern A, et al. Angiographic evolution of coronary artery morphology in unstable angina. J Am Coll Cardiol 1986; 7:472–8.

20. Ambrose JA, Winters SL, Stern A, et al. Angiographic morphology and the pathogenesis of unstable angina pectoris. J Am Coll Cardiol 1985; 5:609–16.

21. Haft JI, Goldstein JE, Niemiera ML. Coronary arteriographic lesion of unstable angina. Chest 1987; 92:609–12.

22. DeZwaan C, Far FW, Janssen JHA, DeSwart HB, Vermeer F, Wellens HJJ. Effects of thrombolytic therapy in unstable angina: Clinical and angiographic results. J Am Coll Cardiol 1988; 12:301–9.

23. Williams AE, Freeman MR, Chisholm RJ, Patt NL. Armstrong PW. Angiographic morphology in unstable angina pectoris. Am J Cardiol 1988; 62:1024–7.

24. Rehr R, Disciascio G, Vetrovec G, Cowley M. Angiographic morphology of coronary artery stenoses in prolonged rest angina: Evidence of intracoronary thrombosis. J Am Coll Cardiol 1989; 14:1429–37.

25. Ambrose JA, Winters SL, Arora RR, Haft JI, Goldstein J, Rentrop KP, Gorlin R, Fuster V. Coronary angiographic morphology in myocardial infarction: A link between the pathogenesis of unstable angina and myocardial infarction. J Am Coll Cardiol 1985; 6:1233–8.

25a. Ambrose JA, Hjemdahl-Monsen CE, Borrico S, Gorlin R, Fuster V. Angiographic demonstration of a common link between unstable angina pectoris and non-Q wave acute myocardial infarction. Am J Cardiol 1988; 61:244–7.

26. Kalbfleisch Sj, McGillem mi, Simon SB, DeBoe SF, Pinto-Ibraim MF, Mancini GBJ. Automated quantitation of indexes of coronary lesion complexity: Comparison between patients with stable and unstable angina. Circulation 1990; 82:439–47.

27. DeWood MA, Spores J, Notske R, Mouser LT, Burroughs R, Golden MS, Lang HT. Prevalence of total coronary occlusion during the early hours of transmural myocardial infarction. N Engl J Med 1980; 303:897–902.

28. Brooks N. Intracoronary thrombolysis in acute myocardial infarction. Br Heart J 1983; 50:397–400.

29. Vetrovec GW, Cowley MJ, Overton H, Richardson DW. Intracoronary thrombus in syndromes of unstable myocardial ischemia. Am Heart J 1981; 102:1202–8.

30. Zack PM, Ischinger T, Oker UT, Dincer B, Kennedy HL. The occurrence of angiographically detected intracoronary thrombus in patients with unstable angina pectoris. Am Heart J 1984; 108:1408–11.

31. Capone G, Wolf N, Meyer B, Mesiter G. Frequency of intracoronary filling defects by angiography in angina pectoris at rest. Am J Cardiol 1985; 56:403–6.

32. Gotoh K, Minamino T, Katoh O, et al. The role of intracoronary thrombus in unstable angina: Angiographic assessment and thrombolytic therapy during ongoing anginal attacks. Circulation 1988; 77:526–34.

33. Vetrovec GW, Leinbach RC, Gold HK, Cowley MJ. Intracoronary thrombolysis

in syndromes of unstable angina: Angiographic and clinical results. Am Heart J 1982; 104:946–52.

34. Sherman CT, Litvak F, Grundfest W, Lee M, Hickey A, Chaux A, Kass R, Blanche C, Matloff J, Morgenstern L, Ganz W, Swan HJC, Forrester J. Coronary angioscopy in patients with unstable angina pectoris. N Engl J Med 1986; 315:913–9.

35. Ramee SR, White CJ, McQueen C, Doyle T, Murgo JP. Percutaneous coronary angioscopy: Clinical results with a coronary microangioscope. Circulation 1989; 80 (Suppl II) II-376 (Abstract).

36. Mizuno K, Yanagida S, Masami S, Arakawa K, Satomura K, Okamoto Y, Arai T, Nakamura H. Angioscopic evaluation of coronary thrombi in patients with acute coronary syndromes. Circulation 1990; 82 (Suppl IV): IV-1225 (Abstract).

37. Nakagawa S, Hanada Y, Koiwaya Y, Tanaka K. Angiographic features in the infarct-related artery after intracoronary urokinase followed by prolonged anti-coagulation. Role of ruptured atheromatous plaque and adherent thrombus in acute myocardial infarction in vivo. Circulation 1988; 78:1335–44.

38. Ellis S, Alderman EL, Cain K, Wright A, Bourassa M, Fisher L. Morphology of left anterior descending coronary territory lesions as a predictor of anterior myocar-dial infarction: A CASS registry study. J Am Coll Cardiol 1989; 13:1481–91.

39. Freeman MR, Williams AE, Chisholm RJ, Armstrong PW. Intracoronary throm-bus and complex morphology in unstable angina: relation to timing of angiography and in-hospital events. Circulation 1989; 80:17–23.

40. Ambrose JA, Alexopoulos D. Thrombolysis in unstable angina: Will the beneficial effects of thombolytic therapy in myocardial infarction apply to patients with unstable angina? J Am Coll Cardiol 1989; 13:1666–71.

41. Tobis JM, Mallery JA, Gessert J, Griffith J, Mahon D, Bessen M, Moriuchi M, Mcleay L, McRae M, Henry WL. Intravascular ultrasound cross-sectional arterial imaging before and after balloon angioplasty in-vitro. Circulation 1989; 80:873–82.

42. Gussenhoven EJ, Essed CE, Lancee CT, Mastik F, Frietman P, Van Egmond FC, Reiber J, Bosch H, Urk HV, Roelandt J, Bom N. Arterial wall characteristics determined by intravascular ultrasound imaging: An in-vitro study. J Am Coll Cardiol 1989; 13:947–52.

43. Holman RL, McGill HC Jr. The natural history of atherosclerosis: the early aortic lesions as seen in New Orleans in the middle of the 20th century. Am J Pathol 1958; 34:209.

44. Strong JP, McGill HC Jr. The natural history of coronary atherosclerosis. Am J Pathol 1962; 40:37.

45. Stary HC. Evolution and progression of atherosclerotic lesions in coronary arteries of children and young adults. Arteriosclerosis 1989; I (Suppl I): 19–32.

46. McGill HC Jr. The geographic pathology of atherosclerosis. Baltimore: Williams & Wilkins, 1968.

47. Faggiotto A, Ross R, Harker L. Studies of hypercholesterolemia in the nonhuman primate. I. Changes that lead to fatty streak formation. Arteriosclerosis 1984; 4:323–40.

48. Mitchinson Mi, Ball RY. Macrophages and atherogenesis. Lancet 1987; 2:147–9.
49. Vikhert AM, Rosinova VM. Endothelial lining of human arteries at genesis of the atherosclerotic plaque. In: Chazov EI, Smirnov VN, eds. Vessel wall in athero- and thromogenesis. Berlin: Springer-Verlag, 1982:4–11.
50. Davies MJ. Thrombosis and coronary atherosclerosis. In: Julian DG, Khbler W, Norris RM, Swan HJ, Collen D, Verstrate M, eds. Thrombolysis in cardiovascular disease. New York: Marcel Dekker, 1989:25–33.
51. Richardson PD, Davies MJ, Born GV. Influence of plaque configuration and stress distribution on fissuring of coronary atherosclerotic plaques. Lancet 1989; 1:941–4.
52. Gorlin R, Fuster V, Ambrose JA. Anatomic-physiologic links between acute coronary syndromes. Circulation 1986; 74:6.
53. Fitzgerald DJ, Roy L, Catella F, Fitzgerald GA. Platelet activation in unstable coronary disease. N Engl J Med 1986; 315:983–9.
54. Theroux P, Latour JF, Leger C, DeLara J. Fibrinopeptide A and platelet factor levels in unstable angina pectoris. Circulation 1987; 75:156.
55. DeWood M, Stifter WR, Simpson CS. Coronary arteriographic findings soon after non-Q-wave myocardial infarction. N Engl J Med 1986; 315:417.
56. Huey Bl, Gheorghiade M, Crampton RS, Beller GA, Kaiser DL, Watson DD, Nygaard TW, Craddock GB, Sayre SL, Gibson RS. Acute non-Q wave myocardial infarction associated with early ST segment elevation: evidence for spontaneous coronary reperfusion and implications for thrombolytic trials. J Am Coll Cardiol 1987; 9:18–25.

4

The Role of Endothelial Injury in Acute Coronary Events and Coronary Restenosis

Lawrence D. Horwitz

University of Colorado Health Sciences Center
Denver, Colorado

INTRODUCTION

Why, in patients with atherosclerotic coronary lesions that have obviously been present for many years, an acute cardiac syndrome should suddenly occur has long been a perplexing mystery. With the advent of coronary angiography in the 1960s, it was commonly believed that the genesis of acute coronary events resulted from the remorseless progression of coronary atherosclerotic lesions until a critical degree of physical obstruction developed. This led to the concept that assessment of the degree of obstruction by angiographers could permit accurate assessment of risk of myocardial infarctions. This attractive myth, which still dominates the approach of the majority of cardiologists in the United States, has been seriously undermined by several observations in recent years.

Various careful pathological studies in patients who died with acute myocardial infarctions demonstrated that, although there was luminal narrowing at the site of occlusive thrombi, the characteristic finding was an acute intimal lesion at the site (1). The typical finding at autopsy is a large thrombus which forms at the locus of a long-standing atherosclerotic lesion that has developed an acute change in the endothelial surface. These acute lesions have been variously described as intimal hemorrhages, fissures, tears, erosions, ulcers, or ruptures (1). Whichever of these descriptive terms is most accurate, the essential point is that the immediate cause of acute myocardial infarction, and its close relative unstable angina, is an acute injury to the intima of the coronary arteries. Without such injury, patients may be subject to chronic angina or ischemia but are not necessarily at high risk for an acute coronary event despite the presence of physical obstruction by plaque.

ANGIOGRAPHY

With the advent of immediate intervention by thrombolysis or angioplasty in acute myocardial infarction, considerable experience was gained with angiography in the early hours of these events. A long-standing controversy about the importance of thrombosis was resolved by the finding that most infarcts were associated with occlusive thrombi. This was true of nearly all infarcts in which new Q waves were noted as well as many non-Q-wave infarcts (2,3). However, angiography in the early hours and within a few weeks of infarctions did not invariably confirm a relationship of these events to the degree of obstruction by the underlying atherosclerotic plaque. Although there was a tendency for thrombotic occlusions to occur at sites where there was a tight underlying atherosclerotic obstruction, this was not always the case. In published series and the personal experience of cardiologists performing catheterizations in the peri-infarct period, there were always cases in which thrombi occurred at sites where there were not severe obstructions. Although some luminal irregularity was almost always seen, it has become apparent that thrombi can form at sites with less than the 50% narrowing of the luminal diameter, which is generally considered to cause hemodynamic impairment and is therefore termed "significant." These observations support the concept that acute events are primarily related to acute local intimal injury, not to the degree of preexisting atherosclerotic obstruction. The high incidence of thrombi at loci with severe fixed obstructions does suggest, however, that tighter stenoses are more prone to acute intimal injury.

Other important evidence has been derived from the study of catheterizations in patients with unstable angina. Studies that examined stable versus unstable angina patients using commonly employed definitions found no distinctive differences in the degree of coronary obstructions between the two groups. However, it became apparent that many patients with unstable angina or other acute syndromes often had obstructions that were eccentric or irregular—a finding associated with the presence of acute rupture and formation of clots that were partially, as opposed to totally, occlusive (4). The involvement of thrombi in unstable angina was also supported by reports of high urine levels of a thromboxane metabolite in this syndrome (5). Finally, direct visualization of coronary lesions judged responsible for the ischemia in patients with unstable angina has revealed that typically these consist of irregular, probably acutely injured, atherosclerotic plaques with overlying thrombi of varying size and configuration (6). It appears that in unstable angina, as in acute myocardial infarction, injury to the intima of the coronary vessel is a crucial mechanism which leads to local platelet aggregation.

DAILY ASPIRIN

The relevance of platelet aggregation and thrombosis to acute coronary syndromes has been dramatically verified by numerous studies in which aspirin effectively prevented or decreased the severity of adverse outcomes. In 1983, a Veterans Administration Cooperative Study on Unstable Angina was published in which a daily aspirin (administered as an "Alka Seltzer" tablet) begun after admission to the hospital reduced mortality and the incidence of acute myocardial infarctions by approximately 50% (7). Aspirin reduces the rate of recurrent infarctions after an initial episode (8). It reduces the mortality when given early in the course of an acute myocardial infarction (9). It also increases the patency rate of coronary artery bypass grafts. There appears to be little doubt that the occurrence of acute intimal lesions leads to local thrombi and these can be successfully treated in part with aspirin or possibly other agents that prevent platelet aggregation.

An entirely separate argument in favor of the importance of endothelial injury in coronary disease or other vascular disorders is based on the extensive knowledge of the biology of the vascular wall that has emerged in the past few years. While the role of vascular smooth muscle in vasoconstriction and vasodilation has long been apparent, little attention was paid to the physiological role of the thin layer of endothelial cells that line the lumen of blood vessels. However, Furchgott reported that endothelial cells were capable of release of a substance he termed "endothelium-derived relaxing factor," which causes vascular smooth muscle relaxation (10). The release of this relaxing factor is essential to the vasodilatation caused by acetylcholine and certain other vasodilators. It activates guanylate cyclase, which in turn causes relaxation. If in various experimental preparations the endothelium is removed or injured, the vessel will no longer respond to acetylcholine and certain other vasodilators. The list of "endothelium-dependent vasodilators," whose activity depends on release of endothelium-dependent relaxing factor, is long. Among them are serotonin, thrombin, bradykinin, adenosine diphosphate, adenosine triphosphate, and the calcium ionophore A23187, as well as acetycholine. There is now overwhelming evidence that endothelial cells are an important modulator of vascular tone in the coronary arteries.

The relaxing factor described by Furchgott appears to be a low-molecular-weight nitrite, possibly nitric oxide. It is released by endothelial cells and causes vasodilatation in the immediate vicinity of the cell that releases it. It does not circulate because it is quickly inactivated in blood. Therefore, local endothelial injury causes a local loss of capacity to vasodilate in response to endothelium-dependent stimuli. If the vascular smooth muscle is not injured at this site, it is still capable of vasodilating in response to certain vasodilators that are not endothelium-dependent. These include nitroglycerin and nitroprusside, which directly activate guanylate cyclase in coronary artery smooth muscle and induce vasodilation even in the presence of local endothelial injury.

In the presence of both acute and chronic coronary disease, endothelial damage or dysfunction may lead to inappropriate vasoconstriction. Loss of normal release of relaxing factor by coronary endothelium in certain settings may lead to loss of the normal vasodilating response. In studies in cardiac catheterization laboratories, vasoconstriction has been noted in response to acetylcholine, serotonin, or exercise at the sites of chronic coronary obstructive lesions (11,12). There is reason to believe that even greater abnormalities may occur with acute endothelial damage. As will be described below, acute ischemia followed by reperfusion in animal models causes local endothelial injury and impaired responsiveness to endothelial-dependent vasodilators. There is considerable reason to believe that coronary spasm is due to endothelial injury and loss of endothelial modulation of local coronary artery tone.

The complexities of endothelial control of arterial vasodilation are still poorly understood. There is evidence that more than one relaxing factor is present in endothelial cells. A factor dependent on potassium channels in vascular smooth muscle has been described (13). This factor may be blocked by agents that alter function of potassium channels such as digitalis glycosides and quinine. Other agents alter vascular tone through adenyl cyclase–controlled mechanisms which may involve the endothelium. Although platelets may be a crucial stimulant, the nature of the pathways that lead to coronary spasm in pathophysiological settings is unknown.

The endothelium also serves as an important defense against local thrombosis. Prostacyclin, other arachidonic acid metabolites, and endothelium-derived relaxing factor all inhibit platelet aggregation and are released by endothelial cells. Therefore, endothelial injury strongly enhances the likelihood of clot formation in a coronary artery. This can increase obstruction directly through the physical mass of the clot or indirectly by inducing vasoconstriction through platelet release of serotonin and other agents that increase vascular smooth muscle tone in the absence of endothelial modulation.

Finally, endothelial injury appears to be an essential element in the restenosis that all too often complicates coronary angioplasty. Damage to the endothelium predisposes to platelet aggregation. It also decreases the availability of growth inhibitors, heparin, and transforming growth factor beta, which are normally present in endothelial cells. Therefore, growth factors released from the aggregating platelets may be free of the usual inhibitory influences. Thus rapid growth of vascular smooth muscle often occurs at sites where the endothelium has been severely damaged by angioplasty (14).

UNSTABLE ANGINA

Unstable angina was originally conceived as a syndrome that is a frequent predecessor to acute myocardial infarction. This concept of impending myocardial infarction, or "preinfarction angina," has been useful in educating physicians regarding patients who deserve aggressive therapy and generally hospitalization. Thus angina at rest, accelerated angina that increases in severity or frequency without an increase in activity, and new-onset angina are all presentations of unstable angina which are characterized by a high risk of infarction. A high percentage of patients with acute myocardial infarction present with a preceding anginal syndrome of this type.

It has also become clear that many patients with acute ischemic syndromes may present without pain. Dyspnea, fatigue, exercise intolerance, or arrhythmia may occur without pain. Unfortunately such presentations are often unrecognized. Certain groups, the elderly, diabetics, heart transplant recipients, and patients with previous infarcts are probably particularly likely to present in this manner. Perhaps a more useful description is severe transient myocardial ischemia (15).

The evidence that unstable angina is related to acute endothelial injury and platelet aggregation at the site of atherosclerosis in the coronary artery wall is convincing. As outlined above, angiographic evidence of thrombi and angioscopic evidence of ruptured plaques on which thrombi form have been described in such patients (4,16). It appears that unstable angina and acute myocardial infarction are part of a spectrum of events involving acute endothelial injury. Patients presenting with such findings probably can either progress to infarction or improve to a stable or even an asymptomatic state, depending on circumstances many of which are poorly understood.

Angioplasty and coronary artery bypass surgery frequently relieve unstable states and are frequently resorted to for therapy. However, aspirin and heparin are also very effective. Probably antianginal drugs, including beta-adrenergic blocking agents, slow calcium blocking agents, and nitrites, are also helpful. However, little is known about the duration of the intimal injury that precipitates this condition and its immediate cause.

POSTINFARCTION ANGINA OR ISCHEMIA

The occurrence of angina or silent ischemia within a few weeks following an acute myocardial infarction is also a highly unstable state that frequently leads to reinfarction. The presence of persistent ischemia can be detected by symptoms, by detection of electrocardiographic ST-segment changes on ambulatory or regular electrocardiograms, or on exercise tests. Several studies have documented that there is a high recurrent infarction rate under such circumstances

(16–18). It is of considerable interest that there is a particular predilection for postinfarction angina to occur in infarctions without Q waves on the electrocardiogram and in patients successfully treated with thrombolytic therapy. Both these settings have early reperfusion as a common thread.

In non-Q-wave infarctions a minority of patients have total occlusions, whereas most patients have infarcts that are caused by a stenosed vessel capable of providing some blood flow (3). Non-Q-wave infarctions generally have early peaking of the blood creatinine phosphokinase levels, a sign of early reperfusion in experimental models (19). At postmortem examinations patients who succumb with non-Q-wave infarctions have considerable amounts of "contraction band necrosis," a distinctive pathological sign of reperfusion injury not usually encountered in Q-wave infarcts (20). These findings suggest that spontaneous early reperfusion occurs in non-Q-wave myocardial infarctions. It is noteworthy that this leads to a much higher rate of both postinfarction angina and recurrent infarctions within 1 year in non-Q-wave than in Q-wave infarctions (17–18,21). It is our thesis that endothelial injury in this setting either is worsened or is precipitated by the early reperfusion characteristic of this syndrome.

The importance of early reperfusion as a cause of postmyocardial ischemia or angina is even more dramatically supported by the findings in patients successfully treated with thrombolytic therapy early in the course of acute myocardial infarctions. Schaer et al. (22) reported that the incidence of postinfarction ischemia was 41% in 41 patients whose occluded artery was successfully reopened by intracoronary streptokinase, but only 10% in 40 patients who continued to be occluded despite intracoronary streptokinase. Thus early reperfusion, which reduces mortality and probably salvages myocardium in acute infarctions, leads to a high predilection for postinfarction angina and probably for recurrent infarction within 1 year.

Studies in animals have clarified the importance of reperfusion in the genesis of coronary endothelial injury. VanBenthuysen, McMurtry, and Horwitz studied canine coronary arteries exposed in vivo to 1 hr of ischemia by ligation (23). Rings excised from these vessels and studied in muscle baths have normal responses to vasoconstrictors and vasodilators and normal endothelial histology if removed immediately after exposure to ischemia (23). However, if, after the ischemic period, the vessel is reperfused for an hour, there is extensive endothelial injury. There is hyperactivity to some vasoconstrictors, most notably ergonovine, when excised coronary rings are studied in muscle baths (23). Responses to endothelium-dependent vasodilators, including acetylcholine, adenosine diphosphate, and A23187, are blunted, although there is a normal response to the endothelium-independent vasodilator nitroprusside (23,24). Finally, the reperfused arteries have extensive endothelial damage on electron microscope studies (23). Thus reperfusion after brief periods of ischemia results in endothelial injury in previously normal vessels, whereas ischemia alone does not. We propose that a similar process occurs in atherosclerotic vessels exposed to ischemia and reperfusion.

The reperfusion injury to the endothelium is probably transient in most cases because endothelium has considerable capacity to regenerate. With mechanical endothelial injury in dogs there is regeneration of endothelium in previously normal coronary arteries within a week (25). In patients with non-Q-wave infarctions, clinical data support the concept of rapid endothelial regeneration after endothelial injury. In the Diltiazem Reinfarction Study, 576 patients with non-Q-wave infarctions were randomized within 3 days to a calcium blocker (diltiazem, 90 mg QID) or placebo (26). The medication was taken for only 14 days. In the diltiazem group the incidence of recurrent infarctions was 5.2%, while in the placebo group it was 9.3% during the 14-day period. Probably this reflects prevention of coronary spasm during a brief time in which transient endothelial injury caused a high susceptibility to this phenomenon.

In summary, there is considerable evidence that early reperfusion can cause endothelial injury leading to platelet aggregation and a propensity to coronary artery spasm. Whether this propensity is also present after angioplasty is unclear. There may be differences in the nature of mechanical endothelial injury from angioplasty and the injury that occurs with ischemia and reperfusion. This could translate into differences in the rate at which endothelium regenerates.

CORONARY RESTENOSIS

Coronary balloon angioplasty has been a highly successful treatment for myocardial ischemia. However, there has been a high rate of "late" restenosis, with estimates ranging from 12 to 48% within 18 months, with most appearing within 6 months. Coronary endothelial injury is involved in this process. Within the first day after angioplasty, there is extensive endothelial injury and denudation and platelets aggregate and adhere at the site (14). Within 2 weeks, there is smooth muscle cell proliferation and migration. Over subsequent months, there is further smooth muscle cell proliferation even though the endothelial cells may be reconstituted and thrombus is not a common feature. Although matrix formation and collagen deposition occur, smooth muscle growth is the fundamental cause of the intimal thickening and restenosis (14). Endothelial injury appears to initiate the process. Platelets are present when the process of smooth muscle growth begins but are not a usual feature week or months later, although smooth muscle growth continues.

Endothelial injury enhances the likelihood of local platelet aggregation. There is evidence that platelets are involved in vascular smooth muscle cell proliferation. After balloon injury, platelet factor 4, which is found in platelet granules, can be detected within 30 min in intima and media (27). In most studies balloon-induced vascular injury in thrombocytopenic animals has resulted in considerably less smooth muscle proliferation than in thrombocytopenic controls (28). Platelets produce "growth factors" that can stimulate vascular smooth muscle cell growth (28). These include platelet-derived growth factor, epidermal growth factor, and several others. There is a strong likelihood that release of such growth factors by adherent platelets causes smooth muscle cell proliferation to commence. The local loss of endothelium also means that certain growth inhibitory factors, which normally counteract the effects of growth factors from platelets or other sources, are also lost. Heparin and other heparin-like agents and transforming growth factor beta are inhibitory factors that are generated in normal endothelial cells and may have an important protective role against restenosis.

In addition to endothelial injury, tears in the smooth muscle during angioplasty have been implicated in the restenosis process. We speculate that once endothelial injury and platelet aggregation initiate the process of smooth muscle proliferation, the damaged smooth muscle cells perpetuate it. After initial stimulation by growth factors released from platelets, damaged smooth muscle cells may, like cancer cells, begin to make their own growth factors. This would explain why growth proceeds even after the endothelium regenerates and platelet aggregation and adherence cease.

CONCLUSIONS

In acute coronary syndromes endothelial injury is the root of all evil. In unstable angina, postinfarction angina, or acute myocardial infarction it is the immediate precipitating cause of the acute event. Platelets are the partners in crime of the damaged endothelial cells. They aggregate at the site of the damage, causing physical obstruction or releasing agents that induce vasoconstriction. Why endothelial damage occurs in unstable angina or acute myocardial infarction is unclear. Accelerated atherosclerosis or severe fixed obstruction may predispose to this phenomenon: the former perhaps because of alterations in the composition or shape of the arterial wall, and the latter perhaps because of increased shear stresses with severe stenosis. In postinfarction angina the injury is related to reperfusion. The most likely mechanism is through release of reactive oxygen metabolites when oxygen and leukocytes are reintroduced during reperfusion.

Endothelial injury and local platelet adherence are probably also the initiating cause of restenosis following coronary balloon angioplasty. Here the cause of the endothelial injury is clearly the direct trauma due to the balloon. The release of growth factors by platelets is probably crucial to the restenosis process. A certain level of injury in the smooth muscle cells may also be necessary to set off production of growth factors in proliferating cells.

REFERENCES

1. Falk E. Plaque rupture with preexisting stenosis precipitating coronary thrombosis. Characteristics of coronary atherosclerotic plaques underlying occlusive thrombi. Br Heart J 1983; 50:127–34.
2. DeWood MA, Spores J, Notske R, Mouser LT, Burroughs R, Golden MS, Lang HT. Prevalence of total coronary occlusion in the early hours of transmural myocardial infarction. N Engl J Med 1980; 303:897–902.
3. DeWood MA, Stifter WF, Simpson CS, Spores J, Eugster GS, Judge TP, Hinnen ML. Coronary arteriographic findings soon after non-Q-wave myocardial infarction. N Engl J Med 1986; 315:417–23.
4. Ambrose JA, Winters SL, Arora RR, Eng A, Ricco A, Gorlin R, Fuster V. Angiographic evolution of coronary artery morphology in unstable angina. J Am Coll Cardiol 1986; 45:411–6.
5. Fitzgerald DJ, Roy L, Catella F, Fitzgerald GA. Platelet activation in unstable coronary disease. N Engl J Med 1986; 315:983–9.
6. Sherman CT, Litvack F, Grundfest ME, Lee M, Hickey A, Chaux A, Kass R, Blanche C, Matloff J, Morgenstern L, Ganz W, Swan HJC, Forrester J. Coronary angioscopy in patients with unstable angina pectoris. N Engl J Med 1986; 315: 913–9.
7. Lewis HD, Davis JW, Archibald DG, Steinke WE, Smitherman TC, Doherty JE III, Schnaper HW, LeWinter MM, Linares E, Pouget JM, Sabharwal SC, Chester E, DeMots H. Protective effects of aspirin against acute myocardial infarction and death in men with unstable angina. N Engl J Med 1983; 309:396–403.
8. Antiplatelet Trialist's Collaboration. Secondary prevention of vascular disease by prolonged antiplatelet treatment. Br Med J 1988; 296:320–31.
9. ISIS-2 Collaborative Group. Randomized trial of intravenous streptokinase, oral aspirin, both, or neither among 17,187 cases of suspected acute myocardial infarction. Lancet 1988; 2:349–60.
10. Furchgott RF. Role of endothelium in responses of vascular smooth muscle. Circ Res 1983; 53:557–73.
11. Ludmer PL, Selwyn AP, Shook TL, Wayne RR, Mudge GH, Alexander RW, Ganz P. Paradoxical vasoconstriction induced by acetylcholine in atherosclerotic coronary arteries. N Engl J Med 1986; 315:1046–51.
12. McFadden EP, Clarke JG, Davis GJ, Haski JC, Haider AW, Maseri A. Effect of intracoronary serotonin on coronary vessels in patients with stable angina and patients with variant angina. N Engl J Med 1991; 324:648–54.
13. Kuriyama H, Suzuki H. The effects of acetylcholine on the membrane and contractiloe properties of the smooth muscle cells of the rabbit superior mesenteric artery. Br J Pharmacol 1978; 64 493–7.
14. Liu W, Roubin GS, King SB III. Restenosis after coronary angioplasty. Potential biologic determinants and role of intimal hyperplasia. Circulation 1989; 79: 1374–87.
15. Braunwald E. Unstable angina: A classification. Circulation 1989; 80:410–4.

16. McQuay NW, Edwards JE, Burchell HB. Types of death in acute myocardial infarction. ARch Intern Med 1955; 96:1–10.
17. Sellier P, Plat F, Corona P, Payen B, Audouin P, Ourbak P. Prognostic significance of angina pectoris recurring soon after myocardial infarction. Eur Heart J 1988; 9: 44–153.
18. Theroux P, Waters DD, Halphen C, Debaisieux J-C, Mizgala HF. Prognostic value of exercise testing soon after myocardial infarction. N Engl J Med 1979; 301: 341–5.
19. Shell We, DeWood MA, Kligerman M, Ganz W, Swan HJC. Early appearance of MB-creatine kinase MB in acute myocardial infarction. Am J Med 1981; 71: 254–62.
20. Kloner RA, Ganote CE, Whalen DA Jr, Jennings RB. Effects of a transient period of ischemia on myocardial cells. II. Fine structure during the first few minutes of reflow. Am J Pathol 1974; 74:399–422.
21. Gibson RS. Non-Q-wave myocardial infarction: Diagnosis, prognosis, and management. Curr Probl Cardiol 1988; 13:1–72.
22. Schaer DH, Ross AM, Wasserman AG. Reinfarction, recurrent angina and reocclusion after thrombolytic therapy. Circulation 1987; 76 (Suppl II): 57–62.
23. VanBenthuysen K, McMurtry I, Horwitz LD. Reperfusion after acute coronary occlusion in dogs impairs endothelium-dependent relaxation to acetyleholine and augments contractile reactivity in vitro. J Clin Invest 1987; 79:265–74.
24. Horwitz LD, VanBenthuysen KYI, Sheridan FM, Lesnefsky EJ, Dauber IM, MeMurtry IF. Coronary endothelial dysfunction from ischemia and reperfusion: Effect of reactive oxygen metabolite scavengers. Free Radical Biol Med 1990; 8: 381–6.
25. Shimokawa H, Aarhus LL, Vanhoutte PM. Porcine coronary arteries with regenerated endothelium have a reduced endothelium-dependent responsiveness to aggregating platelets and serotonin. Circulation Res 1987; 61:256–70.
26. Gibson RS, Boden WE, Theroux P, Strauss HD, et al. Diltiazem and reinfarction in patients with non-Q-wave myocardial infarction. N Engl J Med 1986; 315:423–9.
27. Goldberg ID, Stemmerman MB. Vascular permeation of platelet factor 4 after endothelial injury. Science 1980; 209:611–2.
28. Friedman RJ, Stemmerman FIB, Wenz B, Moore S, Gauldie J, Gent M, Tiell YIL, Spaet TH. The effect of thrombocytopenia on experimental arteriosclerotic lesion formation in rabbits. Smooth muscle cell proliferation and reendothelialization. J Clin Invest 1977; 60:1191–1201.

5

Summary of Pathophysiology of Unstable Angina
Relevance to Therapeutic Options

Douglass Andrew Morrison

Veterans Affairs Medical Center and
University of Colorado Health Sciences Center
Denver, Colorado

THROMBOSIS-PLAQUE RUPTURE

It has been recognized for some time that sudden obstruction of the coronary arteries, usually associated with clot, could produce most of the acute ischemic coronary syndromes (1–8). Based on this conception, Coumadin derivatives were used extensively to treat myocardial infarction and other ischemic syndromes (2–8).

Pathological Support for the Role of Thrombosis

Falk described microscopic examination of autopsy material from 25 patients who died soon after myocardial infarction with sudden death (9). He noted layered thrombi suggesting repeated mural deposits with intermittent fragmentation consistent with peripheral embolization (9). Levin and Fallon correlated postmortem coronary angiography with histological evaluation (10). They showed a strong association between angiographic irregular borders and intraluminal lucencies with histological plaque rupture or hemorrhage with superimposed thrombus (10). Horrie et al. demonstrated that the superimposed thrombus frequently occurs at the site of ruptured plaques (11).

The extent of coronary narrowing does not appear to be different between stable and unstable angina (12). Davies and Thomas reported an autopsy series of 100 patients who died suddenly (<6 hr) of ischemic heart disease (13). They noted intraluminal coronary thrombi in 74 (13). Of the 26 cases without intraluminal thrombi, they found intraintimal thrombi in 21 (13). Subsequently, the same investigators noted that plaque fissuring, by leading to either intraluminal thrombus, intraintimal thrombus, emboli, or spasm, could account for either myocardial infarction, sudden ischemic death, or crescendo angina (14).

Angiographic Data

Alison et al. reported a prospective series of 188 patients with unstable angina (15). The extent of coronary luminal narrowing was the most important factor in determining complications or the need for revascularization (15). Neill et al. provided angiographic evidence to support the pathological concept that intermittent transient coronary artery occlusion is frequently associated with unstable angina (16). Victor and co-workers reported a prospective series with unstable angina that was heavily weighted toward single-vessel lesions (17). Relative to the other series, these single-vessel unstable patients had tight, proximal lesions in large arteries.

Moise et al. reported an important cohort in which they had performed serial angiography (18). They documented marked angiographic progression of coronary narrowing in unstable patients (18). Zack et al. compared the angiograms from 83 patients with unstable angina with the angiograms from 37 patients with stable angina; evidence of intracoronary thrombus was seen in 12% of the unstable patients but none of the stable patients (19). Ambrose and co-workers also compared angiograms from stable versus unstable angina patients (20). They noted qualitative differences, with irregular borders and edges being significantly more frequent in unstable patients (20). In a subsequent study of patients with recent infarction, Ambrose et al. demonstrated angiographically that the irregular stenosis, representing either disrupted plaque, thrombus, or both, suggested a pathophysiological link between unstable angina and myocardial infarction (21). Capone and co-workers extended these findings by subgrouping unstable patients according to how recently they had rest angina (22). Patients with more recent unstable angina were found to have the highest likelihood of angiographic thrombus (22).

Ambrose and co-workers synthesized the findings of Moise et al. regarding angiographic progression with their work on the qualitative appearance of plaque rupture and/or thrombus (23). Specifically, unstable patients appear to have progression angiographically by means of plaque rupture and thrombosis (23).

Haft et al. provided confirmation of the qualitative observations of Ambrose and co-workers (24). Ambrose and Hjelmdahl-Monsen summarized the angiographic observations and the relationship of the plaque-rupture, thrombosis sequence with alternative pathophysiological mechanisms (such as spasm) in a 1987 editorial (25).

Although Ambrose and many other workers had confirmed that quantitative angiographic lesion severity was not different between stable and unstable patients (25), Wilson and co-workers applied a quantitative technique (''ulceration index'') to the qualitative observations regarding plaque rupture and thrombosis (26). Williams and co-workers extended the findings of frequent complex morphology in unstable patients by demonstrating that lesion complexity had prognostic significance (27). Rehr and co-workers also showed a strong association between complex lesion angiographic morphology and rest angina (28). Freeman and co-workers provided additional support for Capone et al.'s thesis that the earlier one studies patients after rest pain, the more likely one is to observe complex morphology consistent with plaque rupture and/or clot (29).

Angioscopic Observations

Sherman et al. reported angioscopic results from 10 patients with stable angina and 10 patients with unstable angina (30). They noted that 7/7 arteries from patients with rest angina had evidence of thrombi and 3/3 arteries from patients with accelerated angina had complex plaques (30). Forrester et al. reported angioscopic data, comparing it to the published, histological, and angiographic observations (31). They provided a humorous review of the thrombosis debate in the first half of this century and went on to develop a global paradigm based on endothelial ulceration and thrombosis as the precipitant of unstable periods in the natural history of coronary disease (31). Their paradigm explains many of the features of stable angina as well as the acute ischemic syndromes (31). It also provides rationale for antiplatelet agents, anticoagulants, and thrombolytics in the treatment of unstable ischemic syndromes (31).

BIOCHEMICAL INSIGHTS AND THE ROLE OF THROMBOLYSIS

Moncada and Vane reviewed the biochemistry of arachidonic acid metabolites, which are fatty acids present in the phospholipids of cell membranes (32). These workers demonstrated that prostacyclin prevents platelet aggregation on vessel walls (32). Conversely, aggregation is promoted by thromboxane derived from platelets, especially adjacent to vessels with injured endothelium (32). Fitzgerald and co-workers studied the biochemical interaction of prostacyclin and thromboxane in unstable ischemic patients (33). Their data supported the contention that platelet activation occurs during spontaneous ischemia in patients with unstable angina (33).

Theroux and co-workers used fibrinopeptide A levels to distinguish between stable and unstable angina, thereby demonstrating an activation of the coagulation system in unstable angina (34). Hamm et al. further subdivided an unstable cohort into groups that responded and did not respond to therapy (i.v. nitroglycerin), showing that failure to respond was associated with higher levels of thromboxane production (35). In commenting on the study of Hamm and co-workers, Chesebro and Fuster suggested that biochemical markers might be used for monitoring therapy (36). Gallino et al. provided data supportive of the concept that thrombosis plays a role in all ischemic syndromes (37). Adams and co-workers developed a paradigm that incorporated rheological factors from atherosclerotic/clot stenoses with these chemical insights (38).

Castellot, Cochran, and Karnovsky demonstrated that heparin inhibits vascular smooth muscle cell proliferation and appears to do so via the synthesis of specific proteins (39,40). Marciniak and Gockerman demonstrated that heparin could induce a decrease in endogenous antithrombin III (41).

Verymylen et al. summarized the conceptual framework for thrombogenesis:

1. Platelets are not activated in the normal circulation.
2. The first step in thrombus formation is platelet adhesion.
3. The platelets then change shape and aggregate.
4. Secretion of platelet granules activates the clotting mechanism by means of thrombin and fibrin formation.
5. There are endogenous inhibitors of thrombus formation, namely prostacyclin, protein C, and antithrombin III (42).

Trip and co-workers further extended the concept that platelet aggregability is a marker and thus potential mechanism for further morbid cardiac events in a cohort of postinfarction patients (43).

Vane et al. summarized the data that support the concept that vascular endothelium functions as an endocrine organ, producing and metabolizing a host of vasoactive and platelet-active substances (44).

Kruskal and co-workers examined fibrin-related antigen in a variety of coronary artery disease subsets (45). Their data supported the concept of an active thrombotic process in unstable angina or myocardial infarction (45). Fuster et al. synthesized the existing pathological/angiographic data base regarding plaque rupture/endothelial injury with the biochemistry of platelet aggregation activation of the coagulation system and thrombosis (46). These concepts provide the conceptual framework for the use of antiplatelet agents such as aspirin, anticoagulation (intravenous heparin or oral Coumadin), and, most recently, thrombolytic agents.

A number of investigations of the use of thrombolytic therapy in unstable angina have been based on this database (47–50). deZwaan et al. reported a high frequency of intraluminal clot in unstable angina patients and used either streptokinase or TPA to effect an improvement in luminal size (47). Ambrose et al. reported the feasibility of using streptokinase in unstable syndromes, but only a minority of their patients showed angiographic improvement (48). Gotoh et al. observed that unstable patients with residual thrombus fared less well than patients without thrombus (49). They also noted some individual improvements after urokinase (49). Mandelkorn and colleagues reported some significant improvements in an unstable cohort given streptokinase (50).

VASOSPASM

Maseri et al. reported a landmark study of 187 patients with rest angina who were evaluated with hemodynamic monitoring, thallium scintigraphy during rest angina, and, in some cases, coronary angiography (51). In all, they documented evidence for a vasospastic mechanism contributing to ischemia in 76/187 patients (51). A further report by the same group documented that pain was a late phenomenon usually not preceded by an increase in the determinants of myocardial O_2 demand (52). Angiographic vasospasm was demonstrated in 37/37 patients studied during an anginal episode (52). deServi et al. reported three patients who had coronary spasm documented during rest angina but increased demand during exercise-induced angina, consistent with the notion that multiple mechanisms may be at work in the same patients (53). Synthesizing these concepts, Maseri proposed a pathogenetic classification incorporating the ideas of both fixed and dynamic stenoses (54).

MYOCARDIAL SUPPLY VERSUS DEMAND

Figueras et al. studied 23 patients during rest angina with electrocardiographic and hemodynamic monitoring (55). The data were consistent with acute left ventricular failure and ischemic electrocardiographic changes without alteration in the determinants of myocardial oxygen demand, thereby supporting the primacy of reduced supply (55). Guazzi and co-workers reported hemodynamic and electrocardiographic data during multiple episodes of rest angina from 11 patients and inferred that rest angina usually accrued from a supply problem (56). This conclusion was also supported by the hemodynamic and great cardiac vein oxygen data obtained by Chierchia et al. from six patients with angina at rest (57). Regardless of whether ischemia was associated with ST depression or elevation, it was not preceded by hemodynamic changes indicative of increased myocardial O_2 demand (56). Alternatively, Roughgarden had documented cases where increases in heart rate and/or blood pressure preceded both electrocardiographic changes and pain (58). As stated previously, deServi et al. reported three patients who had rest anginal episodes without prior increases in the determinants of myocardial oxygen consumption and exertional episodes preceded by increases in myocardial O_2 determinants (53). Accordingly, it can be concluded that both mechanisms can occur even in the same patients. Nevertheless, the majority of rest anginal episodes appear to be primarily a function of decreased supply, with thrombosis and plaque rupture and vasospasm being the most common precipitants.

SILENT ISCHEMIA

Gottlieb et al. reported the results of Holter monitoring in 70 patients with unstable angina (59). Despite vigorous medical therapy, over 50% of the patients manifest silent ischemia (59). In a subsequent study of 2-year follow-up on such patients by the same group, myocardial infarction was found to be much more frequent in patients with silent ischemia than in those without it (60). Nademanee and co-workers also demonstrated an adverse prognosis in unstable angina patients who continued to have episodes of silent ischemia despite medical therapy as opposed to patients who did not have silent ischemia (61). Alternatively, Wilcox et al. looked prospectively at an unstable angina cohort of 66 patients and concluded that recurrent symptoms despite therapy was a far more sensitive predictor of adverse events than silent ischemia despite therapy (62).

THERAPEUTIC IMPLICATIONS

Although increased myocardial oxygen demand does not appear to be primary in most cases of rest angina, therapeutic attempts to reduce demand are often helpful and quite safe. It is to this end that patients are put at bed rest, and this is the major rationale for beta blockade, in particular, and for aiming pharmacological therapy toward target heart rates and/or blood pressures, in general.

Although likely to have some salutary effect on myocardial oxygen demand, the major rationale for both nitrates and calcium blockers is the relief of coronary

Table 1 Pathophysiology of Unstable Angina and Therapeutic Options

Pathophysiological mechanisms of rest angina	Therapeutic implication
Increased myocardial O_2 demand	Bed rest
	Beta blockers
	Pharmacotherapy directed to target HR and/or BP
Decreased myocardial O_2 supply	O_2 therapy
	Intraaortic balloon counterpulsation
Vasospasm	Calcium blockers
	Nitrates
Plaque rupture/thrombosis	Aspirin
	Heparin
	Coumadin
	Thrombolytics
Impaired collateral flow	i.v. nitroglycerin?

vasospasm, both endothelial dependent and independent. Nitrates may also have some beneficial effects on coronary collateral flow.

As emphasized previously, the major new pathogenetic insight in unstable or rest angina is the ubiquitous role of plaque rupture and/or hemorrhage with superimposed intraintimal or intraluminal thrombosis. It is against these problems that antiplatelet therapy (supported by two large prospective randomized trials), anticoagulant therapy, and thrombolytic therapy are all directed.

REFERENCES

1. Herrick JB. Clinical features of sudden obstruction of the coronary arteries. JAMA 1912; 59:2015–20.
2. Nichol ES, Fassett DW. An attempt to forestall acute coronary thrombosis. South Med J 1947; 40:631–7.
3. Beamish RE, Storrie VM. Impending myocardial infarction recognition and management. Circulation 1960; 21:1107–15.
4. Mounsey P. Prodromal symptoms in myocardial infarction. Br Heart J 1951; 13:215.
5. Sampson JJ, Eliaser M Jr. The diagnosis of impending acute coronary artery occlusion. Am Heart J 1937; 13:675–86.
6. Vakil RJ. Intermediate coronary syndrome. Circulation 1961; 24:557–71.
7. Feil H. Preliminary pain in coronary thrombosis. Am J Med Sci 1937; 193:42–8.
8. Wood P. Acute and subacute coronary insufficiency. Br Med J 1961; 1179–1782.
9. Falk E. Unstable angina with fatal outcome: Dynamic coronary thrombosis leading to infarction and/or sudden death. Circulation 1985; 71:699–708.
10. Levin DC, Fallon JT. Significance of angiographic morphology of localized coronary stenoses: Histopathologic correlations. Circulation 1982; 66:316–20.
11. Horie T, Sekiguchi M, Hirosawa K. Relationship between myocardial infarction and pre-infarction angina. Am Heart J 1978; 95:81–8.
12. Guthrie RB, Vlodaver Z, Nicoloff DM, Edwards JE. Pathology of stable and unstable angina pectoris. Circulation 1975; 51:1059–63.
13. Davies MJ, Thomas A. Thrombosis and acute coronary-artery lesions in sudden cardiac ischemic death. N Engl J Med 1984; 310:1137–40.
14. Davies MJ, Thomas AC. Plaque fissuring—The cause of acute myocardial infarction, sudden ischaemic death, and crescendo angina. Br Heart J 1985; 53:363–73.
15. Alison HW, Russell RO Jr, Mantle JA, et al. Coronary anatomy and arteriography in patients with unstable angina pectoris. Am J Cardiol 1978; 41:204–9.
16. Neill WA, Wharton TP, Jr, Fluri-Lundeen J, Cohen IS. Acute coronary insufficiency—coronary occlusion after intermittent ischemic attacks. N Engl J Med 1980; 302:1157–62.
17. Victor MF, Likoff MJ, Mintz GS, Likoff W. Unstable angina pectoris of new onset: A prospective clinical and arteriographic study of 75 patients. Am J Cardiol 1981; 47:228–32.

18. Moise A, Theroux P, Taeymans Y, et al. Unstable angina in progression of coronary atherosclerosis. N Engl J Med 1983; 309:685–9.

19. Zack PM, Ischinger T, Aker UT, Dincer B, Kennedy HL. The occurence of angiographically detected intracoronary thrombus in patients with unstable angina pectoris. Am Heart J 1984; 108:1408–12.

20. Ambrose JA, Winters SL, Stern A, et al. Angiographic morphology and the pathogenesis of unstable angina pectoris. J Am Coll Cardiol 1985; 5:609–16.

21. Ambrose JA, Winters SL, Arora RR, et al. Coronary angiographic morphology in myocardial infarction: A link between the pathogenesis of unstable angina and myocardial infarction. J Am Coll Cardiol 1985; 6:1233–8.

22. Capone G, Wolf NM, Meyer B, Meister SG. Frequency of intracoronary filling defects by angiography and angina pectoris at rest. Am J Cardiol 1985; 56:403–6.

23. Ambrose JA, Winters SL, Arora RR, et al. Angiographic evolution of coronary morphology in unstable angina. J Am Coll Cardiol 1986; 7:472–8.

24. Haft JI, Goldstein JE, Niemiera ML. Coronary arteriographic lesion of unstable angina. Chest 1987; 92:609–12.

25. Ambrose JA, Hjemdahl-Monsen CE. Arteriographic anatomy and mechanisms: Myocardial ischemia and unstable angina. J Am Coll Cardiol 1987; 6:1397–402.

26. Wilson RF, Holida MD, White CW. Quantitative angiographic morphology of coronary stenoses leading to myocardial infarction or unstable angina. Circulation 1986; 73:286–93.

27. Williams AE, Freeman MR, Chisholm RJ, Patt NL, Armstrong PW. Angiographic morphology in unstable angina pectoris. Am J Cardiol 1988; 62:1024–7.

28. Rehr R, Disciascio G, Vetrovec G, Cowley M. Angiographic morphology of coronary artery stenoses in prolonged rest angina: Evidence of intracoronary thrombosis. J Am Coll Cardiol 1989; 14:1429–37.

29. Freeman MR, Williams AE, Chisholm RJ, Armstrong PW. Intracoronary thrombus and complex morphology in unstable angina. Circulation 1989; 80:17–23.

30. Sherman CT, Litvack F, Grundfest W, et al. Coronary angioscopy in patients with unstable angina pectoris. N Engl J Med 1986; 315:913–9.

31. Forrester JS, Litvack F, Grundfest W, Hickey A. A perspective of coronary disease seen through the arteries of living man. Circulation 1987; 75:505–13.

32. Moncada S, Vane JR. Arachidonic acid metabolites and the interactions between platelets and blood-vessel walls. N Engl J Med 1979; 20:1142–7.

33. Fitzgerald DJ, Roy L, Catella F, Fitzgerald GA. Platelet activation in unstable coronary disease. N Engl J Med 1986; 315:983–9.

34. Theroux P, Latour JG, Liger-Gauthier C, DeLara J. Fibrinopeptide A and platelet factor levels in unstable angina pectoris. Circulation 1987; 75:156–62.

35. Hamm CW, Lorenz RL, Bleifeld W, Kupper W, Wober W, Weber PC. Biochemical evidence of platelet activation in patients with persistent unstable angina. J Am Coll Cardiol 1987; 10:998–1004.

36. Chesebro JH, Fuster V. Editorial: Platelet activation in unstable angina: Role of thromboxane A_2 and other mediators of vasocontriction. J Am Coll Cardiol 1990; 15:727–9.

37. Gallino A, Haeberli A, Baur HR, Straub PW. Fibrin formation and platelet aggrega-

tion in patients with severe coronary artery disease. Relationship with the degree of myocardial ischemia. Circulation 1985; 72:27–30.

38. Adams PC, Fuster V, Badimon L, Badimon JJ, Cheseboro JH. Platelet/vessel wall interactions, rheologic factors and throbogenetic substrate in acute coronary syndromes: preventive strategies. Am J Cardiol 1987; 60:9G–16G.

39. Castellot JJ, Cochran DL, Karnovsky MJ. Effect of heparin on vascular smooth muscle cells I. Cell metabolism. J Cell Physiol 1985; 124:21–8.

40. Cochran DL, Castellot JJ, Karnovsky MJ. Effect of herapin vascular smooth muscle cessl II. Specific protein synthesis. J Cell Physiol 1985; 124:29–36.

41. Marciniak E, Gockerman JP. Heparin induced decrease in circulatory antithrombin. III. Lancet 1977; 581–584.

42. Vermylen J, Verstraete M, Fuster V. Role of platelet activation and fibrin formation in thrombogenesis. J Am Coll Cardiol 1986; 8:2B–9B.

43. Tripp MD, Cats VM, can Capelle FJL, Vreeken J. Platelet hyperreactivity and prognosis in survivors of myocardial infarction. N Engl J Med 1990; 322:1549–54.

44. Vane JR, Anggard EE, Boltering RM. Regulatory functions of the vascular endothelium. N Engl J Med 1990; 323:27–36.

45. Kruskal JB, Commerford PJ, Franks JJ, Kirsch RE. Fibrin and fibrinogen related antigens in patients with stable and unstable coronary artery disease. N Engl J Med 1987; 317:1361–5.

46. Fuster V, Badimon L, Cohen M, Ambrose JA, Badimon JJ, Chesebro J. Insights into the pathogenesis of acute ischemic syndromes. Circulation 1988; 77:1213–20.

47. deZwaan C, Bar FW, Janssen JHA, et al. Effects of thrombolytic therapy in unstable angina: Clinical and angiographic results. J Am Coll Cardiol 1988; 12:301–9.

48. Ambrose JA, Hjemdahl-Monsen CE, Borrico S, et al. Quantitative and qualitative effects of intracoronary streptokinase in unstable angina and non Q-wave infarction. J Am Coll Cardiol 1987; 9:1156–65.

49. Gotoh K, Minamino T, Katoh O, et al. The role of intracoronary thrombus in unstable angina: Angiographic assessment of thrombolytic therapy during ongoing anginal attacks. Circulation 1988; 77:526–34.

50. Mandelkorn JB, Wolf NM, Singh S, et al. Intracoronary thrombus in non transmural myocardial infarction and unstable angina pectoris. Am J Cardiol 1983; 52: 1–6.

51. Maseri A, L'Abbate A, Baroldi G, et al. Coronary vasospasm as a possible cause of myocardial infarction. Aconclusion derived from the study of "preinfarction" angina. N Engl J Med 1978; 299:1271–7.

52. Maseri A, Severi S, De Nes M, et al. "Variant" angina: One aspect of a continuous spectrum of vasospastic myocardial ischemia. Am J Cardiol 1978;42: 1019–33.

53. deServi S, Specchia G, Ardeseno D, et al. Angiographic demonstration of different pathogenetic mechanisms in patients with spontaneous and exertional angina associated with ST segment depression. Am J Cardiol 1980; 45:1285–90.

54. Maseri A. Pathogenetic classification of unstable angina as a guideline to individual patient management and prognosis. Am J Med 1986; 80:48–55.

55. Figueras J, Singh BN, Ganz W, Charuzi Y, Swan HJC. Mechanism of rest and

nocturnal angina: observations during continuous hemodynamic and electrocardiographic monitoring. Circulation 1979; 59:955–68.

56. Guazzi M, et al. Left and right heart—hemodynamics during spontaneous angina pectoris. Br Heart J 1975; 37:401–13.

57. Chierchia S, Brunelli C, Simonetti I, Lazzari M, Maseri A. Sequence of events in angina at rest: Primary reduction in coronary flow. Circulation 1980; 61:759–68.

58. Roughgarden JW. Circulatory changes associated with spontaneous angina pectoris. Am J Med 1966; 41:947–61.

59. Gottlieb SO, Weisfeldt ML, Ouyang P, Melits ED, Girstenblith G. Silent ischemia as a marker for early unfavorable outcomes in patients with unstable angina. N Engl J Med 1986; 314:1214–9.

60. Gottlieb SO, Weisfeldt ML, Ouyang P, Mellits D, Gerstenblith G. Silent ischemia predicts infarction and death during 2 year follow-up of unstable angina. J Am Coll Cardiol 1987; 10:756–60.

61. Nademanee K, Intarachot V, Josephson MA, et al. Prognostic significance of silent myocardial ischemia in patients with unstable angina. J Am Coll Cardiol 1987; 10:1–9.

62. Wilcox I, Freedman B, Kelly DR, Harris PJ. Clinical significance of silent ischemia in unstable angina pectoris. Am J Cardiol 1990; 65:1313–6.

III
MEDICAL THERAPY
FOR UNSTABLE ANGINA

6

Medical Therapy for Unstable Angina Supported by Controlled Studies

H. Daniel Lewis, Jr.

Veterans Affairs Medical Center
Kansas City, Missouri, and
University of Kansas School of Medicine
Kansas City, Kansas

INTRODUCTION

In the 1950s and 1960s patients with unstable angina (referred to as preinfarction syndrome, coronary insufficiency, intermediate coronary syndrome, etc.) were considered to be at high risk, but were not a well-defined group. After the advent of coronary care units in the late 1960s and early 1970s, identification of these patients was facilitated. This permitted evaluation of the natural history of unstable angina and led to controlled studies of therapy for unstable angina.

Now unstable angina is defined as new onset or sudden worsening of angina characterized by increased frequency, prolonged duration, or occurrence at rest or during minimal activity. This syndrome is associated with increased risk of acute myocardial infarction or death. Between 1974 and 1984 the mortality and myocardial infarction rate at 1–4 months after diagnosis of unstable angina were 5% and 8–10%, respectively (1). The mortality at 1 year was about 10%. These rates are about half as high as those found in the early 1970s (2,3). The lower rates of death and myocardial infarction were probably primarily related to selection of patients. Prior to the development of coronary care units, patients with unstable angina were not admitted to the hospital unless they had persistent pain and ST-T changes on the electrocardiogram. As a consequence, only the sickest patients were admitted. Subsequently, criteria for admission to coronary care units became less restrictive, resulting in admission of patients with lower risk of infarction and death.

It has been known since the 1960s that the characteristic pathophysiological mechanism in acute myocardial infarction is ruptured atherosclerotic plaque with platelet aggregation at the site of exposed collagen leading to thrombus formation (4). However, the prevalence of this pathophysiological process in acute myocardial infarction, unstable angina, and sudden death was not fully recognized until the 1980s. Intravascular thrombus has been demonstrated to be present in these acute coronary artery syndromes in 70–90% of the cases. Hence, the rationale for antiplatelet and anticoagulant therapy in unstable angina is well established. Coronary artery spasm may sometimes be associated with this process and may rarely be the sole cause of unstable angina.

Unstable angina may be precipitated by conditions that increase myocardial oxygen consumption or that decrease oxygen delivery to the myocardium. In these cases the risk may be different from that noted above because of different pathophysiology. The risk may be decreased by treatment of the underlying precipitating factor, such as tachyarrhythmia, hypertension, congestive heart failure, thyrotoxicosis, anemia, or hypoxia. Exacerbation of stable angina by increased physical activity or by noncompliance with antianginal medications should not necessarily be considered unstable angina.

Patients with unstable angina should be admitted to a coronary care unit or other monitored bed for several reasons. Acute myocardial infarction should be ruled out with serial electrocardiograms and cardiac enzyme determinations. Acute infarction occurring before or after admission can be recognized and treated promptly. Placing the patient at bed rest and removing him from a stressful environment will decrease myocardial work and myocardial oxygen consumption. The patient's vital signs and clinical status can be observed and an electrocardiogram obtained when there is a recurrence of pain. This can be helpful in determining whether the pain is due to myocardial ischemia. If the pain is due to unstable angina, these observations may guide further medical therapy toward controlling heart rate or blood pressure. The observations may also be helpful in determining prognosis and, therefore, if and when to intervene with revascularization. Most patients soon become free of pain in the coronary care unit with bed rest and medications that decrease myocardial oxygen demand or increase myocardial perfusion. Continued angina and ischemic ST-segment or T-wave changes demonstrated on the electrocardiogram while in the coronary care unit indicate higher risk that may require more aggressive management (2). If the patient does not have ischemic electrocardiographic changes or continued chest pain, he may safely be risk-stratified electively by a stress test (5,6) or coronary arteriography.

The results of randomized, controlled clinical trials in patients with unstable angina have provided guidelines for therapy. The most common problems affecting the validity of results of clinical trials are biased selection of patients and assignment of therapy, biased evaluation of outcomes, and inadequate study size. Randomization of treatment assignment is the basis for providing that the treatment groups are comparable. Blinding of treatment and of assessment of outcomes prevents bias. Having a large enough sample size assures that randomization will provide comparable treatment groups. Importantly, a large enough sample size provides an adequate number of end-point events to ensure recognition of moderate, but clinically important, treatment effects.

ANTIPLATELET AND ANTICOAGULANT THERAPY
Anticoagulant Therapy (see Table 1)

In the 1950s enthusiasm was high for anticoagulant therapy for unstable angina (preinfarction syndrome, coronary insufficiency, intermediate coronary syndrome) as well as for acute myocardial infarction. The initial studies used varying definitions for unstable angina and therefore evaluated patients with varying risks. All these studies also suffered from lack of controls or inadequate controls.

The first attempt at a randomized clinical trial of anticoagulant therapy for unstable angina was carried out by Wood, who in 1961 reported on 150 patients with acute and subacute coronary insufficiency (7). Patients treated with anticoagulants, primarily phenindione, for at least 6 weeks were compared with patients treated conservatively. Of the first 40 patients entered, alternate patients received anticoagulant therapy. The study was not blinded. When it "became obvious, however, that the controls were faring worse than the treated cases," the last 30 patients in the control group were selected because of a contraindica-

Table 1 Anticoagulant Therapy

		n	Death	MI	UA			
Wood, 1961 (7)	Control	50	30%	22%				
150 pts; 2 months	Anticoagulant	100	6	3				
Telford, 1981 (9)	Control	114	2%	15%				
400 pts; 7 days	Heparin	100	0	3				
Williams, 1986 (10)	Control	51	8%	6%	20%			
102 pts; 6 months	Heparin + warfarin	51	2	4	6			
						IABP	PTCA	CABG
Zwerner, 1987 (11)	Control	29	3%	10%		14%	14%	45%
62 pts; 8 days	Heparin	33	9	12		12	15	39

pts = patients; *n* = number of patients; MI = myocardial infarction; UA = unstable angina; IABP = intraaortic balloon pump; PTCA = percutaneous transluminal coronary angioplasty; CABG = coronary artery bypass graft surgery.

tion to anticoagulants, physician bias, and so forth. The trial was then completed with 100 patients treated with anticoagulants and 50 controls. Within 2 months myocardial infarction occurred in 3% of the treated cases and 22% of the controls. Death occurred in 6% of the treated patients and 30% of the controls.

These dramatic results led to the general acceptance of anticoagulant therapy for unstable angina. However, the trial was not randomized. It can only be considered a concurrent control trial. The lack of blinding led to bias in selection of patients and therapy and was associated with an inordinately high mortality rate in the control group. When anticoagulant therapy for acute myocardial infarction fell out of favor about 1970, the deficiencies in Wood's study were pointed out. Subsequently, anticoagulant therapy for unstable angina became less routine.

Interest in anticoagulant therapy was renewed by the Netherlands Sixty Plus Reinfarction Study in 1980 (8) and, in particular for unstable angina, by Telford and Wilson's Northern Ireland study reported in 1981 (9). The latter was a randomized, double-blind, double-placebo-controlled, 2×2 factorial design study of heparin and atenolol therapy (heparin, atenolol, heparin and atenolol, and placebo) in 214 patients with intermediate coronary syndrome. Some of the patients had elevated cardiac enzymes on admission and therefore had non-Q-wave myocardial infarctions at entry. Since there was no interaction between heparin and atenolol, all the patients who received heparin can be compared with all who did not. Patients received this randomly assigned treatment for 7 days. Subsequently, all treated and control patients who did not have a contraindication received warfarin for an additional 7 weeks. During the first week 15% of the placebo group had myocardial infarctions and there were two deaths, in contrast to only 3% with infarctions ($p = 0.024$) and no deaths in the heparin group. The benefit persisted; between 1 and 8 weeks the placebo group had three infarctions and three deaths, compared to four infarctions and no deaths in the heparin group. The frequency of recurrent chest pain was not significantly reduced by heparin. This study was highly acclaimed as a very well-designed study. However, it had a major flaw. Of 400 patients randomly assigned to therapy, 186 were subsequently withdrawn from the study for various reasons, usually failure to meet entry criteria or evidence of transmural infarction at baseline. Consequently, the randomization was invalidated, and the study can only be considered a concurrent control study.

In 1986 Williams et al reported a randomized trial of 102 patients with unstable angina (10). Fifty-one patients were treated initially with intravenous heparin for 48 hr and warfarin for 6 months. There were four deaths, three myocardial infarctions, and 10 patients with recurrent unstable angina in the control group in comparison with one death, two infarctions, and three cases of recurrent unstable angina in the treated group (combined events 34% compared with 12%; $p < 0.05$). Most of the difference was in recurrent unstable angina, and the trial was not blinded. Patients who showed elevation of initial cardiac enzymes were withdrawn and their trial number reallocated to the next patient entering the trial. Perhaps this irregularity in random allocation of therapy led to an unbalanced distribution of baseline characteristics. More control patients received beta blocker therapy because of more severe anginal symptoms. The study was clearly too small to detect a difference in myocardial infarction or death. The results should be considered inconclusive.

In 1987 Zwerner et al. reported the results of a randomized trial of up to 8 days of intravenous heparin plus standard therapy compared with standard therapy alone in 62 patients with unstable angina (11). There were no significant differences between the treatment groups (33 patients assigned to heparin and 29 to control) for myocardial infarction, death, aortocoronary bypass surgery, or percutaneous transluminal angioplasty. However, since the study was too small to have detected any differences, it must also be considered inconclusive.

Antiplatelet Therapy (see Table 2)

The Veterans Administration Cooperative Study on Aspirin Therapy and Unstable Angina was started in 1973. During the time it was conducted six large multicenter, randomized trials of aspirin therapy after myocardial infarction showed trends of decreased mortality or recurrent infarction, but none showed statistically significant results. The VA study reported by Lewis et al. in 1983 was a randomized, placebo-controlled, double-blind, multicenter trial of aspirin treatment (324 mg in buffered solution daily) for 12 weeks in 1266 men with unstable angina (12). Treatment was begun within 51 hr of admission to the hospital, with 625 patients assigned aspirin and 641 placebo. Death or acute myocardial infarction was 51% lower in the aspirin treatment group: 31 patients (5%) compared with 65 controls (10.1%); $p = 0.0005$. Nonfatal infarction was 51% lower in the aspirin group; 21 patients (3.4%) compared with 44 controls (6.9%); $p = 0.005$. Mortality was also 51% lower in the aspirin group: 10 patients (1.6%) compared with 21 controls (3.3%), although the difference was of marginal statistical significance; $p = 0.054$. Although the study medication was discontinued at 12 weeks, follow-up at 1 year was available in 86% of the patients. At 1 year mortality was still 43% lower in the aspirin group (9.6% compared with 5.5%; $p = 0.008$). The benefit persisted. There was no difference in gastrointestinal symptoms or evidence of blood loss between the treated and control groups.

The VA Cooperative Study showed that aspirin has an important protective effect against myocardial infarction (51% reduction) in men with unstable angina. It was the first study to show statistically significant benefit of aspirin therapy in patients with coronary artery disease. It suggested a similar beneficial

Table 2 Antiplatelet and Anticoagulant Therapy

	n	Death	Nonfatal MI (Q)	(Non-Q)	Death or MI	Risk reduction
VA Cooperative Study (12)						
Lewis, 1983						
1266 pts; 12 weeks						
Control	641	3.3%	6.9%		10.1%	
Aspirin	625	1.6	3.4***		5.0****	51% d or MI
Canadian Multicenter (13)						
Cairns, 1985						
555 pts; 18 months						
Control	279	11.7%			17.0%	
Aspirin	276	3.0***			8.6	51% d or MI
Théroux, 1988 (14)						
479 pts; 7 days						
Control	118		12.0%			
Aspirin	121		3.0**			71% MI
Aspirin + heparin	122		1.6***			88%
Heparin	118		0.8*****			94%
Charvat, 1989 (15)						
266 pts; 72 hr (15)						
Control	105	2.0%	19.0%	21.9%		
Aspirin + dipyridamole	100	3.0	20.0	24.0		
Heparin	61	1.6	3.2**	29.5		
Cohen, 1989 (16)						
99 pts; 12 weeks						
Aspirin, 325 mg		0%	3%		3%	
Heparin + coumadin		0(4)†	4(4)		4(8)	
Aspirin, 80 mg, + heparin + coumadin		0(3)	0(3)		0(6)	
					Risk ratio for MI or death	
Wallentin, 1989 (17)						
794 pts; 90 days						
Control	198					
Aspirin + heparin	210				0.23***	
Aspirin	187				0.41***	
Heparin	199				0.87	

*p < 0.05. **p < 0.01. ***p < 0.005. ****p < 0.001.

VA = Veterans Administration; pts = patients; n = number of patients; MI = myocardial infarction; d = death; †( ) during or after percutaneous angioplasty or coronary artery bypass surgery.

effect on mortality. In the dosage used, 324 mg in buffered solution daily for 12 weeks, there was no evidence of adverse effects.

In 1985 Cairns et al. reported the results of the Canadian randomized, placebo-controlled, double blind, multicenter trial of antiplatelet therapy in 555 patients with unstable angina (13). Within 8 days of admission to the hospital, patients were assigned to aspirin, 325 mg four times daily, sulfinpyrazone, 200 mg four times daily, both, or neither, and treated for up to 2 years (mean 18 months). Aspirin therapy was associated with a risk reduction of 51% in cardiac death or nonfatal myocardial infarction, from 36 patients (17.0%) in the controls to 17 (8.6%) in the group treated with aspirin; $p = 0.008$. Cardiac death alone was reduced 71% from 22 patients (11.7%) to 6 (3.0%); $p = 0.004$. By intention-to-treat analyses, the reduction by aspirin in cardiac death or nonfatal infarction was 30% ($p = 0.072$), and for cardiac death alone 56% ($p = 0.009$). There was no benefit seen with sulfinpyrazone for any outcome event. There was no evidence of an interaction between sulfinpyrazone and aspirin. Although major bleeding was not a problem, minor gastrointestinal side effects were more common in the aspirin-treated patients.

The results of the Canadian trial were remarkably similar and complementary to those of the VA Cooperative Study. The Canadian trial confirmed the efficacy of aspirin in preventing myocardial infarction in patients with unstable angina, and it demonstrated a statistically significant reduction in mortality. It showed this with a much larger dose of aspirin, dispelling concerns of loss of efficacy at higher dosage. The Canadian study included 27% women. Aspirin demonstrated at least as much benefit in the women as in the men, dispelling concerns of lack of efficacy in women. In the Canadian study, aspirin therapy did not start until up to 8 days after admission to the hospital, in contrast to within 51 hr in the VA study. Even so, the effects of aspirin therapy were quite similar, and the benefits persisted during up to 2 years of treatment. The mortality curves of the aspirin and the control groups continued to diverge throughout the study. The benefits of aspirin treatment were seen in the Canadian study, in which coronary artery bypass surgery occurred in 31.5% of the patients as well as in the VA study, with only 3.5% of the patients having bypass surgery. The VA Cooperative Study demonstrated the advantage of the once-daily lower dosage aspirin therapy through better compliance and lack of adverse effects of aspirin.

Antiplatelet and Anticoagulant Therapy

In 1988 Théroux et al. reported a randomized, placebo-controlled, double-blind trial in 479 patients with unstable angina (14). The patients were randomly assigned to aspirin, 325 mg twice daily, heparin, 1000 units/hr intravenously, the combination of aspirin and heparin, or double placebo. Treatment was started 7.9 ± 8.0 hr after the last episode of pain and continued for 6 ± 3 days. Myocardial infarction occurred in 12% of the 118 patients receiving placebo, but was significantly reduced in the patients receiving heparin (0.8%; $p < 0.001$), aspirin (3%; $p = 0.01$), and aspirin plus heparin (1.6%; $p = 0.003$). Although there was a trend favoring benefit of heparin over aspirin, there were no statistically significant differences between the three treatment groups. The combination of heparin and aspirin was no more effective then heparin alone in the prevention of infarction. However, the combination was associated with slightly more frequent serious bleeding episodes, 3.3% compared with 1.7%. Myocardial infarction was associated with Q waves in 86% of the control patients and 29% of the treated patients ($p < 0.01$). No deaths occurred in any of the treated patients, compared to 1.7% in the controls, but the number of deaths was too small to evaluate. Refractory angina occurred in 23% of the control patients and was reduced by 69% in the heparin-treated patients and by 60% in those treated with the combination of heparin and aspirin. Aspirin alone was not associated with a reduction in refractory angina.

This trial confirmed the efficacy of aspirin therapy in preventing myocardial infarction acutely in patients with unstable angina. It clearly established the efficacy of intravenous heparin therapy in preventing myocardial infarction acutely in patients with unstable angina. It showed a trend suggesting an advantage of heparin over aspirin in preventing infarction, but showed no advantage in combining the two therapies. It seemed to show that heparin reduced the incidence of refractory unstable angina, whereas aspirin did not.

In 1989 Charvat and Kuruvilla reported the results of a randomized study of heparin, 1000 IU/hr; aspirin, 100 mg daily, plus dipyridamole, 75 mg twice daily, plus 5% dextrose in water infusion; and dextrose in water infusion alone (in 61, 100, and 105 patients, respectively) for 3 days in 266 patients with unstable angina (15). There was no difference in total number of myocardial infarctions in the three groups. However, there were significantly fewer Q-wave infarctions in the heparin-treated patients (3.2%) compared to the antiplatelet-treated (20%) and the control patients (19%); $p = 0.006$. It is not clear why there were only 61 patients in the heparin-treated group. It suggests that about 40 patients were removed from that group after random assignment. The results must be considered inconclusive.

In 1989 Cohen et al. presented a pilot trial of antithrombotic therapy in 94 patients with unstable angina or non-Q-wave infarction (16). Patients were randomly assigned to aspirin, 325 mg daily, full-dose heparin followed by Coumadin, or the combination of aspirin, 80 mg daily, plus heparin followed by Coumadin started within 12.4 ± 10.4 hr and continued for 12 weeks. In this small pilot study no significant differences between the groups were noted with respect to recurrent ischemia, revascularization, myocardial infarction, death, or major bleeding. In spite of antithrombotic therapy, including combination therapy, a substantial percentage of patients had recurrent angina and subsequent percutaneous transluminal coronary angioplasty or coronary artery bypass graft surgery. With antithrombotic therapy and early intervention there was a very low rate of death and myocardial infarction.

In 1989 Wallentin et al. reported the results of the RISK study of 794 men with unstable angina or non-Q-wave myocardial infarction (17). The study was a 2×2 factorial trial, with patients randomly assigned to aspirin, 75 mg daily for at least 3 months, and/or intravenous heparin, 30,000 IU/24 hr for 5 days. Between 24 and 72 hr after hospital admission, the patients were started on intravenous heparin and aspirin ($n = 210$), intravenous heparin and oral placebo ($n = 199$), intravenous placebo and aspirin ($n = 187$), or intravenous placebo and oral placebo ($n = 198$). At 5 days, 30 days, and 90 days, the patients treated with heparin and aspirin had significantly decreased risk ratios for myocardial infarction or death relative to those treated with intravenous and oral placebos (0.14, 0.20, and 0.23, respectively). The risk ratios were significantly decreased for aspirin alone at 30 days and 90 days (0.34 and 0.41), but not at 5 days. Heparin alone did not show any significant reduction in risk, but when added to aspirin, it conferred decreased risk at 5 days and seemed to contribute to long-term benefit. Incapacitating angina leading to coronary angiography also occurred less frequently in the 397 patients randomly assigned to aspirin therapy (18).

This study confirmed the efficacy of aspirin in preventing myocardial infarction or death in patients with unstable angina and showed the effectiveness of a dosage of only 75 mg. It is not clear why it did not confirm Théroux's results of the efficacy of heparin in preventing myocardial infarction and refractory angina. The difference could be related to starting therapy later, 1–3 days after admission to the hospital compared to within hours in Théroux's study. This is the only study to suggest that aspirin reduces angina.

Other Antiplatelet Therapy

Ticlopidine is an antiplatelet drug that differs from aspirin in that it does not block cyclooxygenase. It appears to interfere with the ADP-mediated platelet activation mechanism and the platelet fibrinogen receptor. In 1990 Balsano et al. reported the results of a randomized, unblinded trial of ticlopidine therapy in 652 patients with unstable angina (19). Evaluation of the end-point results were blinded. In 314 patients treated with ticlopidine, there were eight deaths and 15 who had myocardial infarction (7.3% events) within 6 months, compared with 16 deaths and 30 who had myocardial infarction (13.6% events) in the control group of 338 patients. This represented a reduction in risk of vascular death or nonfatal infarction of 46% ($p = 0.009$), of nonfatal infarction of 46% ($p = 0.039$), and of death of 47% ($p = 0.139$). Ticlopidine appears to be equally effective as aspirin in patients with unstable angina. When the study was stopped, however, the difference in mortality was not statistically significant.

Summary

There is clear evidence that aspirin decreases the risk of myocardial infarction and death by about one-half in patients with unstable angina. It is effective acutely and is of continued benefit chronically. There is reasonable evidence that ticlopidine has a similar effect to that of aspirin. There is no evidence that sulfinpyrazone or dipyridamole is of any benefit in patients with unstable angina. There is reasonable evidence that acute heparin therapy decreases the risk of myocardial infarction by at least as much as aspirin, although one large study does not confirm this. The data suggest that heparin may relieve angina.

BETA-BLOCKER AND CALCIUM CHANNEL BLOCKER THERAPY

Beta Blocker Therapy (see Table 3)

Sublingual nitroglycerin is frequently effective in giving immediate relief from angina and ischemic electrocardiographic changes. Consequently, long-acting nitrates in the form of nitroglycerin paste and oral nitroglycerin in large doses were the standard therapies for unstable angina in the early 1970s. The initial reports of beta-blocker therapy for unstable angina were uncontrolled. In 1970, Mizgala reported on 15 patients with acute coronary insufficiency refractory to nitrates and heparin therapy (20). With increasing doses of propranolol, 13 of 15 patients had complete relief of symptoms. Another uncontrolled study, reported by Fischl et al. in 1973, was also thought to show dramatic results (21). Of 20 patients with refractory intermediate coronary syndrome treated with rapidly increasing oral doses of propranolol, 17 had prompt relief of pain, usually within 12 hr. They noted increases in heart rate and blood pressure during episodes of pain and significant lowering of heart rate and blood pressure with propranolol

Table 3 Beta-Blocker Therapy

		n	Death	MI	Q-wave MI
Norris, 1978 (22)	Control	23	0	22	8
43 pts; 27 hr	Propranolol	20	0	11	2
Yusuf, 1980 (23)	Control	44	9	27	
79 pts; hospital stay	Atenolol	35	4	11	
Telford, 1981 (9)	Control	105	2	10	
214 pts; 7 days	Atenolol	109	0	10	

pts = patients; n = number of patients; MI = myocardial infarction.

therapy. They concluded that the therapy was safe and effective in most patients, and would allow consideration of revascularization surgery on an elective basis. Randomized trials were finally reported in 1978. Most of these trials evaluated patients with unstable rest angina.

In 1978 Norris et al. reported on 43 patients who, within 4 hr of onset of pain of suspected acute myocardial infarction without ST elevation or pathological Q waves, were randomly assigned to intravenous and then oral propranolol (20 patients) compared with no additional therapy (23 patients) for 27 hr (22). Two patients in the treated group developed pathological Q waves, compared with eight patients in the control group. Eleven of nineteen treated patients (one patient's enzymes were lost) developed elevated serum levels of creatine kinase, compared with 22 of 23 in the control group. Apparently, many of these patients had a non-Q-wave infarction at entry.

In 1980 Yusuf et al. reported on early intravenous atenolol followed by oral atenolol in 135 patients with electrocardiographic (ECG) evidence of acute myocardial infarction and 79 patients with threatened myocardial infarction but no definite ECG evidence of infarction (no ST elevation) at entry (23). In the latter group, 35 patients were randomly assigned to atenolol and 44 to control. In the antenolol group there were 11 myocardial infarctions and four deaths, compared to 27 infarctions and nine deaths in the control group. There were two nonfatal cardiac arrests in the atenolol group, compared to six in the control group. Again, a significant number of these patients must have had a non-Q-wave infarction at entry into the study.

In 1981 Telford et al. reported the results of a 2×2 factorial randomized, placebo-controlled trial of heparin, atenolol, heparin and atenolol, and placebo (9). Since there was no interaction between atenolol and heparin, the results in all patients who received atenolol can be compared with results in all those who did not. The 214 patients consisted of patients with preinfarction angina (increasing severe angina without further ECG changes), acute coronary insufficiency (cardiac pain associated with ST-segment changes and/or T-wave inversion without significant cardiac enzyme elevation), and subendocardial infarction (ST-segment and/or T-wave changes with elevated cardiac enzymes). Patients were randomly assigned to initial intravenous atenolol followed by oral atenolol for 7 days (109 patients) or to intravenous and oral placebo (105 patients). At 7 days there was no difference in results, with 10 myocardial infarctions in each group and two deaths in the control group. During another 7 weeks of follow-up there were five additional infarcts and three deaths in the atenolol group and two infarcts and no deaths in the control group. Unfortunately, the 214 patients were derived from 400 patients randomly assigned to therapy, with 186 patients subsequently removed from the study for various reasons. This invalidated the random allocation of therapy, so the study should be considered a concurrent control study.

Calcium Channel Blocker with Beta-Blocker Therapy

Although Fischl et al. in 1973 had noted elevated blood pressure and heart rate consistent with increased myocardial oxygen consumption in patients with unstable angina, investigators later found evidence for decreased coronary artery flow. The earlier findings fit well with the typical pathophysiology in stable exertional angina. Consequently, the treatment would seem to have a similar basis as that for stable angina, and beta-blocker therapy seemed quite appropriate. In 1980 Neill et al. (24), Smitherman et al. (25), and Chierchia et al. (26) each reported evidence supporting limitations in coronary flow in unstable angina. Maseri et al. promulgated the importance of coronary vasospasm in stable and unstable angina (26a). This led to concern that beta-blocker therapy could possibly aggravate unstable angina and suggested that there may be greater benefit from calcium-channel blocker therapy. Calcium-channel blockers without negative chronotropic effect, however, could be associated with reflex tachycardia and, like nitrate therapy, increased myocardial oxygen consumption. This led to several studies to compare beta blockers and calcium-channel blockers in patients with unstable angina.

Calcium Channel Blocker with Negative Chronotropic Effects (see Table 4)

In 1983 Andre-Fouet et al. randomly assigned 70 patients with unstable angina to increasing dosages of diltiazem or propranolol therapy (27). The randomization was stratified within a group of 29 patients with ST-segment elevation only and a

Table 4 Diltiazem and Propranolol Therapy

		n	Death	MI	CABG	Complete relief of pain	
Andre-Fouet, 1983 (27) 70 pts; CCU stay	Diltiazem	34				23	
	Propranolol	36				18	
							Chest pain (episodes/day)
Théroux, 1985 (28) 100 pts; 5.1 months	Before (Control)						0.75
	Diltiazem	50	2	5	21	14	0.26*
	Propranolol	50	2	4	19	13	0.29*

$*p < 0.05$.
pts = patients; n = number of patients; MI = myocardial infarction; CABG = coronary artery bypass graft surgery.

group of 41 with other ST-segment or T-wave changes. At least two-thirds of the 34 diltiazem-treated patients had complete relief of chest pain, compared to only half the 36 patients treated with propranolol. Similar results were seen within the subgroup with ST-segment elevation only. Similarly, of 24 patients with angina exclusively at rest, there were nine successes and four failures with diltiazem, while there was no symptomatic relief in the 11 patients treated with propranolol. This study was probably heavily weighted with patients with coronary artery spasm. Unfortunately, it was also a single-blind study where the events of note were all based on subjective symptomatology.

In 1985 Théroux et al. reported a randomized study of diltiazem and pro-pranolol therapy in 100 patients with unstable angina, excluding Prinzmetal's angina patients with ST-segment elevation (28). There was no placebo group, and the study was single blind. In the first month of follow-up, the number of chest pain episodes was reduced from 0.75 per day overall to 0.26 per day in the 50 diltiazem-treated patients and to 0.29 per day in the 50 propranolol-treated patients. Fourteen patients receiving diltiazem and 13 receiving propranolol became free of symptoms. In a mean of 5.1 months of follow-up there were two deaths, five infarctions, and 21 coronary artery bypass surgeries in the diltiazem group and two deaths, four infarctions, and 19 bypasses in the propranolol group. Nine diltiazem- and six propranolol-treated patients were without symptoms. The comparability of the results in the two groups suggested that coronary artery spasm was not the main factor involved in unstable angina when Prinzmetal's angina patients were excluded, and that diltiazem could be used as an alternative to the usual treatment with beta-blocking drugs.

In 1986 Parodi et al. reported a randomized, double-blind, multiple-cross-over, placebo-controlled trial of verapamil and propranolol in 10 patients with frequent episodes of rest angina with associated ST-segment shifts (29). Three patients were said to have variant angina, five had both ST elevation and depression, and two had ST depression only. During the 16 days of the trial, a continuous ECG recording revealed only 2.6 ST-segment shifts per 24 hr during verapamil periods compared to 11.9 per 24 hr during corresponding placebo periods. There was no difference in the number of ST-segment shifts per 24 hr during propranolol therapy compared to during placebo therapy (11.9 compared to 12.0, respectively). There were statistically significant reductions in number of angina attacks and number of nitroglycerin tablets used with verapamil therapy, but not with propranolol therapy. Of a total of 1602 episodes of transient ST-segment shifts, 1309 were ST-segment elevation. No patient had previously documented myocardial infarction. Consequently, these patients probably were predominantly Prinzmetal's angina patients.

Nifedipine (see Table 5)

In 1982 Gerstenblith et al. compared nifedipine plus conventional treatment to conventional treatment alone, which then consisted of propranolol and long-

Table 5 Nifedipine and Beta-Blocker Therapy

Study	Treatment	n	Death	MI	Q-Wave MI	Angina	CABG	CABG or PTCA for Symptoms	CABG or PTCA for Anatomy	Ischemia or MI	Risk ratio
Gerstenblith, 1982 (30) 138 pts; 4 months	Control	70	5	12			27				
	Nifedipine	68	7	11		Decreased	18				
Muller, 1984 (31) 125 pts; 14 days	Control	63		9			13				
	Nifedipine	63		9		Unchanged	14				
Gottlieb, 1986 (32) 81 pts; 4 weeks	Control	39	0	3				15	2		
	Propranolol	42	1	6		Decreased		10	4		
HINT, 1986 (33) 338 pts; 48 hr	Placebo	84		13	9					31	
No pretreatment with beta-blocker	Nifedipine	89		25	14					42	1.15
	Metoprolol	79		13	6	Decreased				22	0.76
	Combination	35		12	7	Decreased				28	0.80
177 pts; 48 hr	Placebo	81		16	6					41	
Pretreatment with beta-blocker	Nifedipine	91		13	6	Decreased				29	0.68

pts = patients; n = number of patients; MI = myocardial infarction; CABG = coronary artery bypass graft surgery; PTCA = percutaneous transluminal coronary angioplasty.

acting nitrates (30). The trial was placebo-controlled, double-blind, with 138 patients randomly assigned to therapy, 68 to nifedipine and 70 to placebo, for 4 months. The end-points of the study were sudden death, myocardial infarction, and aortocoronary bypass surgery. Any of these three represented failure of therapy. Only 30 nifedipine-treated patients compared to 43 placebo patients failed therapy ($p = 0.03$). The study was heavily weighted with patients with transient ST-segment elevation, but the results were similar in this subgroup. There were nine failures of 25 patients with ST elevation in the nifedipine group, compared to 18 who failed of 27 in the placebo group. At the time, this was interpreted as an advantage of the calcium-channel blocker in patients with superimposed coronary artery spasm. In fact, many of these patients may have had more severe (subtotal) coronary artery obstruction due to thrombus leading to transmural myocardial ischemia (4).

Overall the results of the study were interpreted as evidence that nifedipine prevented sudden death and myocardial infarction as well as relieving anginal pain. However, in the nifedipine group there was one sudden death and 11 infarcts compared to two sudden deaths and 12 infarcts in the conventional treatment group. The difference between the groups was in the frequency of bypass surgery. When left main coronary artery stenosis was excluded, there were 13 bypass surgeries out of 63 patients in the nifedipine group and 24 surgeries out of 63 patients in the placebo group; $p = 0.02$. Since the study was double blind as well as randomized, the data appear valid. Nifedipine was effective in relieving unstable anginal pain and myocardial ischemia.

In 1984 Muller et al. reported a randomized, double-blind clinical trial of conventional therapy compared to nifedipine therapy in 126 patients (31). Nifedipine and conventional therapy were each titrated to increasing levels as dictated by recurrence of angina. The patients were followed for 14 days with primary end-points of control of pain and occurrence of myocardial infarction. In comparing the 63 patients treated with nifedipine with the 63 treated with conventional therapy, there was no difference in time to relief of anginal pain, number of angina attacks per 24 hr during the first 2 days, number of sublingual nitroglycerin tablets used, number of patients requiring morphine, or incidence of myocardial infarction. Fourteen patients failed to respond to nifedipine therapy and 13 failed to respond to conventional therapy. When beta-blocker was added to the therapy of the former group and nifedipine was added to the latter group, five patients in each group became pain free.

The randomization was stratified within two subgroups, 34 patients who had a relative contraindication to beta-blocker (whose conventional therapy therefore consisted only of isosorbide dinitrate) and 92 patients without contraindication to beta-blocker (whose conventional therapy consisted of propranolol and isosorbide dinitrate). The study showed the therapies were equivalent when nifedipine was compared with conventional therapy for both groups combined as well as when the treatments were compared separately within each group.

However, significant differences did appear to exist between nifedipine and conventional therapy when time to control of pain was compared in the subgroups receiving and/or not receiving prior beta-blockers. Patients who had received prior beta-blocker therapy appeared to benefit more from nifedipine than from increasing beta-blocker and nitrate therapy. Patients who had not received prior beta-blocker appeared to benefit more from propranolol and nitrate therapy than from addition of nifedipine. However, this was from post hoc subgroup analyses, and other measures of angina control did not reflect these differences.

In 1986 Gottlieb et al. reported a randomized, double-blind trial of propranolol compared with placebo for 4 weeks in 81 patients with unstable angina (32). All patients also received nifedipine, 80 mg daily, and long-acting nitrates. There was no difference in the occurrence of cardiac death, myocardial infarction, and aortocoronary bypass surgery between the two groups (18 of 39 placebo and 16 of 42 propranolol-treated patients). However, in the propranolol-treated patients there was statistically significant benefit in controlling angina as measured by recurrent resting angina, number of episodes of angina during the first 4 days, duration of angina, sublingual nitroglycerin requirement, and, as recorded on 24-hr continuous ECG, the number and duration of ST-segment changes during ischemic episodes. The study did not support any detrimental effect of beta-blocker therapy by possible potentiation of any coronary vasopastic component. It showed that propranolol reduces the frequency and duration of symptomatic and silent myocardial ischemic episodes.

The largest randomized trial was the Holland Interuniversity Nifedipine/Metoprolol Trial (HINT), reported in 1986 (33). In this study 338 patients not previously treated with beta-blocker were randomly assigned to nifedipine (89 patients), metoprolol (79 patients), nifedipine and metoprolol (86 patients), or placebo (84 patients). Another 177 patients, who had been pretreated with beta-blocker, were randomly assigned to nifedipine or placebo (96 and 81 patients, respectively). The primary event outcome was recurrent ischemia or myocardial infarction within 48 hr. In the patients not previously on beta-blocker therapy, the event rate ratios relative to placebo were 1.15 for nifedipine, 0.76 for metoprolol, and 0.80 for nifedipine and metoprolol combined (a 24% and a 20% reduction in events for the latter two groups, respectively). In patients already on a beta-blocker, the addition of nifedipine was beneficial (event rate ratio 0.68).

These results suggest that in patients not on previous beta-blockade, metoprolol has a beneficial short-term effect on unstable angina, that a fixed combination with nifedipine provides no further gain, and that nifedipine alone may be detrimental. On the other hand, the addition of nifedipine to beta-blockade existing at the time when the patient's condition became unstable seems beneficial.

Summary

The initial studies of beta-blocker therapy for unstable angina were uncontrolled in patients refractory to nitrates. Three randomized trials of beta-blocker compared with placebo included some patients with non-Q-wave infarction at entry. The two smaller trials (43 and 79 patients) showed a lower incidence of myocardial infarction, and one of these a lower mortality in the treated group. The largest of these three trials (214 patients) revealed no difference in infarctions or deaths. In this trial the randomization was invalidated, and the study could have suffered from type II error with too few end-point events to avoid missing a moderate, but important effect. An overview (metanalysis) of the randomized trials of beta-blocker therapy suggests only 13% reduction in the risk of developing myocardial infarction (34).

In two studies heavily weighted with Prinzmetal's angina, calcium-channel blockers with negative chronotropic effects were more effective than propranolol in relieving pain in patients with unstable angina. The first was a randomized study of diltiazem in 70 patients. The second was a double-blind, multiple-crossover, placebo-controlled trial of verapamil in 10 patients. In a randomized trial of 100 patients excluding Prinzmetal's angina, diltiazem and propranolol were equally effective in relieving pain and no difference was seen in subsequent events.

There are three randomized trials of nifedipine, a calcium-channel blocker without heart-rate-slowing effects, compared with placebo or beta-blocker therapy in patients with unstable angina. There is one randomized trial of propranolol or placebo added to conventional therapy including nifedipine. In 138 patients treated with nifedipine or placebo added to conventional therapy including beta-blockers and nitrates, nifedipine was effective in relieving unstable anginal pain and myocardial ischemia, thereby decreasing the frequency of aortocoronary bypass surgery. There was no difference in the incidence of myocardial infarction or death. In 126 patients randomly assigned to nifedipine or to conventional therapy titrated to increasing dosages, the two treatments were equivalent in relief of pain, including when treatment failures were crossed over to the other therapy. In 81 patients randomly assigned to the addition of propranolol or placebo to conventional therapy including nifedipine and long-acting nitrates, there was no difference between treatments in the number of end-points of death, myocardial infarction, and coronary bypass surgery, and no difference in controlling symptomatic and silent ischemic episodes from continuous ECG recordings. In the largest study of 338 patients not previously treated with a beta-blocker, metoprolol and metoprolol plus nifedipine in fixed combination were equally effective compared to placebo in preventing recurrent ischemia or myocardial infarction, while nifedipine alone was not at all effective or possibly detrimental. An overview (metanalysis) of the randomized trials of nifedipine therapy in patients with unstable angina indicates there was no difference in mortality or myocardial infarction rate between treatment and control (35).

However, in 177 patients who were already receiving beta-blocker when their unstable angina developed, the addition of nifedipine compared to control appeared to be quite beneficial. These findings are probably related to reflex tachycardia with nifedipine and heart rate control with beta-blocker. The evidence supports relief of anginal pain and myocardial ischemia with beta-blocker and calcium-channel-blocker therapy in patients with unstable angina. There is no convincing evidence by adequately sized, well-controlled, randomized trials of prevention of myocardial infarction or death by these therapies.

NITRATE THERAPY

Intravenous Nitroglycerin

Like the initial reports of the use of beta-blockers in patients with unstable angina, most studies of intravenous nitroglycerin have been uncontrolled. They simply evaluated giving a progressively larger dose until pain was relieved or adverse effects occurred. The assumption was that the treatment caused the pain relief. Though uncontrolled, the results of these studies carried out in patients with unstable rest angina refractory to beta-blocker and nitrates by other routes of administration have usually been dramatic enough that intravenous nitroglycerin therapy has become nearly universally accepted for refractory unstable angina.

In 1979 Dauwe et al. presented a series of 14 patients with refractory unstable angina treated with intravenous infusion of nitroglycerin (36). The dose was increased progressively to relief of pain or until adverse effects occurred. Angina disappeared in 12 patients and headache caused discontinuance of the infusion in one patient. In three patients whose nitroglycerin was transiently discontinued, angina recurred within 1 hr.

In 1979 Page et al. reported 17 patients with unstable angina refractory to medical management who were treated with intravenous nitroglycerin infusion (37). The treatment was effective in decreasing or stopping angina attacks in all the patients except one. It appeared to be effective and well tolerated by the patients.

In 1980 Brodsky et al. reported 14 patients with unstable angina refractory to propranolol and conventional nitrate preparations who were treated with intravenous infusion of nitroglycerin (38). Control of angina was achieved in five patients. Hypotension occurred in six patients, but was corrected with fluid in three of them. Intraaortic balloon pump was required in seven nonresponders.

In 1980 Mikolich et al. reported a retrospective study of 75 patients who received continuous intravenous infusion of nitroglycerin for prolonged chest pain due to myocardial ischemia (39). Subsequent to this infusion it was determined that 30 of the patients had acute myocardial infarction. Pain relief with the infusion was obtained in 40 of the 45 unstable angina patients. In 22 patients, relief occurred immediately and in 18 it occurred with titration. Prior to the infusion, 28 of these patients had received no relief from sublingual nitroglycerin. Similarly 19 of the 30 patients with infarction had relief of pain with intravenous nitroglycerin. The data suggested that intravenous nitroglycerin is useful adjunctive therapy for ischemic chest pain even when it is refractory to sublingual nitroglycerin.

Less optimistic results were presented by Squire et al. in 1982 (40). Continuous intravenous nitroglycerin for 105 ± 12 hr was given to 42 patients with unstable angina refractory to beta-blocker and standard nitrate therapy. In 19 patients angina was decreased, but intravenous nitroglycerin failed to alter the attack rate in 23 patients in spite of higher nitroglycerin doses (393 versus 227 μg/min). The nonresponders had a higher frequency of myocardial infarction (10/23 versus 0/19) and death (9/23 versus 1/19), suggesting to Squire et al. that these patients should be considered for immediate revascularization. Tachyphylaxis, known to occur with nitrates in less than 24 hr, could have been a factor in this study (41).

In 1982 Roubin et al. reported on 16 patients with refractory unstable angina treated with intravenous nitroglycerin (42). All 16 patients had significant relief of pain, with six patients obtaining complete relief. The problem of nitroglycerin adsorption to polyvinylchloride tubing had been recognized in 1978. Roubin et al. measured an 85% decrease in concentration between the glass intravenous bottle and the patient's vein. They suggested this as an explanation for larger-than-expected doses of intravenous nitroglycerin and for failure to relieve pain. The rate of adsorption varies with the type and length of the tubing, and with the rate and duration of the infusion. They thought that from a practical standpoint, the adsorption of nitroglycerin should not be a serious problem, since individual variations in metabolism required titrating the drug anyway. Profound hypotension and bradycardia seen during infusion in some patients with acute myocardial infarction had not been reported in unstable angina. Reflex tachycardia was seldom a problem, since the patients were usually already on beta-blocker therapy. By 1982 intravenous nitroglycerin infusion had become the mainstay of treatment for refractory unstable angina.

DePace et al. reported in 1982 on 20 patients with refractory unstable angina treated with intravenous nitroglycerin (mean dose 72.4 μg/min, range 15–225 μg/min) (43). Considerable reduction or abolition of ischemic episodes occurred in 85% of the patients without substantial change in blood pressure, heart rate, or pulmonary capillary wedge pressure. In some patients in whom blood pressure or wedge pressure was high, there was a substantial reduction, suggesting that intravenous nitroglycerin may relieve rest angina by different pathophysiological mechanisms. In some patients it favorably altered hemodynamic determinants of myocardial oxygen consumption, while in others its effect must have been directly on the coronary circulation.

In 1983 Kaplan et al. reported 35 patients with refractory unstable angina treated with intravenous nitroglycerin (44). Complete relief of rest angina was obtained in 25 patients, and partial relief (greater than 50% decrease in the number of episodes per day) occurred in eight more patients.

In 1979 Distante et al. studied intravenous infusion of isosorbide dinitrate in 12 patients with frequent rest angina of short duration (less than 10 min) refractory to medical management (45). The patients had variable coronary anatomy, and the angina was thought to be primarily of vasospastic origin because of ST-segment elevation, good exercise tolerance, and the results of ergonovine maleate provocative test. They were studied by double crossover design with alternating treatment and placebo periods. The number of transient ischemic episodes, as measured by ST-segment changes on continuous ECG, was reduced from 100, 104, and 91 during baseline and two placebo control periods to 13 and 20 during the two treatment periods. The ischemic attacks were abolished in both treatment periods in four patients and in one of the treatment periods in three patients and were significantly reduced in the other five patients. Intravenous nitrate therapy appeared quite effective and with negligible side effects in patients with unstable angina of vasospastic origin refractory to conventional medical therapy.

Summary

In summary, there is no randomized clinical trial of intravenous nitroglycerin therapy in patients with unstable angina. There are several small (14–45 patients) uncontrolled trials and one double crossover trial in 12 patients. All were conducted in patients with unstable angina refractory to the usual medical therapy. Most patients obtained relief of pain with intravenous nitroglycerin over a variable length of time, usually short, and sometimes dramatic. Intravenous nitroglycerin appears to be effective in obtaining relief of pain and ischemia in refractory unstable angina, but this has not been demonstrated by well-controlled trials. There are no data to evaluate its effect on prevention of myocardial infarction or death. There are, in fact, no randomized trials of nitrate therapy by any route in patients with unstable angina.

OTHER VASODILATOR THERAPY

In 1988 Lichstein et al. reported the results of a randomized, placebo-controlled, double-blind trial of prostacyclin infusion for 72 hr in 111 patients with unstable angina (46). At 30 days they found no difference in mortality, incidence of myocardial infarction, incidence of revascularization, or severity of angina between the treated and placebo groups.

CONCLUSION

Randomized clinical trials have clearly documented that aspirin decreases mortality and myocardial infarction rate by about one-half in patients with unstable angina. Ticlopidine appears to have an effect similar to that of aspirin, but it is more expensive and has more serious adverse effects. There is reasonable evidence that heparin also decreases myocardial infarction rate by at least one-half in these patients.

Randomized trials have shown the efficacy of beta-blockers and of calcium-channel blockers in relieving angina and myocardial ischemia in patients with unstable angina. An overview (metanalysis) of the randomized trials of beta-blocker therapy in patients with unstable angina suggested only a small reduction in the risk of developing myocardial infarction. An overview of the randomized trials of the calcium channel blocker nifedipine showed no effect on mortality or infarction rate. Although nitrates appear effective in relieving symptoms, randomized clinical trials of nitrate therapy have not been performed in patients with unstable angina. There is no evidence that they decrease infarction or death rate in these patients.

The evidence supports treating all patients with unstable angina with aspirin initially and continuing it indefinitely. A dosage of 160 mg daily, found effective in acute myocardial infarction in ISIS-2 (47) and for primary prevention in the Physician's Health Study (48) should be adequate. This dose is not available in the United States, so 325 mg daily, the only enteric-coated dose, is appropriate. If the enteric-coated preparation is used, the initial dose should be chewed, as in ISIS-2, to achieve blood levels quickly.

Patients with persistent or recurrent angina at rest after admission to the hospital are appropriate candidates for intravenous heparin infusion. Although Théroux's study showed no additional benefit from the combination, use of aspirin in addition to heparin should be considered, because of the conflicting results on efficacy of heparin in Wallentin's study, and because the two drugs inhibit different thrombotic mechanisms. Aspirin and anticoagulants should not be used together for chronic outpatient therapy, but the risk of bleeding is small during a few days of treatment in the hospital.

Although beta-blockers may have some effect in decreasing the incidence of myocardial infarction in patients with unstable angina, the evidence clearly supports the use of beta-blockers, calcium-channel blockers, or nitrates only for relief of anginal pain and myocardial ischemia. Usually at least two of these drugs are used. If more than one drug is used, one of them should be a beta-blocker or a calcium-channel blocker with negative chronotropic effects. Patients who have persistent anginal pain or recurrent rest pain, particularly when accompanied by ischemic ST-segment or T-wave changes, are appropriate candidates for intravenous nitroglycerin infusion.

Successful management of angina should be followed by elective risk stratification with a stress test or coronary arteriography. Failure of the above measures to provide relief of myocardial ischemic pain constitutes refractory unstable angina, a particularly high-risk problem, necessitating prompt evaluation for revascularization.

REFERENCES

1. Rahimtoola SH. Coronary bypass surgery for unstable angina. Circulation 1984; 69:842–8.
2. Gazes, PC, Mobley EM Jr, Farris HM Jr, Duncan RC, Humphries, GB. Preinfarctional (unstable) angina—A prospective study—Ten year follow-up. Circulation 1973; 48:331–7.
3. Russel RO Jr, Rackley CE, Kouchoukos NT. Unstable angina pectoris: Management based on available information. Circulation 1982; 65(Suppl II):II-72–7.
4. Fuster V, Badiman L, Cohen M, Ambrose JA, Badiman JJ, Chesebro J. Insights into the pathogenesis of acute ischemic syndromes. Circulation 1988; 77:1213–20.
5. Nixon JV, Hillert MC, Shapiro W, Smitherman TC. Submaximal exercise testing after unstable angina. Am Heart J 1980; 99:772–8.
6. Butman SM, Olson HG, Gardin JM, Piters KM, Hullett M, Butman LK. Submaximal exercise testing after stabilization of unstable angina pectoris. J Am Coll Cardiol 1984; 4:667–73.
7. Wood, P. Acute and subacute coronary insufficiency. Br Med J 1961; 1:1779–82.
8. Sixty Plus Reinfarction Study Research Group. A double-blind trial to assess long-term oral anticoagulant therapy in elderly patients after myocardial infarction. Lancet 1980; 2:989–94.
9. Telford, AM, Wilson C. Trial of heparin versus atenolol in prevention of myocardial infarction in intermediate coronary syndrome. Lancet 1981; 1:1225–8.
10. Williams DO, Kirby MG, McPherson K, Phear DN. Anticoagulant treatment in unstable angina. Br J Clin Pract 1986; 40:114–6.
11. Zwerner PL, Gore JM, Corrao JM, et al. Heparin in the treatment of unstable angina: A randomized prospective trial. Circulation 1987; 76(Suppl IV):IV-180 (Abstract).
12. Lewis HD Jr, Davis JW, Archibald DG, et al. Protective effects of aspirin against acute myocardial infarction and death in men with unstable angina: results of a Veterans Administration Cooperative Study. N Engl J Med 1983; 309:396–403.
13. Cairns JA, Gent M, Singer J, et al. Aspirin, sulfinpyrazone, or both in unstable angina: Results of a Canadian multicenter trial. N Engl J Med 1985; 313:1369–75.
14. Théroux P, Ouimet H, McCans J, et al. Aspirin, heparin, or both to treat acute unstable angina. N Engl J Med 1988; 319:1105–11.
15. Charvat J. Kuruvilla T. Comparative study of heparin and antiplatelets in treatment of preinfarction angina. Cardiologia 1989; 34:149–54.
16. Cohen M, Adams PC, Hawkins L, Bach M, Fuster V. Antithrombotic therapy in rest angina prevents death and infarction but not recurrent ischemia. Circulation 1989; 80(Suppl II):II-419 (Abstract).

17. Wallentin L, for the RISK study group. ASA 75mg and/or heparin after an episode of unstable coronary artery disease—Risk for myocardial infarction and death in a randomized placebo-controlled study. Circulation 1989; 80(Suppl II):II-419 (Abstract).

18. Wallentin L, for the RISK study group. ASA 75mg after an episode of unstable coronary artery disease—Effects on angina and need for revascularization. Circulation 1989: 80(Suppl II):II-419 (Abstract).

19. Balsano F, Rizzon P, Violi F, et al., and the Studio della Ticlopidine nell'Angina Instabile Group. Antiplatelet treatment with ticlopidine in unstable angina: A controlled multicenter clinical trial. Circulation 1990; 82:17–26.

20. Mizgala HF. Reflections on the use of propranolol in angina pectoris. Am Heart J 1970; 80:428–30.

21. Fischl SJ, Herman MV, Gorlin R. The intermediate coronary syndrome: Clinical angiographic and therapeutic aspects. N Engl J Med 1973; 288:1193–8.

22. Norris RM, Clarke ED, Sammel NL, Smith WM, Williams B. Protective effect or propranolol in threatened myocardial infarction. Lancet 1978; 2:907–9.

23. Yusuf S, Ramsdale D, Peto R, et al. Early intravenous atenolol treatment in suspected acute myocardial infarction. Lancet 1980; 2:273–6.

24. Neill WA, Wharton TP Jr, Fluri-Lundeen J, Cohen IS. Acute coronary insufficiency—Coronary occlusion after intermittent ischemic attacks. N Engl J Med 1980; 302:1157–62.

25. Smitherman TC, Hillert MC Jr, Narahara KA, et al. Evidence for transient limitations in coronary blood flow during unstable angina pectoris: Hemodynamic changes with spontaneous pain at rest versus exercise-induced ischemia following stabilization of angina. Clin Cardiol 1980; 3:309-16.

26. Chierchia S, Brunelli C, Simonetti I, Lazzari M, Maseri A. Sequence of events in angina at rest: primary reduction in coronary flow. Circulation 1980; 61:759–68.

26a. Maseri A, Severi S, DeNes M, et al. "Variant" angina: One aspect of a continuous spectrum of vasospastic myocardial ischemia. Pathogenic mechanisms, estimated incidence and clinical and coronary arteriographic findings in 138 patients. Am J Cardiol 1978; 42:1019–35.

27. Andre-Fouet X, Usdin JP, Gayet Ch, et al. Comparison of short-term efficacy of diltiazem and propranolol in unstable angina at rest—A randomized trial in 70 patients. Eur Heart J 1983; 4:691–8.

28. Théroux P, Taeymans Y, Morisette D, Bosch X, Pelletier GB, Water DD. A randomized study comparing propranolol and diltiazem in the treatment of unstable angina. J Am Coll Cardiol 1985; 5:717–22.

29. Parodi O, Simonetti I, Michelassi C, et al. Comparison of verapamil and propranolol therapy for angina pectoris at rest: A randomized, multiple-crossover, controlled trial in the coronary care unit. Am J Cardiol 1986; 57:899–906.

30. Gerstenblith G, Ouyang P, Achuff SC, et al. Nifedipine in unstable angina: A double-blind, randomized trial. N Engl J Med 1982; 306:885–9.

31. Muller JE, Turi ZG, Pearle DL, et al. Nifedipine and conventional therapy for unstable angina pectoris: A randomized, double-blind comparison. Circulation 1984; 69:729–39.

32. Gottlieb SO, Weisfeldt ML, Ouyang P, et al. Effect of the addition of propranolol

to therapy with nifedipine for unstable angina pectoris: A randomized, double-blind, placebo-controlled trial. Circulation 1986; 73:331–7.

33. The Holland Interuniversity Nifedipine/Metoprolol Trial (HINT) Research Group. Early treatment of unstable angina in the coronary care unit: A randomized, double-blind, placebo controlled comparison of recurrent ischaemia in patients treated with nifedipine or metoprolol or both. Br Heart J 1986; 56:400–13.

34. Yusuf S. The use of beta-blockers in the acute phase of myocardial infarction. In: Califf RM, Wagner GS, eds. Acute coronary care. Boston: Martinus Nijhoff, 1986.

35. Held PH, Yusuf S, Furberg CD. Calcium channel blockers in acute myocardial infarction and unstable angina: An overview. Br Med J 1989; 299:1187–92.

36. Dauwe F, Affaki G, Waters DD, Théroux P, Mizgala HF. Intravenous nitroglycerin in refractory unstable angina. Am J Cardiol 1979: 43:416 (Abstract).

37. Page A, Huret JF, Roudaut R, et al. La trinitrine intraveineuse dans le traitement du syndrome de menace: Résultats préliminaires [Intravenous trinitroglycerin in the treatment of pre-infarction syndrome: Preliminary results]. Nouv Presse Med 1979; 8:266–70.

38. Brodsky SJ, Halperin JL, Klein MD, Ryan TJ. Intravenous nitroglycerin infusion in unstable angina. Clin Res 1980; 28:608A (Abstract).

39. Mikolich JR, Nicoloff NB, Robinson PH, Logue RB. Relief of refractory angina with continuous intravenous infusion of nitroglycerin. Chest: 1980; 77:375–9.

40. Squire A, Cantor R, Packer M. Limitations of continuous intravenous nitroglycerin prophylaxis in patients with refractory angina at rest. Circulation 1982; 66(Suppl II):II-120 (Abstract).

41. Parker JO. Intermittent transdermal nitroglycerin therapy in the treatment of chronic stable angina. Editorial comment. J Am Coll Cardiol 198; 13:794–5.

42. Roubin GS, Harris PJ, Eckhardt I, Hensley W, Kelly DT. Intravenous nitroglycerine in refractory unstable angina pectoris. Aust NZ J Med 1982; 12:598–602.

43. DePace NL, Herling IM, Kotler MN, Hakki A-H, Spielman SR, Segal BL. Intravenous nitroglycerin for rest angina: Potential pathophysiologic mechanisms of action. Arch Intern Med 1982; 142:1806–9.

44. Kaplan K, Davison R, Parker M, Przybylek J, Teagarden JR, Lesch M. Intravenous nitroglycerin for the treatment of angina at rest unresponsive to standard nitrate therapy. Am J Cardiol 1983; 51:694–8.

45. Distante A, Maseri A, Severi S, Biagini A, Chierchia S. Management of vasospastic angina at rest with continuous infusion of isosorbide dinitrate: A double crossover study in a coronary care unit. Am J Cardiol 1979; 44:533–9.

46. Lichstein E, Mendizabel R, Théroux P, et al. Epoprostenol (prostacyclin) in unstable angina. J Clin Pharmacol 1988; 28:300–5.

47. ISIS-2 (Second International Study of Infarct Survival) Collaborative Group. Randomized trial of intravenous streptokinase, oral aspirin, both or neither among 17,187 cases of suspected acute myocardial infarction: ISIS-2. Lancet 1988; 2: 349–60.

48. Steering Committee of the Physicians' Health Study Research Group. Final report on the aspirin component of the ongoing Physicians' Health Study, N Engl J Med 1989; 321:129–35.

7

What Constitutes Medically Refractory?

Douglass Andrew Morrison

Veterans Affairs Medical Center and
University of Colorado Health Sciences Center
Denver, Colorado

WHY ATTEMPT TO DEFINE MEDICALLY REFRACTORY?

Most patients with unstable angina can be medically stabilized (1–10). In patients who are medically stabilized, there are no data to support the contention that acute (emergent) coronary artery bypass graft surgery (CABG) or percutaneous transluminal coronary angioplasty (PTCA) prolongs life or prevents infarction. Since CABG and PTCA are more dangerous in unstable patients, it makes sense to try to stabilize these patients (66,84,88).

Although there is no debate that patients with medically refractory symptoms should undergo coronary angiography so as to consider either CABG or PTCA, there is no uniformly accepted definition of "medically refractory." Defining medically refractory would allow us to identify a subset for whom either CABG or PTCA would be appropriate. Given the high risk for either PTCA or CABG of medically refractory patients, a trial of PTCA versus CABG in such patients could likely have hard end-points (death or infarction). All currently ongoing trials of PTCA versus CABG are soft-end-point trials (relief of angina, treadmill test or thallium test results) (11; Table 1).

Table 1 Prospective Trials of Angioplasty Versus Surgery

Trial	Location	Entry criteria	Unstable angina included	Follow-up	End-points
BARI	14 US centers	Multivessel	Yes, not medically refractory	1, 3, 5 years	5-year mortality and MI ETT Relief of angina
CABRI	European centers	Revascularization indicated		6 months 2 years	Relief of angina
DUAST	10 Dutch centers	Multivessel suitable for both	Yes	6 months 1, 2, 3, 5 years	Relief of angina Exercise capacity
EAST	Emory University	Revascularization indicated, multivessel	Yes	1, 3 years	Angiography Thallium ETT
GABI	German centers	Class III	No	3, 6, 12 months	Angina, ETT, MI, death
RITA	14 British Cardiac Society centers	Revascularization indicated, single vessel indicated	Yes	1, 6 months 1, 2, 3, 4, 5 years	Symptomatic relief Complications Prognosis

BARI = Bypass Angioplasty Revascularization Investigation; CABRI = Coronary Angioplasty Bypass Revascularization Investigation; DUAST = Dutch Angioplasty Surgery Trial; EAST = Emory University Surgery Trial; RITA = Randomized Interventional Treatment of Angina.

MEDICALLY REFRACTORY: WHICH MEDICINES?

Table 2 is a list of studies of patients with unstable angina which included a stated or implied definition of medically refractory. Most of these studies used some combination of therapeutic agents as their definition of medically refractory. None required reaching arbitrary target dosages. Most simply mentioned drug categories. For example, nearly all included only patients who were taking some beta-blocker. *Far fewer specified* intravenous nitroglycerin, heparin, or antiplatelet agents such as aspirin. Although there are reports of the use of thrombolytic agents, no study to date has included "failure to stabilize in response to thrombolytic therapy" as part of the definition of "medically refractory."

Table 2 Medically Refractory Unstable Angina

First author	Ref	β-blocker	Ca²⁺ blocker	Nitrates	i.v. NTG	Heparin	ASA	Target HR	Target BP	ECG changes
Lewis	12	−	−	+	−	−	±	−	−	−
Luchi, S	13, 14	−	−	+	−	−	−	−	−	+
Russell	16–19	+	−	+	−	±	−	+	+	+
Vakil	20	−	−	−	−	±	−	−	−	+
Krauss	21	−	−	−	−	±	−	−	−	−
Gazes	22	+	−	+	−	±	−	−	−	+
Conti	23	+	−	+	−	+	−	−	−	+
Bertolasi	24	+	−	+	−	±	−	−	−	+
Duncan	25	+	−	+	−	−	−	−	−	+
Heng	26	+	−	+	−	−	−	−	−	−
Day	27	±	−	+	−	−	−	−	−	−
Mulcahy	28	±	−	+	−	±	−	−	−	−
Ouyang	29	+	+	+	−	±	±	−	−	+
Selden	30	+	−	+	−	−	−	?	?	+
Cairns	31	±	−	+	−	−	±	−	−	+
Theroux	32	±	±	+	+	+	+	−	−	−
Mikolich	33	−	−	+	+	−	−	−	+	−
Kaplan	34	+	−	+	+	−	−	−	−	+
DePace	35	−	−	+	+	−	−	+	+	+
Roubin	36	+	+	+	+	−	−	−	−	−
Squire	37	+	−	+	+	−	−	−	−	−
Dauwe	38	+	−	+	+	−	−	−	−	−
Brodsky	39	+	−	+	+	−	−	−	−	−
Curfman	40	+	−	−	+	−	−	+	+	−
Parodi	41	−	+	+	−	−	−	−	−	+
Mehta	42	−	+	+	−	−	−	−	−	+

Table 2 Medically Refractory Unstable Angina (*Continued*)

First author	Ref	β-blocker	Ca^{2+} blocker	Nitrates	i.v. NTG	Heparin	ASA	Target HR	Target BP	ECG changes
HINT	43	±	±	±		±	±	−	−	−
Theroux	44	+	+	+		−	−	−	−	+
Gottlieb	45	+	+	+	+	−	−	−	−	+
Muller	46	+	+	+	+	−	−	−	−	+
Gerstenblith	47	+	+	+		−	±	−	−	+
Norris	48	+	±	±		±	−	−	−	−
Telford	49	+	−	+		+	+	−	−	+
Shapiro	50	±	±	±	±	−	−	−	−	+
Rentrop	51	−	+	+	±	+	+	−	−	−
Vetrovec	52	+	−	+		+	−	−	−	+
deZwaan	53	−	−	−	+	+	−	−	−	+
Douglas	54	+	−	+		−	−	?	?	−
Ambrose	55	±	±	+	+	+	−	−	−	+
Pugh	56	+	−	+		−	−	?	?	−
Brown	57	+	−	+		−	−	+	+	+
Gotoh	58	+	+	+	+	+	Coumadin	−	−	+
Hultgren	59	+	−	+		−	−	?	?	+
Jones	60	+	−	+	+	−	−	−	−	+
Hultgren	61	+	−	+		−	−	−	−	−
Edwards	62	+	+	+	+	+	−	−	?	?
Weintraub	63	+	−	+		−	−	+	+	+
Bardet	64	+	−	+		+	−	−	−	+
Singh	65	+	+	+		−	−	−	−	±
Jones EL	66	+	−	+	+	−	−	−	−	±
Levine	67	+	−	+	+	−	−	+	+	−
Brundage	68	+	−	+		−	−	+	+	±

108

Author	69–96	1	2	3	4	5	6	7	8
Jones RN	69	+	+	+	+	−	−	−	−
Langou	70	+	+	+	−	−	−	?	?
Olinger	71	−	−	+	−	+	−	?	?
Ahmed	72	+	+	+	+	+	−	−	−
Rankin	73	+	+	+	−	−	−	?	?
Cohn	74	+	+	+	+	+	−	−	−
Hatcher	75	+	+	+	+	?	−	?	−
Firth	76	?	?	?	?	?	−	−	−
Wohlgelertner	77	±	±		+	+	?	−	−
Perry	78	±	+		+	±	?	−	−
Plokker	79	−	±		+	−	+	−	−
Holt	80	+	+	−	−	+	±	−	±
Steffenino	81	+	+	+	−	+	+	−	±
Quigley	82	+	+	+	+	+	−	−	±
Williams	83	−	−	+	+	+	−	−	−
Meyer	84	+	+	+	+	+	+	−	−
deFeyter	85	+	+	+	±	+	−	−	+
Timmis	86	−	+	+	+	−	−	−	+
Myler	87	+	+	+	+	+	+	−	±
Meyer	88	+	+	+	±	−	−	−	+
deFeyter	89	+	+		+	+	−	−	+
Sharma	90	−	+	+	+	+	+	−	−
deFeyter	91	+	+	+	+	+	−	+	+
Hopkins	92	−	+	+	−	+	+	−	−
Gottlieb	93	−	+	−	−	−	+	−	+
Leeman	94	72%	96%	96%		54%	65%	−	±
Grover	95	±	±	±	±	+		−	±
Nicklas	96	+	+	+	±	+	+	−	+

MEDICALLY REFRACTORY: PHYSIOLOGICAL TARGET END-POINTS?

Although no studies use arbitrary minimal dosages to *define* medically refractory, some authors have titrated medicines toward physiological target heart rates and/or blood pressures. In the citations listed in Table 2, eight specifically mentioned target heart rates and seven mentioned target blood pressures.

Plotnick tells us in Chapter 9 of this book that the National Cooperative Study of unstable angina used the beta-blocker propanolol with physiological targets of a systolic blood pressure < 120 mmHg and a heart rate < 60 beats/min through the day. In contrast, although 62.1% of the patients in the VA Cooperative Study comparing medical and surgical therapy for unstable angina were taking propanolol, Scott et al. reported no such use of target heart rates and blood pressures (Chapter 8 and Refs. 13–15).

Although there is limited support for this approach in the literature, this has been pervasive in our institution (Denver VA Medical Center). Patients are not considered medically refractory if they continue to have a blood pressure at rest > 140 mmHg or a resting heart rate > 60–70 beats/min.

PROBLEM WITH THE PHYSIOLOGICAL END-POINT OF MEDICAL THERAPY

An impressive array of data has been gathered to support the hypothesis that unstable angina accrues primarily from a limitation of myocardial oxygen supply (3–7). This limitation occurs against the background of a maximally locally vasodilated coronary tree. It accrues most commonly from a flow-limiting stenosis that has a translesional pressure gradient. Accordingly, reducing the driving pressure of the bloodstream below a critical point (depending on the severity of the gradient) is fraught with hazard. If one pharmacologically reduces the pressure head of blood in all patients with unstable angina prior to catheterization and PTCA and CABG, the risks of all three of these procedures may well be increased.

MEDICALLY REFRACTORY: DURATION OF THERAPY?

In an attempt to give medical therapy a chance to work, some studies have insisted on a finite period, for example 24–48 hr, in the intensive care unit at bed rest, before angina is declared medically refractory. Like the definition of infarction pain versus postinfarction angina, this is (a) arbitrary and (b) not always practical.

Table 3   Therapeutic Algorithm

Rest Angina

1. Is it myocardial ischemic?
   ECG with pain
   Reversible thallium
   Reversible wall motion: echo TE or 2D
   MUGA or contrast

2. Anginal equivalent

3. Silent ischemia

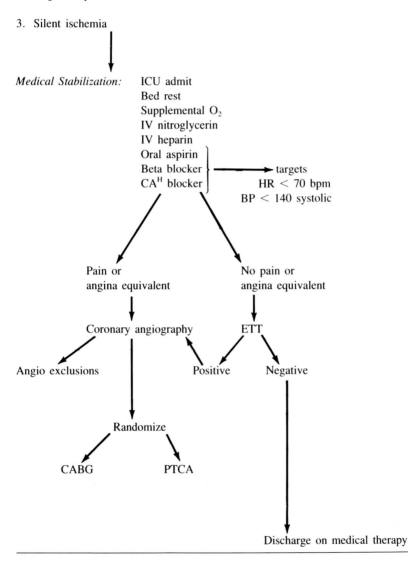

Medical Stabilization: ICU admit
Bed rest
Supplemental O_2
IV nitroglycerin
IV heparin
Oral aspirin
Beta blocker
CA^H blocker

$\rightarrow$ targets
HR < 70 bpm
BP < 140 systolic

Pain or
angina equivalent

No pain or
angina equivalent

Coronary angiography   ETT

Angio exclusions   Positive   Negative

Randomize

CABG   PTCA

Discharge on medical therapy

MEDICALLY REFRACTORY: OBJECTIVE EVIDENCE OF ISCHEMIA

Insisting on electrocardiographic (ECG) changes with pain will clearly eliminate most nonischemic etiologies. Unfortunately, because the ECG is imperfect, it will also eliminate some legitimate ischemia, especially from the circumflex or right coronary artery distributions. Most of the cited studies include this requirement.

MEDICALLY REFRACTORY: PROPOSED DEFINITION (TABLE 3)

We propose that chest discomfort or angina equivalent (dyspnea, fullness, etc., consistent with the patient's prior episodes) that is accompanied by reversible ECG changes, echo or MUGA wall motion, or thallium perfusion changes is "medically refractory" if:

1. The patient is on some dose of intravenous nitroglycerin preferably $\geq$ 50 mg/min.
2. The patient is on aspirin $\geq$ 80 mg/day, preferably 325 mg *po qd*.
3. The patient is on heparin such that PTT $\geq$ 60 sec.
4. The patient is on some combination of beta-blocker and/or calcium blocker so that resting heart rate is < 70 beats/min, resting systolic blood pressure is < 150 mmHg.

Criterion 4 may be waived if rest heart rate $\leq$ 60 beats/min *or* resting systolic blood pressure is <120 mmHg.

REFERENCES

1. Bernard R, Corday E, Eliasch H, et al. Report of the Joint International Society and Federation of Cardiology/World Health Organization Task Force on Standardization of Clinical Nomenclature: Nomenclature and criteria for diagnosis of ischemic heart disease. Circulation 1979; 59:607–8.
2. Braunwald E. Unstable angina. A classification. Circulation 1989; 80:410–4.
3. Conti CR, Hill, JA, Mayfield WR. Unstable angina pectoris: Pathogenesis and Management. Curr Probl Cardiol 1989; 14:553–623.
4. Farhi JI, Cohen M, Fuster V. Editorial: The broad spectrum of unstable angina pectoris and its implications for future controlled trials. Am J Cardiol 1986; 58:547–50.
5. Munger TM, Oh JK. Unstable angina. Mayo Clin Proc 1990; 65:384–406.
6. Fowler NO. Editorial: "Preinfarctional" angina: A need for an objective definition and for a controlled clinical trial of its management. Circulation 1971; 44:755–8.
7. Smitherman TC. Unstable angina pectoris: The first half century: Natural history, pathophysiology, treatment. Am J Med Sci 1986; 292:395–406.

8. Scanlon PJ. The intermediate coronary syndrome. Prog Cardiovasc Dis 1981; 23:351–64.

9. Patterson DLH. Unstable angina. Postgrad Med J 1988; 64:196–200.

10. Hecht HS, Rahimtoola SH. Unstable angina: A perspective. Chest 1982; 82:466–72.

11. Gersh BJ, Robertson T. The efficacy of percutaneous transluminal coronary angioplasty (PTCA) in coronary artery disease—Why we need randomized trials. In Topol EJ, Ed. *Textbook of interventional cardiology.* Chapter 12. 1990 Philadelphia: Saunders, pp. 240–53.

12. Lewis HD Jr, Davis JW, Archibald DG, Steinke WE, Smitherman TC, Doherty JE III, Schnaper HW, LeWinter MM, Linares E, Pouget JM, Sabharawal SC, Chesler E, DeMots H. Protective effects of aspirin against acute myocardial infarction and death in men with unstable angina. N Engl J Med 1983; 309:396–403.

13. Luchi RJ, Scott SM, Deupree RH, and the Principal Investigators and Their Associates of Veterans Administration Cooperative Study No. 28. Comparison of medical and surgical treatment for unstable angina pectoris. N Engl J Med 1987; 316:977–84.

14. Scott SM, Luchi RJ, Deupree RH, and the Veterans Administration Unstable Angina Cooperative Study Group. Veterans Administration Cooperative Study for Treatment of Patients with Unstable Angina. Circulation 1988; 78 (Suppl I):I-113–I-121.

15. Parisi AF, Khuri S, Deupree RH, Sharma GVRK, Scott SM, Luchi RJ. Medical compared with surgical management of unstable angina: 5 year mortality and morbidity in the Veterans Administration study. Circulation 1989; 80:1176–89.

16. Russell RO, Moraski RE, Kouchoukos N, et al. Unstable angina pectoris: National Cooperative Study Group to Compare Medical and Surgical Therapy. I. Report of protocol and patient population. Am J Cardiol 1976 37:896–902.

17. Russell RO, Moraski RE, Kouchoukos N, et al. Unstable angina pectoris: National Cooperative Study Group to Compare Surgical and Medical Therapy. II. In-hospital experience and initial follow-up results in patients with one, two, and three vessel disease. Am J Cardiol 1978; 42:839–48.

18. Russell RO, Moraski RE, Kouchoukos N, et al. Unstable angina pectoris: National Cooperative Study Group to Compare Surgical and Medical Therapy. III. Results in patients with S-T segment elevation during pain. Am J Cardiol 1980; 45:819–24.

19. Russell RO, Moraski RE, Kouchoukos N, et al. Unstable angina pectoris: National Cooperative Study Group to Compare Medical and Surgical Therapy. IV. Results in patients with left anterior descending artery disease. Am J Cardiol 1981; 48:517–24.

20. Vakil RJ. Preinfarction syndrome—Management and follow-up. Am J Cardiol 1964; 14:55–63.

21. Krauss KR, Hutter AM, DeSanctis RW. Acute coronary insufficiency. Arch Intern Med 1972; 129:808–13.

22. Gazes PC, Mobley EM Jr, Faris HM Jr, Duncan RC, Humphries GB. Preinfarctional (unstable) angina—A prospective study—Ten year follow up. Circulation 1973; 48:331–7.

23. Conti CR, Brawley RK, Griffith LSC, Pitt B, Humphries JO, Gott VL, Ross RS.

Unstable angina pectoris: Morbidity and mortality in 57 consecutive patients evaluated angiographically. Am J Cardiol 1973; 32:745–50.

24. Bertolasi CA, Tronge JE, Riccitelli MA, Villamayor RM, Zuffardi E. Natural history of unstable angina with medical or surgical therapy. Chest 1976; 70: 596–605.

25. Duncan B, Fulton M, Morrison SL, Lutz W, Donald KW, Kerr F, Kirby BJ, Julian DG, Oliver MF. Prognosis of new and worsening angina pectoris. Br Med J 1976; 1:981–5.

26. Heng MK, Norris RM, Singh BN, Partridge JB. Prognosis in unstable angina. Br Heart J 1976; 38:921–5.

27. Day LJ, Thibault GE, Sowton E. Acutre coronary insufficiency Review of 46 patients. Br Heart J 1977; 39:363–70.

28. Mulcahy R, Daly L, Graham I, Hickey N, O'Donoghue S, Owens A, Ruane P, Tobin G. Unstable angina: Natural history and determinants of prognosis. Am J Cardiol 1981; 48:525–8.

29. Ouyang P, Brinker JA, Mellits ED, Weisfeldt ML, Gerstenblith G. Variables predictive of successful medical therapy in patients with unstable angina. Selection by multivariate analysis from clinical, electrocardiographic and angiographic evaluations. Circulation 1984; 70:367–76.

30. Selden R, Neill WA, Ritzman LW, Okies JE, Anderson RP. Medical versus surgical therapy for acute coronary insufficiency. N Engl J Med 1975; 293: 1329–33.

31. Cairns JA, et al. Aspirin, sulfinpyrazone, or both in unstable angina. N Engl J Med 1985; 313:1369–75.

32. Theroux P, et al. Aspirin, heparin, or both to treat acute unstable angina. N Engl J Med 1988; 319:1105–11.

33. Mikolich JR, Nicoloff NB, Robinson PH, Logue RB. Relief of refractory angina with continuous intravenous infusion of nitroglycerin. Chest 1980; 77:375–9.

34. Kaplan K, Davison R, Parker M, Przybylek J, Teagarden JR, Lesch M. Intravenous nitroglycerine for the treatment of angina at rest unresponsive to standard nitrate therapy. Am J Cardiol 1983; 51:694–8.

35. DePace NL, Herling IM, Kotler MN, Hakki AH, Spielman SR, Segal BL. Intravenous nitroglycerin for rest angina. Arch Intern Med 1982; 142:1806–9.

36. Roubin GS, Harris PJ, Eckhardt I, Hensley W, Kelly DT. Intravenous nitroglycerin in refractory unstable angina pectoris. Aust NZ J Med 1982; 12:598–602.

37. Squire A, Cantor R, Packer M. Abstract: Limitations of continuous intravenous nitroglycerin prophylaxis in patients with refractory angina at rest. Circulation 1982; 66(Suppl II):120.

38. Dauwe F, et al. Abstract: Intravenous nitrogylercin—Refractory unstable angina. Am J Cardiol 1979; 43:416.

39. Brodsky SJ, et al. Abstract: Intravenous nitroglycerin-fusion in unstable angina. Clin Res 1980; 28:608A.

40. Curfman GD, Heinsimer JA, Lozner EC, Fung HL. Intravenous nitroglycerin in the treatment of spontaneous angina pectoris: A prospective randomized trial. Circulation 1983; 67:276–82.

41. Parodi O, Maseri A, Simonetti I. Management of unstable angina at rest by verapamil. Br Heart J 1979; 41:167–74.
42. Mehta J, Pepine CJ, Day M, Guerrero JR, Conti CR. Short term efficacy of oral verapamil in rest angina. Am J Med 1981; 71:977–82.
43. Holland Interuniversity Nifedipine-Metoprolol Trial Research Group: Early treatment of unstable angina in the coronary care unit: A randomized double-blind placebo controlled comparison of recurrent ischemia in patients treated with nifedipine and metoprolol or both. Br Heart J 1986; 56:400–13.
44. Theroux P, Taeymans Y, Morrissette D, et al. A randomized study comparing propanolol and diltiazem in the treatment of unstable angina. J Am Coll Cardiol 1985; 5:717–22.
45. Gottlieb SO, Weisfeldt ML, Ouyang P, et al. The effect of the addition of propanolol to therapy with nifedipine for unstable angina pectoris: A randomized double-blind placebo controlled trial. Circulation 1986; 73:331–7.
46. Muller JE, Turi ZG, Pearl ED, et al. Nifedipine in conventional therapy for unstable angina pectoris: A randomized double-blind comparison. Circulation 1984; 69:728–39.
47. Gerstenblith G, Ouyang P, Achuff SC, et al. Nifedipine in unstable angina. N Engl J Med 1982; 306:885–9.
48. Norris RM, Sammel NL, Clark ED, Smith WN, Williams B. Protective effect of propanolol on threatened myocardial infarction. Lancet 1978; 2:907–9.
49. Telford AM, Wilson C: Trial of heparin vs. atenolol in prevention of myocardial infarction in intermediate coronary syndrome. Lancet 1981; 2:1225–8.
50. Shapiro EP, Brinker JA, Gottlieb SO, Guzman PA, Bulkley BH. Intracoronary thrombolysis 3–13 days after acute myocardial infarction for postinfarction angina pectoris. Am J Cardiol 1985; 55:1453–8.
51. Rentrop P, Blanke H, Karsch KR, et al. Selective intracoronary thrombolysis in acute myocardial infarction and unstable angina pectoris. Circulation 1981; 63:307–17.
52. Vetrovec GW, Leinbach RC, Gold HK, Cowley MJ. Intracoronary thrombolysis in syndromes of unstable ischemia: Angiographic and clinical results. Am Heart J 1982; 104:946–52.
53. Douglas BC, Adelman AG, Huckell VF, et al. Unstable angina: A clinical, angiographic and surgical profile. Cardiovasc Med 1978; 167–76.
54. Ambrose JA, Hjemdahl-Monsen CE, Borrico S, et al. Quantitative and qualitative effects of intracoronary streptokinase in unstable angina and non Q-wave infarction. J Am Coll Cardiol 1987; 9:1156–65.
55. deZwaan C, Bar FW, Janssen JHA, et al. Effects of thrombolytic therapy in unstable angina: Clinical and angiographic results. J Am Coll Cardiol 1988; 12:301–9.
56. Pugh B, Platt MR, Mills LJ, et al. Unstable angina pectoris: A randomized study of patients treated medically and surgically. Am J Cardiol 1978; 41:1291–8.
57. Brown CA, Hutter AM Jr, DeSanctis RW, et al. Prospective study of medical and urgent surgical therapy in randomizable patients with unstable angina pectoris: Results of in-hospital and chronic mortality and morbidity. Am Heart J 1981; 102:959–64.

58. Gotoh K, Minamino T, Katoh O, et al. The role of intracoronary thrombus in unstable angina: Angiographic assessment of thrombolytic therapy during ongoing anginal attacks. Circulation 1988; 77:526–34.

59. Hultgren HN, Pfeiffer JF, Angell WW, Lipton MJ, Bilisoly S. Unstable angina: Comparison of medical and surgical management. Am J Cardiol 1977; 39:734–40.

60. Jones EL, Waites TF, Craver JM, et al. Unstable angina pectoris: Comparison with the National Cooperative Study. Ann Thorac Surg 1982; 34:427–34.

61. Hultgren HN, Sheitigar UR, Miller DC. Medical versus surgical treatment of unstable angina. Am J Cardiol 1982; 50:663–70.

62. Edwards FH, Bellamy R, Burge JR, et al. True emergency coronary artery bypass surgery. Ann Thorac Surg 1990; 49:603–11.

63. Weintraub Rm, Avoesty JM, Paulin S, et al. Medically refractory unstable angina pectoris. I. Long term follow-up of patients undergoing intraaortic balloon counterpulsation and operation. Am J Cardiol 1979; 43:877–82.

64. Bardet J, Rigaud M, Kahn JC, et al. Treatment of post myocardial infarction angina by intraaortic balloon pumping and emergency revascularization. J Thorac Cardiovasc Surg 1977; 74:299–305.

65. Singh AK, Rivera R, Cooper GN Jr, Karlson KE. Early myocardial revascularization for post infarction angina: Results and long term follow-up. J Am Coll Cardiol 1985; 6:1121–5.

66. Jones EL, Waites TF, Craver JM, et al. Coronary bypass for relief of persistent pain following acute myocardial infarction. Am Thorac Surg 1981; 32:33–43.

67. Levine FH, Gold HF, Leinbach RC, Daggett Wm, Austen G, Buckly MJ. Safe early revascularization for continuing ischemia after acute myocardial infarction. Circulation 1979; 60(Suppl I):I-5–I-8.

68. Brundage BH, Ullyot DJ, Winoker S, Chaterjie K, Ports TA, Turkey K. The role of aortic balloon pumping in postinfarction angina. Circulation 1980; 62(Suppl I): I-119–I-123.

69. Jones RN, Pifarre R, Sullivan HJ, et al. Early myocardial revascularization for post infarction angina. Ann Thorac Surg 1987; 44:159–63.

70. Langou RA, Geha AS, Hammond GL, Cohen LS. Surgical approach for patients with unstable angina pectoris: Role of the response to initial medical therapy and intraaortic balloon pumping and perioperative complications after aortocoronary bypass grafting. Am J Cardiol 1978; 42:629–32.

71. Olinger GN, Bonchek LI, Keelan MH, et al. Unstable angina: The case for operation. Am J Cardiol 1978; 42:634–40.

72. Ahmed M, Thompson R, Searbra-Gomes R, et al. Unstable angina: A clinical arteriographic correlation and long term results of early myocardial revascularization. J Thorac Cardiovasc Surg 1980; 79:609–16.

73. Rankin JS, Newton JR, Jr., Califf RM, et al. Clinical characteristics and current management of medically refractory unstable angina. Ann Surg 1984; 200:457–64.

74. Cohn LH, Alpert J, Koster JK, Mee RBB, Collins JJ Jr. Changing indications for the surgical treatment of unstable angina. Arch Surg 1978; 113:1312–6.

75. Hatcher CR Jr, King SB III, Kaplan A. Surgical management of unstable angina. World J Surg 1978; 2:689–700.

76. Firth BG, Hillis LD, Willerson JT. Unstable angina pectoris: Medical versus surgical treatment. Herz 1980; 5:16–24.

77. Wohlgelertner D, Cleman M, Highman H, et al. Percutaneous transluminal angioplasty of the "culprit lesion" for management of unstable angina pectoris in patients with multivessel coronary disease. Am J Cardiol 1986; 58:460.

78. Perry RA, Seth A, Hunt A, Shier MF. Coronary angioplasty in unstable angina and stable angina: A comparison of success and complications. Br Heart J 1988; 60: 367–72.

79. Plokker HWT, Ernst SMPG, Bal ET, et al. Percutaneous transluminal coronary angioplasty in patients with unstable angina pectoris refractory to medical therapy. Cathet Cardiovasc Diag 1988; 14:15–8.

80. Holt GW, Sugrue DD, Bresnahan JF, et al. Results of percutaneous transluminal coronary angioplasty for unstable angina pectoris in patients 70 years of age and older. Am J Cardiol 1988; 61:994–7.

81. Steffino G, Meier B, Finci L, Rutishauser W. Follow up results of treatment of unstable angina by coronary angioplasty. Br Heart J 1987; 57:416–9.

82. Quigley PJ, Erwin J, Maurer BJ, Walsh MJ, Geary GF. Percutaneous transluminal coronary angioplasty in unstable angina. Br Heart J 1986; 55:227–30.

83. Williams DO, Riley RS, Singh AK, Gewirth H, Most AS. Evaluation of the role of coronary angioplasty in patients with unstable angina pectoris. Am Heart J 1981; 102:1–9.

84. Meyer J, Schmitz H, Erbel R, et al. Treatment of unstable angina pectoris with percutaneous transluminal coronary angioplasty (PTCA). Cathet Cardiovasc Diag 1981; 7:361–71.

85. deFeyter PJ, Serruys PW, Arnold A, et al. Coronary angioplasty of the unstable angina related vessel in patients with multi-vessel disease. Eur Heart J 1986; 7: 460–7.

86. Timmis AD, Griffin B, Crick JCP, Sowton E. Early percutaneous transluminal coronary angioplasty in the management of unstable angina. Int J Cardiol 1987; 14:25–31.

87. Myler RF, Shaw RE, Stertzer SH, et al. Unstable angina and coronary angioplasty. Circulation 1990; 82 (Suppl II):II-88–II-95.

88. Meyer J, Schmitz HJ, Kiesslich T, et al. Percutaneous transluminal coronary angioplasty in patients with stable and unstable angina pectoris: Analysis of early and late results. Am Heart J 1983; 106:973–80.

89. deFeyter PJ, Serruys PW, Suryapranata H, Beatt K, Van den Brand M. Coronary angioplasty early after diagnosis of unstable angina. Am Heart J 1987; 114:48–54.

90. Sharma B, Wyeth RP, Kolath GS, Gimenez HJ, Franciosa JA. Percutaneous transluminal coronary angioplasty of one vessel for refractory unstable angina pectoris: Efficacy and single end multi-vessel disease. Br Heart J 1988; 59:280–6.

91. deFeyter PH, Serruys PW, Soward A, et al. Coronary angioplasty for early post-infarction/unstable angina. Circulation 1986; 74:1365–70.

92. Hopkins J, Savage M, Zalewski A, et al. Recurrent ischemia in the zone of prior myocardial infarction: Results of coronary angioplasty of the infarct related artery. Am Heart J 1988; 115:14–19.

93. Gottlieb SO, Walford GD, Ouyang P, et al. Initial and late results of coronary angioplasty for early postinfarction-unstable angina. Cathet Cardiovasc Diag 1987; 13:93–9.

94. Leeman DE, McCabe CH, Faxon DP, et al. Use of percutaneous transluminal

coronary angioplasty and bypass surgery despite improved medical therapy for unstable angina pectoris. Am J Cardiol 1988; 61:36G–44G.

95. Grover FL, Hammermeister KE, Burchfiel C, and the cardiac surgeons of the Department of Veterans Affairs. Initial report of the Veterans Administration Preoperative Risk Assessment for Cardiac Surgery. Ann Thorac Surg 1990; 50:12–28.

96. Nicklas JM, Topol EJ, Kander N, et al. Randomized, double-blind, placebo-controlled trial of tissue plasminogen activator in unstable angina. J Am Coll Cardiol 1989; 13:434–41.

IV
SURGICAL THERAPY
FOR UNSTABLE ANGINA

8

Veterans Administration Cooperative Study Comparing Medical and Surgical Therapy for Unstable Angina

Stewart M. Scott

Duke University Medical Center and
Veterans Affairs Medical Center
Asheville, North Carolina

Robert J. Luchi

Baylor College of Medicine and
Veterans Affairs Medical Center
Houston, Texas

Robert H. Deupree

Veterans Affairs Medical Center
West Haven, Connecticut

INTRODUCTION

In 1970 the most common cause of death among American men was myocardial infarction. Angina almost always preceded infarction, sometimes by as little as 12 hr or as long as 4 weeks. The treatment of preinfarction angina consisted of bed rest, analgesics, long-acting nitrates, anticoagulants, and propranolol. Calcium-channel-blocking agents were not available and antiplatelet drugs were infrequently used. Coronary artery bypass surgery using an autologous saphenous vein was a new operation for patients with chronic stable angina, although some physicians considered bypass surgery to be the treatment of choice for patients with preinfarction angina. The definition of preinfarction angina was not precise, for, in fact, not all patients progressed to myocardial infarction. The term ''unstable angina'' was proposed by Fowler as best describing the various subsets of angina included in this syndrome (1). The mortality associated with the medical treatment of unstable angina was high, and the risks of coronary arteriography and surgery in these patients were unknown. In 1972, the National Institutes of Health (NIH) initiated a prospective, randomized study to compare coronary artery bypass surgery with conventional medical therapy for patients with unstable angina. The study failed to demonstrate significant differences in either mortality or nonfatal myocardial infarction between the group of patients treated medically and the group treated with surgery (2).

Because surgical technique was rapidly improving and the medical care for patients with unstable angina was expanding to include new drugs and new devices, a Veterans Administration (VA) study was designed to compare medicine and surgery used to treat patients with unstable angina (3). Unlike the NIH study, patients were stratified prospectively by clinical presentation and by left ventricular function before being randomly assigned to treatment. Patients with significant narrowing of the left main coronary artery were excluded from both the NIH study and the VA study. Approximately 10% of patients with unstable angina have significant left main coronary artery disease, and in 1976 the VA study of surgery for chronic stable angina confirmed that patients with left main coronary artery disease had significantly better survival when randomized to coronary artery bypass surgery rather than to medicine (4).

STUDY DESIGN

Between June 1, 1975, and June 30, 1982, 468 men with unstable angina pectoris were entered into a study designed to compare the results of medical and surgical treatment (Fig. 1). This study was a cooperative effort of investigators from 12 university-affiliated VA hospitals and the VA Center for Cooperative Studies in West Haven, Connecticut. A Data Monitoring Board, consisting of five consultants, monitored the study throughout patient intake and follow-up (Appendix). Male patients less than 70 years of age who were admitted to any of the participating hospitals with chest pain were screened for inclusion in the study. Unstable angina was defined according to severity of symptoms and by clinical presentation. Type I unstable angina included patients with angina pectoris that had been present for more than 2 months during which the progression of symptoms had accelerated, as manifested by an increase in severity (doubling of nitrate requirement) or an increase in frequency of episodes (doubling of the number of attacks per day). Type I unstable angina also included patients with angina at rest occurring within 8 weeks of the time the patient was first considered for the study. Symptoms had to have been present within 10 days of entry. Also considered type I disease was angina pectoris of 2 months' or less duration in which pain was produced by less than ordinary activity (NYHA class

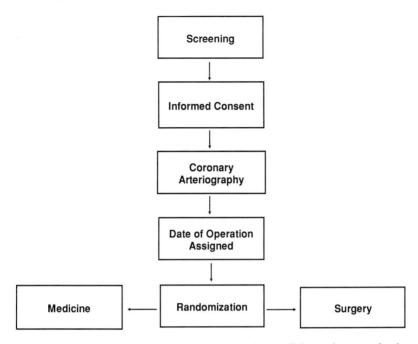

Figure 1 Prospective, randomized study comparing medicine and surgery for the treatment of unstable angina.

III) or angina of recent onset with recurrent chest pain at rest. With resting chest pain, electrocardiographic changes consisting of ST-segment depression of at least 1 mm or T-wave inversion had to be present. A positive exercise test was required of patients who did not have recurring chest pain at rest.

Type II unstable angina was defined as recurring episodes of prolonged chest pain that were incompletely relieved by nitrates. One such episode of chest pain should have occurred within 10 days of entering the study. During at least one episode of pain, ST-segment depression or elevation of at least 1 mm or T-wave inversion should be documented.

Acute myocardial infarction was excluded by serial electrocardiography and serum creatine kinase measurements.

The reasons for excluding patients from the study at the time of screening are listed in Table 1. Informed consent was obtained for coronary arteriography, randomization, treatment, and all follow-up studies. Coronary arteriography included left ventriculography and was done prior to randomization and again at 1 year after treatment was begun.

Table 1 Reasons for Excluding Patients at Screening Before Entry

	Patients (*n*)
Outcome of screening	
Patients screened	3159
Patients screened but excluded	2433
Patients included	726 (23%)
Reason for exclusion	
Acute myocardial infarction	609
Character of pain did not qualify	615
Onset or change in angina 8 weeks or more before this hospitalization	53
Pain of unstable angina not present within 10 days of admission	17
Exercise tolerance test performed and found to be negative	105
Acute infarction less than 3 months before date of screening	130
Previous operation for angina pectoris	190
Current participation in another study of unstable angina or another clinical trial	19
Question of likelihood of cooperation	73
Refusal of consent	344
Death before randomization	6
Other	272

Randomization was performed at the Coordinating Center. Patients were stratified according to left ventricular function and type of unstable angina. Left ventricular function was considered normal if the ejection fraction was 0.50 or greater and the end-diastolic pressure was less than 16 mmHg. Patient follow-up began with the date assigned to start therapy.

DATA ANALYSIS AND SAMPLE SIZE

Death and myocardial infarction were the primary and secondary end-points of this study. Operative mortality included any death occurring within 30 days of surgery. A perioperative myocardial infarction was any infarction occurring with Q waves within 10 days after surgery. Myocardial infarction was defined by the appearance of Q waves or QS deflections lasting 0.04 sec or longer, with evolutionary ST-T wave changes on the electrocardiogram and accompanied by a compatible history or an increase in myocardial (MB) creatine kinase 1.5 times normal. A non-Q-wave myocardial infarction was defined by persistent ST depression or T-wave inversion and appropriate history or enzyme changes. A myocardial infarction was considered fatal if death occurred within 30 days of onset. All electrocardiograms were interpreted with a centrally located Hewlett-Packard 5000 ECG Management System and edited by the same cardiologist. All angiograms were reviewed by a panel of cardiologists.

Life table methods were used to calculate cumulative survival and morbidity rates beginning with the date of assigned start of treatment. The Mantel-Haenszel chi-square test was used to compare overall cumulative curves (5). The primary analysis was performed according to treatment assigned at randomization, regardless of adherence. The effects of baseline variables on survival were examined using multiple logistic regression analysis (6). Maximum-likelihood estimates were computed by the Newton-Raphsen method (7). Sample sizes were estimated separately for type I and type II patients in order to detect in each group, with a power of 0.95, a 50% reduction in the 5-year mortality rate for surgical compared with medical therapy. All p values reflect two-sided tests of significance.

PATIENT POPULATION

A total of 468 patients were randomized; 237 patients were assigned to medical therapy and 231 to surgery. There were 374 type I patients and 94 type II patients. Randomization distributed patients to treatment groups equally according to their clinical presentation and left ventricular function (Table 2). The clinical characteristics of patients at the time they were entered into the study are summarized in Table 3.

Table 2 Stratification of Patients by Clinical Presentation of Angina Pectoris, Left Ventricular Function, and Type of Treatment

Presentation of angina/ ventricular function	Medical treatment	Surgical treatment	Total
Type I			
Normal	133	134	267
Abnormal	57	50	107
	190	184	374
Type II			
Normal	36	31	67
Abnormal	11	16	27
	47	47	94
Total			
Normal	169	165	334
Abnormal	68	66	134
	237	231	468

Table 3 Clinical Characteristics of Patients at Time of Randomization

	All patients		Type I		Type II	
	Medicine ($n = 237$)	Surgery ($n = 231$)	Medicine ($n = 190$)	Surgery ($n = 184$)	Medicine ($n = 47$)	Surgery ($n = 47$)
Age (years)	56.3 ± 6.9	55.7 ± 7.1	56.2 ± 6.9	56.0 ± 7.0	56.3 ± 7.1	54.8 ± 7.7
History of myocardial infarction	42.6	41.7	40.5	42.9	51.1	37.0
Diabetes	17.9	16.2	17.0	16.4	21.3	15.6
Systolic blood pressure	129.4 ± 17.7	132.5 ± 21.2	128.9 ± 17.2	133.1 ± 21.2	131.2 ± 19.6	130.3 ± 21.3
Diastolic blood pressure	79.4 ± 10.3	80.7 ± 11.1	79.2 ± 10.3	81.2 ± 10.5	80.1 ± 10.4	78.3 ± 13.0
Abnormal left ventricular function	28.7	28.6	30.0	27.2	23.4	34.0
Ejection fraction	62.7 ± 12.6	63.5 ± 13.8	62.6 ± 12.5	63.3 ± 14.0	63.1 ± 13.1	64.2 ± 12.9
Vessels diseased						
One	18.6	18.8	17.5	18.6	23.4	19.6
Two	33.1	36.7	31.7	36.6	38.3	37.0
Three	48.3	44.5	50.8	44.8	38.3	43.5

Values are mean ± SD where applicable.

CORONARY ARTERIOGRAPHY

Of the 726 patients who had coronary arteriography when screened for entry into the study, 255 patients were excluded for reasons listed in Table 4. A total of 303 patients entering the study had coronary arteriograms after 1 year of follow-up. The complication rate for screening coronary arteriography was 0.7% and included two fatal myocardial infarctions, two nonfatal myocardial infarctions, and one cerebrovascular accident. Only one complication, a nonfatal myocardial infarction, occurred during 1-year follow up angiography, a complication rate of 0.3%.

MEDICAL TREATMENT

Investigators were free to select what they considered appropriate medical therapy, with the exception that patients were not to be given drugs for long-term anticoagulation. In the medical cohort 62.9% of patients received long-acting nitrates, 62.1% received propranolol, and 18.1% received aspirin. Only 15% adhered to diet and weight management and 12% followed an exercise program. Two percent of patients were taking calcium-channel-blocking agents at the time of 2-year follow-up.

Table 4 Reasons for Excluding Patients After Arteriographic Examination

Reason for exclusion	Patients (*n*)
Lesion in left main artery	90
Normal coronary arteries	51
Coronary artery disease without critical stenoses	38
Distal diffuse coronary artery disease	15
Left ventricular aneurysm	10
Ejection fraction less than 0.30	8
Patient's refusal or ineligibility	8
Complication of coronary arteriography (myocardial infarction, cerebrovascular accident, death)	4
Other	31
Patients examined but excluded	255
Patients examined	726
Patients included	471[a] (65%)

[a]Three patients were found to have a left ventricular ejection fraction less than 0.30 after the central committee reviewed the arteriograms. These patients were observed but not included in the analyses. Thus, 468 patients constituted the study population.

SURGERY

Reversed autologous saphenous vein bypass, as described by Favaloro (8), was the specified surgical procedure, although one patient did receive an internal mammary artery graft. The mean and median intervals between randomization and operation were 9.3 and 5 days, respectively. No deaths occurred during this interval. Nine deaths occurred within 30 days of surgery. The overall operative mortality was 4.1%; the operative mortality for patients with type I angina was 4.3% but for type II patients the operative mortality was only 2.1%. For unexplained reasons, the operative mortality for medical failures was 10.3%

The average number of grafts for each patient was 2.7. When compared to the number of diseased arteries present, this number indicated that 90% of patients had been completely revascularized. At 1 year 140 patients, or 67% of the 209 surgical patients eligible for coronary arteriography, were studied. A total of 273 of the 365 grafts were visualized (74.8%), suggesting that 58.8% of the patients were still completely revascularized. Twenty-seven percent of the surgical patients were receiving aspirin, 40% were taking propranolol, and 31% were receiving long-acting nitrates. Not all patients were able to complete their assigned therapy. Eleven patients (4.8%) randomized to surgery did not receive an operation. Two had a myocardial infarction after randomization but before being assigned a date for surgery.

TREATMENT FAILURE

The most common reason for patients not adhering to assigned treatment was failure of medical treatment. Eight years after randomization 45% of the medical patients had received surgery (Fig. 2). This was true for both type I and type II patients. Patients with three-vessel disease had the highest rate of crossover, 57%. During the first 30-day period immediately following randomization, medical failure was greatest among patients with type II disease, 19.1% compared to 5.8% for type I patients.

Characteristics of patients failing medical treatment were determined by logistic regression analysis. Significant independent predictors were age, three-vessel disease, systolic blood pressure above 90 mmHg, and propranolol dependence. The younger patients were more likely to crossover, as were patients with three-vessel disease. Patients on 240 mg or more of propranolol a day and still having at least one episode of angina were unlikely to adhere to medical treatment.

SURVIVAL

The primary end-point of this study was survival, yet throughout follow-up there has never been a significant difference between the two major treatment groups

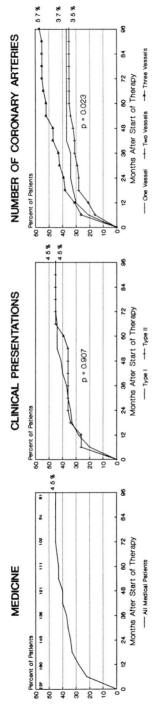

Figure 2 The cumulative occurrence of all medical treatment failures is shown in the left panel. Medical treatment failure according to clinical presentation is shown in the middle panel. Medical treatment failure by number of major coronary arteries involved is shown in the right panel.

when survival was analyzed by the life table method. After 8 years, 72% of the surgical patients and 71% of the medical patients are still alive (Fig. 3). When survival is analyzed according to clinical presentation, that is type 1 or type II, the difference in survival is still not significant (Fig. 4). The smaller-than-expected number of type II patients entered into the study resulted in a power insufficient to show a statistically significant difference between survival of medical and surgical patients, although the survival of surgical patients is greater than that of medical patients. If the type II patients are further stratified according to left ventricular function, there is a significant difference between medical and surgical patients. Survival of type II patients with impaired left ventricular function is improved with surgery (Fig. 5) (9).

The number of coronary arteries involved did not influence survival during the first 2 years after randomization to treatment. After five years, however, survival of patients with three-vessel coronary artery disease receiving surgery was significantly better than survival of patients with three-vessel coronary artery disease treated medically (10). This has remained true after 8 years of follow-up. The survival of patients with single- or double-vessel disease is the same whether randomized to medicine or to treatment with surgery (Fig. 6).

The effect of abnormal left ventricular function (EF < 0.5 and/or LVEDP 16 mmHg or greater) on survival has been inconsistent. During the first 2 years of follow-up, there were no significant differences between the two treatment groups, but after 3 years, there was a 65% reduction in mortality for patients with

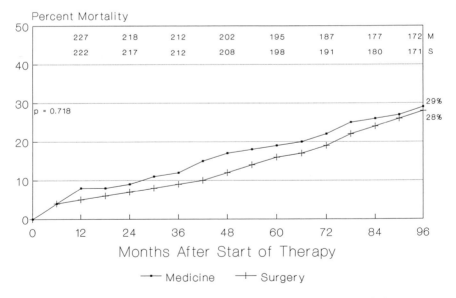

Figure 3 Cumulative mortality of all patients assigned to medical or surgical treatment.

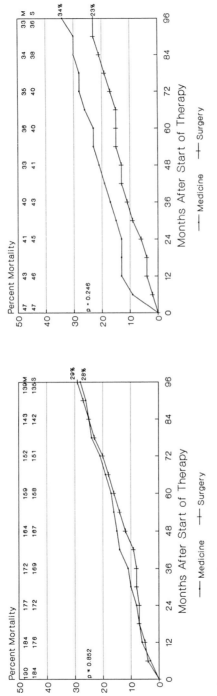

Figure 4 Cumulative mortality of patients according to clinical presentation. Type I is shown in the left panel and type II is shown in the right panel.

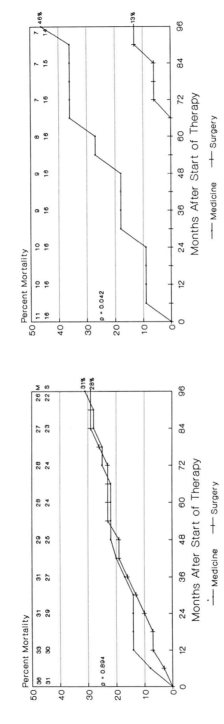

Figure 5 Cumulative mortality of type II patients with normal left ventricular function (left panel) and type II patients with abnormal left ventricular function (right panel).

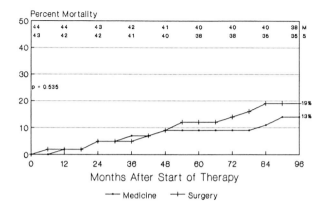

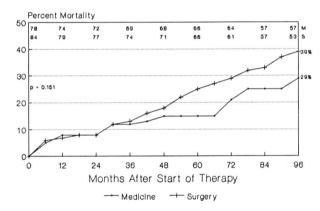

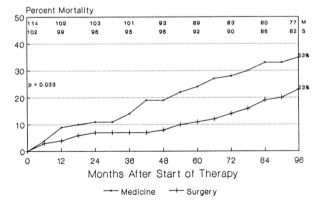

Figure 6 Cumulative mortality of patients with one-vessel coronary artery disease (top panel), two-vessel coronary artery disease (middle panel), and three-vessel coronary artery disease (bottom panel).

abnormal left ventricular function assigned to surgery, and survival was significantly better for surgical patients with ejection fractions less than 0.5 (11). This improved survival with surgery was not sustained at 5 years or at 8 years (Fig. 7). An ejection fraction of less than 0.5 was no longer significant at 5 years, but if patients were arbitrarily grouped into thirds, the surgical patients in the lower tercile of ejection fraction (30–58) did have improved survival (Fig. 8).

After 2 years and again after 5 years of patient follow-up, life table analyses failed to show any significant differences between medical and surgical treatment groups overall, by clinical presentation, or by left ventricular function. It was observed, however, that curves reflecting mortality as a function of left ventricular ejection fraction were significantly different from each other (3). Logistic multiple regression analyses relating pretreatment LVEF treated as a continuous, rather than a categorical, independent variable were performed for medical and surgical groups (Table 5). The relation between each patient's ejection fraction and mortality at 2 years was determined. The logistic curve with the best fit was calculated with the equation for estimated mortality $= 1/[1 + e^{-(a + b\,\text{LVEF})}]$, in which the values of coefficients a and b were obtained by an iterative process. The slope for the curve for the medical group was significantly different from zero, while the slope for the surgical group was not significantly different from zero. These observations have been consistent throughout the follow-up period and strongly support the premise that there is a significant interaction between treatment and LVEF as these variables affect survival in patients with unstable angina. This is further supported by life table analysis of patients with low ejection fractions (Fig. 8).

It has been shown, therefore, that survival is significantly improved in patients assigned to surgery rather than medicine if the patients have three-vessel coronary artery disease or if their left ventricular ejection fraction is compromised. Survival of patients with one- or two-vessel disease and normal or abnormal left ventricular function is not significantly different when medical and surgical groups are compared. Survival of surgical patients with three-vessel disease and normal left ventricular function is better than that of medical patients, but this difference is not significant ($p = 0.28$). For patients with three-vessel coronary artery disease and abnormal left ventricular function, the difference is significant ($p = 0.04$). Survival of the type II patients with abnormal LVF is significantly better with surgery (Fig. 5).

When analyses were made not only by treatment assigned but by treatment received and by treatment assigned with treatment-failure patients withdrawn at the time of failure, the results were the same.

MYOCARDIAL INFARCTION

Nonfatal myocardial infarction has been documented in 85 patients (Table 6). Since the study began, the incidence of myocardial infarction has been similar in

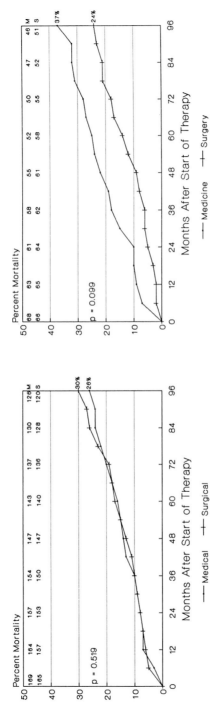

Figure 7 Cumulative mortality of patients with normal ventricular function (left panel) and abnormal left ventricular function (right panel).

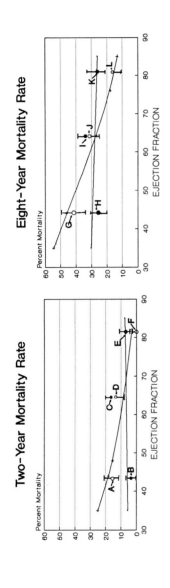

Two-Year Mortality Rate

Eight-Year Mortality Rate

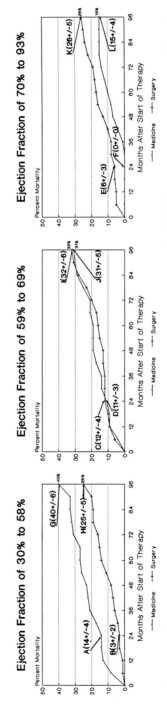

Figure 8 The curves in the upper panels were computed by logistic regression analysis in which LVEF was used as a continuous variable. The relation between each patient's LVEF and mortality was determined. The logistic curve with best fit was calculated with the equation: Estimated mortality $= 1/[1 + e^{-(a + b\ \text{LVEF})}]$, when a is the intercept and b is the slope. The values for these coefficients are shown in Table 6. The lower panels are life table plots of patients in three tercils based on ejection fraction at time of entry into the study. Corresponding points representing mortality from the life table curves are shown on the regression analysis curves (A–L) including the standard error for each point.

Table 5 Values Used to Plot Logistic Regression Analysis Curves in Figure 8

Logistic regression analysis		2-year results		8-year results	
		Coefficient	p-value	Coefficient	p-value
Medical	Intercept	−0.6746	0.5326	1.6298	0.0276
	slope	−0.0503	0.0074	−0.0414	0.0006
Surgical	Intercept	−3.0377	0.0192	−0.6885	0.3205
	slope	−0.0061	0.7573	−0.0042	0.6929
All patients	The interaction of treatment and ejection fraction was statistically significant at 2 years and at 8 years. In a logistic model containing treatment, ejection fraction, and treatment by ejection fraction interaction, the p-value for a test of interaction was 0.0300 at 2 years and 0.0214 at 8 years.				

Table 6 Number of patients with One or More Nonfatal Myocardial Infarctions During the First 10 Days and During the First 8 Years of Follow-up by Clinical Presentation and by Left Ventricular Function

		Nonfatal myocardial infarction rate (%)			
		During first 10 days		During first 8 years	
	Subgroup	Medicine (n = 237)	Surgery (n = 231)	Medicine (n = 237)	Surgery (n = 231)
Clinical presentation	Type I	2.1% (4/190)	8.7% (16/184)	19.5% (37/190)	16.3% (30/184)
	Type II	6.4% (3/47)	14.9% (7/47)	17.0% (8/47)	21.3% (10/47)
Left ventricular function	Normal LVF	3.0% (5/169)	10.9% (18/165)	20.1% (34/169)	17.6% (29/165)
	Abnormal LVF	2.9% (2/68)	7.6% (5/66)	16.2% (11/68)	16.7% (11/66)
Total		3.0% (7/237)	10.0% (23/231)	19.0% (45/237)	17.3% (40/231)

the medical and surgical groups. Nineteen percent of the medical patients and 17.3% of the surgical have had myocardial infarctions. Three patients assigned to surgery had a myocardial infarction before surgery could be performed. Two of these patients never had surgery and one patient had surgery after a 7.7-month delay. Five patients assigned to medicine had a myocardial infarction before treatment was begun.

Twenty-three patients experienced perioperative myocardial infarction, all occurring within 10 days of surgery. This was 10.0% of the 231 patients assigned to surgery and 10.0% of 220 patients (22/220) who actually received surgery. The perioperative infarction rates of 8.7% (16 of 184) for type I patients and 14.9% (7 of 47) for type II patients were not significantly different ($p = 0.2053$). For medical patients during the same period, 10 days from start of therapy, the rate of myocardial infarction was 3.0% (7 of 237 patients). The rate of 2.1% (4 of 190) for type I patients did not differ significantly from the rate of 6.4% (3 of 47) for type II patients ($p = 0.1209$).

If the incidence of nonfatal myocardial infarction is determined from the date of randomization rather than from the start of therapy date, the rate of nonfatal myocardial infarction for medical patients is 21.1% (50/237) and for surgical patients is 18.6% (43/231).

QUALITY OF LIFE

Quality of life was based on the number of new hospitalizations for angina or cardiac events, the severity of each individual's angina as determined from an angina questionnaire, the amount of medication each patient required for control of angina, the patient's ability to return to work, and exercise tolerance measured on a treadmill (12).

New Hospitalizations

There were significantly fewer new hospitalizations for the surgical patients compared to medical patients during the first 6 months after randomization (52 versus 78). Subsequently the number of hospitalizations were similar for medical and surgical patients (Fig. 9).

When hospitalizations for cardiac events only were compared, they were found to be twice as frequent in medical patients in the first 6 months after randomization (30% versus 14%). At 1 year this difference was 43% versus 25% and at 5 years, 68% versus 51% ($p = 0.001$). The differences were similar when comparisons were made for type I and for type II patients.

Ninety-eight of 340 cardiovascular hospitalizations (29%) in the medical group during the first 5 years of follow-up were for coronary artery bypass surgery. Only 2 of 231 (1%) readmissions among surgical patients were for

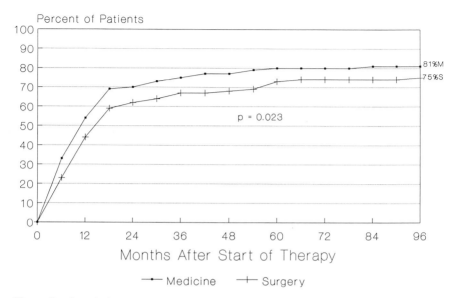

Figure 9 Cumulative percentage of patients in each treatment group with new hospitalizations.

coronary artery bypass surgery. Medical patients spent an average of 4.1 days in the hospital whereas surgical patients averaged 2.6 days.

Subjective Response to Treatment

The patient's own evaluation of the treatment he received was assessed at 3 months. Most of the patients who had received surgery said they felt improved (146 of 183, or 79.8%). Only 116 of the 200 medical patients (58%) believed they were better, $p < 0.01$. Six percent of the patients felt worse after surgery and 14.6% of the medical patients were subjectively worse.

Surgery resulted in significantly less chest pain (angina) at 3 months. After 5 years, 54.8% of the surgical patients had no angina compared to 32.9% of medical patients ($p < 0.01$). Fewer surgery patients were using nitroglycerine (58% versus 47.7%; $p = 0.05$).

Medications

When this study began, calcium channel blockers were not available and their subsequent use was not documented. The numbers of medical and surgical patients taking β-blockers when randomized were similar. For the first 3 years after treatment was begun, significantly fewer surgical patients required

Table 7 Duration of Treadmill Performance in Minutes at Six Periods of Follow-up Assigned Treatment

	6 months		1 year		2 years		3 years		4 years		5 years	
	M	S	M	S	M	S	M	S	M	S	M	S
P_{10}	2.0	3.0	2.7	3.2	3.2	2.7	3.5	3.4	3.1	3.8	3.1	3.7
P_{25}	3.3	4.5	3.8	5.0	4.2	4.6	4.7	5.0	4.8	5.8	4.5	5.5
P_{50}	5.0	6.3	6.0	7.0	6.1	6.8	6.3	7.5	6.4	7.0	6.2	6.8
P_{75}	7.0	9.0	7.5	9.1	7.8	9.2	8.1	9.7	8.5	9.0	8.0	9.0
P_{90}	9.0	10.0	10.0	10.6	10.0	12.0	10.4	12.0	10.0	11.0	9.2	11.0
n	140	133	147	131	117	99	107	95	81	85	83	82
Mean	5.4	6.6	6.0	7.2	6.2	7.1	6.5	7.5	6.6	7.4	6.3	7.1
SE	0.24	0.24	0.23	0.24	0.24	0.33	0.25	0.31	0.29	0.29	0.25	0.31

n = number of patients; M = medical patients; S = surgical patients. Percentile estimates are shown for 10th (P_{10}), 25th (P_{25}), median (P_{50}), 75th (P_{75}), and 90th (P_{90}) percentiles. All measurements of duration are in minutes.

β-blockers, but by 5 years the difference between medical and surgical patients taking β-blockers was no longer significant. The number of surgical patients taking long-acting nitrates was significantly less than the number of medical patients taking long-acting nitrates throughout 5 years of follow-up (195/227, 85.9% versus 179/235, 76.2%, $p = 0.01$).

Ability to Work

The number of patients able to return to work was not improved with surgery. Throughout follow-up, the difference between the number of medical and surgical patients working was not significant.

Treadmill Performance

Patients were asked to perform a Bruce multistage treadmill test at 6 months and thereafter at 12-month intervals. Compliance at 5 years was 53%. A statistical summary of the treadmill performance of each treatment group is given in Table 7. In addition to mean values, medians (P_{50}) and percentile estimates are shown. Treadmill duration was significantly increased in surgical patients compared to medical patients at 6 months and after 5 years ($p < 0.01$). Percentile estimates were also used to compare the two treatment groups. At the end of 5 years 90% of surgical patients remained on the treadmill for 11.0 min or less ($P_{90} = 11.0$) while 90% of the medical patients remained on the treadmill for 9.2 min or less ($P_{90} = 9.2$). Heart rate and double product responses were improved in surgical patients at 6 months but were no different from responses in medical patients at 3- and 5-year follow-up. Some improvement in treadmill performance of medical patients was observed during follow-up and was attributed to the addition of calcium-channel blockers and to medical crossover. When censored crossover analysis was made, that is, removing nonadherers from the study at the time of crossover, results did not change.

ACKNOWLEDGMENT

We are indebted to Mrs. Margaret Garrison of the Asheville VA Medical Center for her help in preparing this manuscript and to Ms. Lisa Garland for the preparation of the graphics used to illustrate this manuscript.

APPENDIX: PARTICIPANTS IN VETERANS ADMINISTRATION COOPERATIVE STUDY
Participating Hospitals and Investigators

Buffalo, NY: Aziz-ur-Rahim Masud, M.D., and Joginder Bhayana, M.D. Durham, NC: Kenneth Morris, M.D., Neal Shadoff, M.D., Andrew Wechsler,

M.D., Richard Stack, M.D., Harry R. Phillips III, M.D., Thomas Bashore, M.D., and Michael Hindman, M.D. Houston, TX: James K. Alexander, M.D., Alfredo Montero, M.D., Gene A. Guinn, M.D., and Robert A. Chahine, M.D. Lexington KY: Anthony N. Demaria, M.D., John Zeok, M.D., John Slack, M.D., and Henry Hanley, M.D. Long Beach, CA: Harold Olson, M.D., Edward A. Stemmer, M.D., and Jack Ferlinz, M. D. Oklahoma City, OK: Eliot Schecter, M.D., and Ronald Elkins, M.D. Asheville, NC: Thomas Maley, M.D., Gulshan K. Sethi, M.D., Thomas Pinto, M.D., Paravasth Seshachary, M.D., and Vassil Prokov, M.D. Palo Alto, CA: Herbert N. Hultgren, M.D., and Craig Miller, M.D. West Roxbury, MA: Alfred Parisi, M.D., Shukri F. Khuri, M.D., G. V. R. K. Sharma, M.D., and Ernest Barsamian, M.D. Ann Arbor, MI: Richard Foster, M.D., and Lucy Goodenday, M.D. Cleveland, OH: Berian Davis, M.D. Madison, WI: Vincent Yap, M.D.

Executive Committee

Robert J. Luchi, M.D., Medical Cochairman, Houston, TX; Stewart M. Scott, M.D., Surgical Cochairman, Asheville, NC; Alfred Parisi, M.D., West Roxbury, MA; Edward A. Stemmer, M.D., Long Beach, CA; Andrew Wechsler, M.D., Durham, NC; and Robert H. Deupree, PhD, Biostatistician, West Haven, CT.

Data Monitoring Board

John A. Waldhausen, M.D., Chairman, Hershey, PA; Lawrence W. Shaw, Biostatistician, Gainesville, FL; John Michael Criley, M.D., Torrance, CA; Paul Ebert, M.D., Chicago, IL: and Richard O. Russell Jr., M.D., Birmingham, AL.

Human Rights Subcommittee

Edward R. Ryan, Ph.D., Chairman, West Haven, CT; Jack H. Evans, New Haven, CT; Richard C. Feldman, New Haven, CT; Barbara A. Kathe, R.S.M., Ph.D., New Hartford, CT; Mary Joan Cook, R.S.M., Ph.D., W. Hartford, CT; William Field, M.D., New Haven, CT; formerly, Hugh L. Dwyer, M.D., Woodbridge, CT; James M. Solomon, M.D., Guilford, CT; Sarah McCue Horwitz, Ph.D., Hamden, CT; Willis Pritchett, R.Ph, New Haven, CT; and Frank Votto, Cheshire, CT.

Cooperative Studies Program Central Administration (Washington, DC)

Daniel Deykin, M.D., Chief.

Statistical Assistants

Lynn Durant; formerly Patricia Danner, Cynthia Cushing, Katherine Newvine, Victoria Zappone, Anne Malloy, Mary Ann Cosharek, and Jo-Anne Falcigno.

Programmers

Katherine Newvine; formerly, Margaret Lee, Gary Johnson, Cynthia Johnson, Joanne Kelly, and Mary Ann O'Brien.

REFERENCES

1. Fowler, NO. Preinfarctional Angina. A need for an objective definition and for a controlled clinical trial of its management. Circulation 1971; 44:755–58.
2. Unstable Angina Pectoris Study Group. Unstable angina pectoris national cooperative study group to compare surgical and medical therapy. II. In-hospital experience and initial follow-up results in patients with one, two and three vessel disease. Am J Cardiol 1978; 42:839–48.
3. Luchi RJ, Scott SM, Deupree RH, and the unstable angina study principal investigators and their associates. Comparison of medical and surgical treatment for unstable angina pectoris. N Engl J Med 1987; 316:977–84.
4. Takaro T, Hultgren HN, Lipton MJ, Detre KM, and participants in the VA Study Group. The VA Cooperative randomized study of surgery for coronary arterial occlusive disease. II. Subgroup with significant left main lesions. Circulation 1976; 54(Suppl III):107.
5. Mantel, N, Haenszel W. Statistical aspects of the analysis of data from retrospective studies of diseases. J Natl Cancer Inst 1959; 22:719.
6. Walker SH, Duncan DB. Estimation of the probability of an event as a function of several independent variables. Biometrika 1967; 54:167.
7. Ralston A, Wilf HS. Mathematical methods for digital computers. New York: Wiley, 1967.
8. Favaloro RG. Saphenous vein graft in the surgical treatment of coronary artery disease: Operative technique. J Thorac Cardiovasc Surg 1969; 58:178.
9. Sharma GVRK, Deupree RH, Khuri SF, Parisi AF, Luchi RJ, Scott SM, and the Veterans Administration Unstable Angina Cooperative Study Group. Coronary bypass surgery improves survival in high-risk unstable angina: Results of a Veterans Administration cooperative study with an 8-year follow-up (in press).
10. Parisi AF, Khuri S, Deupree RH, Sharma GVRK, Scott SM, Luchi RJ. Medical compared with surgical management of unstable angina. 5-year mortality and morbidity in the Veterans Administration study. Circulation 1989; 80:1176–89.
11. Scott SM, Luchi RJ, Deupree RH, and the Veterans Administration Unstable Angina Cooperative Study Group. Veterans Administration cooperative study for treatment of patients with unstable angina. Results in patients with abnormal left ventricular function. Circulation, 1988; 78:(Suppl I):I-113–I-212.
12. Booth DC, Deupree RH, Hultgren HN, DeMaria AN, Scott SM, Luchi RJ, and the Investigators of Cooperative Study No. 28. Quality of life after bypass surgery for unstable angina: 5-year follow-up results of a VA Cooperative Study. Circulation 1991; 83:87–95.

9

National Cooperative Study of Unstable Angina

Gary D. Plotnick

*University of Maryland School of Medicine and
The Johns Hopkins University School of Medicine
Baltimore, Maryland*

INTRODUCTION

The National Cooperative Study of Unstable Angina sponsored by the National Heart, Lung, and Blood Institute (NHLBI) examined the impact of urgent coronary artery bypass surgery (CABG) and is considered by many the prototype of prospective cooperative randomized trials (1–4). This NHLBI trial was being completed just as the Veterans Administration (VA) Cooperative trial was starting. Identification of the strengths and weaknesses of this early trial led to design modifications that have strengthened subsequent randomized trials. Thus, it is appropriate that this first large, randomized study of unstable angina be described in detail. In the early 1970s, as CABG was experiencing its first major surge in popularity, emergency coronary bypass surgery was being touted as necessary therapy for patients with unstable angina. At that time, it was believed that urgent coronary artery bypass graft surgery would reduce the anticipated high mortality and morbidity thought to be associated with "unstable angina pectoris" and thus could prevent death and myocardial infarction and improve the quality of life. However, some clinicians favored medical therapy, not being convinced of either the grim prognosis of unstable angina or the major therapeutic advantages of urgent CABG. Valid arguments could be made for either of two courses of action (medical management or urgent surgical management). With no clear evidence as to which is a better choice, it is both logical and ethical to choose therapy on a randomized basis. With this approach, if one form of therapy is in fact better than another, at least half the patients will receive the better therapy. Under the direction of Dr. Richard S. Ross and Dr. Richard C. Conti of the Johns Hopkins Medical Institutions, the NHLBI agreed to sponsor a large, multicenter, randomized cooperative study investigating this question. The institutions that agreed to participate included: University of Alabama at Birmingham, University of Chicago, Cornell, Duke, Johns Hopkins Medical Institutions, the Massachusetts General Hospital, the University of Rochester, and Stanford. The University of Florida at Gainesville was added when Richard Conti moved to Florida. These nine university medical centers evaluated and randomized patients with unstable angina, assigning either current medical therapy alone or medical therapy plus urgent CABG (defined as surgery within 7 days) (1,2).

CRITERIA FOR INCLUSION

Criteria for inclusion in the study were both clinical and angiographic (Table 1). In this study, unstable angina was clinically defined as changing angina pectoris with new onset or an accelerating pattern occurring either ''on effort'' or ''at rest.'' Most patients had prolonged rest pain episodes that necessitated admission to the coronary care unit, a pattern sometimes designated as ''impending myocardial infarction.'' However, patients who developed evidence of an acute

Table 1 Criteria for Inclusion in the NIH-Sponsored National Cooperative Randomized Trial to Compare Medical and Surgical Therapy of Unstable Angina Pectoris

Clinical
   CCU admission
   Episode of ''unstable angina''
   Transient ST-T changes with pain
   No new Q-wave or enzyme rise in first 24 hr
   Age < 70 years, general condition life expectancy ≥ 5 years
   No evidence of MI within previous 3 months
   Not considered previous medical failure
   Informed consent

Angiographic
   70% or greater narrowing of one or more major coronary arteries
   Less than 50% narrowing of left main coronary artery
   Distal vessel ≥ 1mm
   ''Salvageable'' left ventricular function
     Ejection fraction ≥ 0.30
     End-diastolic volume < 125 ml/m^2

myocardial infarction on admission were excluded (Table 2). For inclusion, at least one episode of pain needed to be associated with documented transient ST-segment shifts (either upward or downward), T-wave changes, or both, which returned to normal or toward control (baseline) pattern shortly after abatement of pain. This criterion was believed necessary to ensure that only those with objective evidence of "myocardial ischemia" would be included. Following informed consent, the patients who agreed to participate in the study were taken to the catheterization laboratory, usually within 72 hr of admission. For continued inclusion in the trial, the angiogram had to demonstrate one or more lesions in a major coronary artery of 70% narrowing or greater with distal circulation thought to be adequate to accept a graft, i.e., suitable for CABG. In addition, patients with poor left ventricle function (ejection fraction < 0.30) or end-diastolic volume > 125 ml/m^2 were excluded. Of the patients who met the clinical criteria, approximately 9% were excluded because of insignificant disease, 15–20% were excluded due to left main coronary artery disease and were treated surgically, and 15% were excluded because they were not thought to be good surgical candidates (poor distal vessels or poor left ventricular function), and were treated medically. It should be noted that these were the relatively early days of CABG; it is likely many patients excluded for CABG because of poor distal vessels or moderate ventricular dysfunction would be eligible for surgery today.

If the patient was considered "randomizable," the patient was assigned either medical therapy or urgent surgery (to be performed within 8 days).

The clinical and angiographic characteristics of the 288 patients randomized between 1972 and 1977 are shown in Table 3. Of the 147 who were randomized

Table 2 Criteria for Exclusion in the NIH-Sponsored National Cooperative Randomized Trial to Compare Medical and Surgical Therapy

---

Clinical
  Age equal to or greater than 70 years
  Life expectancy less than 5 years from noncoronary artery disease
  Myocardial infarction within 3 months
  Appearance of new Q waves or enzyme elevation during 24 hr

Angiographic
  Absence of coronary disease
  Left main coronary disease ($\geq 50\%$ stenosis)
  Poor left ventricular function
    Ejection fraction < 0.30
    End-diastolic volume ≥ 125 ml/m^2
  Severe distal vessel disease unacceptable for bypass graft
  Requirement for valve replacement or aneurysmectomy

Table 3 Comparison of NHBLI Trial and VA Trial

	NHBLI		VA	
	Medical ($n = 147$)	Surgical ($n = 141$)	Medical ($n = 237$)	Surgical ($n = 231$)
Age (years)	53	53	56	56
Males	82%	86%	100%	100%
Prior MI	27%	35%	43%	42%
Smokers	73%	75%	87%	93%
Diabetes	14%	10%	18%	16%
Angiographic findings				
Triple-vessel disease	39%	43%	48%	44%
Double-vessel disease	37%	33%	33%	37%
Single-vessel disease	24%	24%	19%	19%
Ejection fraction (30–49%)	23%	23%	18%	17%
Survival				
1 year	92%	95%	95%	92%
2 years	91%	93%	91%	90%
Crossover to surgery				
At 24 months	31%		34%	
At 42[a]–60[b] months	45%[a]		43%[b]	
Nonfatal MI				
At 24[a]–30[b] months	11%[a]	13%[a]	12%[b]	12%[b]

to medicine and 141 randomized to surgery, most were men with rest angina, most had previous ischemic symptoms, manifested by ST-segment depression with pain, and the majority had multiple-vessel disease. There were no baseline differences between the medical and surgical cohorts (2). Comparisons between the patients entered into the NHLBI study and into the VA study (5,6) are shown in Table 3. The similarities between clinical, angiographic, and early outcome characteristics of the 468 patients randomized in the VA study and those of the 288 patients randomized in the NHLBI study are remarkable. It had been argued that the NHLBI study involved a select patient population, that many patients were excluded and only good risk patients remained. Similar criticisms could be made of the VA cooperative study.

RESULTS

The National Cooperative Study of Unstable Angina failed to demonstrate a survival advantage of acute surgical therapy over medical therapy (Table 4). Of the 147 randomized to medical therapy, there were four (3%) in-hospital deaths compared with seven (5%) in-hospital deaths among the 141 patients assigned to

Table 4 Mortality and Morbidity Results: National Cooperative Randomized Trial of Unstable Angina

	Medical (n = 147)	Surgical (n = 141)	p
In-hospital			
Deaths	4 (3%)	7 (5%)	NS
MI	12 (8%)	24 (17%)	<0.05
Long-term			
Average follow-up	68 months	65 months	
Deaths	24 (16%)	21 (15%)	NS
MI	27 (18%)	47 (33%)	<0.05

acute surgery therapy. At long-term follow-up, an additional 20 patients had died in the medical group and 14 in the surgical group. No differences in mortality were found between urgent surgery and aggressive medical therapy. There was a difference, however, in the myocardial infarction rate, with more patients in the surgical group suffering myocardial infarctions. Symptomatic status was evaluated during follow-up, and 40% of the patients randomized to medical therapy had New York Heart Association class 3–4 angina at least once during follow-up, compared with 15% of those randomized to surgical therapy. The results of the National Cooperative Study, like those of the VA study, suggest no survival advantage for urgent surgery over medical therapy. In fact, the myocardial infarction rate was higher in those with urgent surgery, whereas long-term symptomatic relief appeared better in the surgical group.

From the scientific standpoint, interpretation, particularly of long-term results, was severely compromised by the large percentage of patients randomized to medical therapy who eventually underwent "elective" CABG due to recurrent symptoms. These "crossovers" represent patients in whom there was psychological pressure to maintain medical therapy, but due to unacceptable symptoms surgical therapy was employed. Of patients initially randomized to medicine, 36% had crossed over to surgical therapy by 30 months and 43% by 68 months. These crossovers limit interpretation of long-term results and emphasize that the study really compared patients treated with urgent surgery versus those initially treated with medicine who had the option of later surgery.

SUBGROUP ANALYSIS OF PATIENTS WITH TRANSIENT ST-SEGMENT ELEVATION

Subsequent to the initial report of results, further analysis was carried out and was the subject of two subsequent reports. The first analyzed the results in patients who demonstrated transient ST-segment elevation during pain (3). Of the total of 288 randomized patients, 79 (27%) had episodes of transient ST-segment elevation with episodes of pain. Hospital mortality rate was 4.8% in the 42 patients randomized to medicine and 5.4% in the 37 patients randomized to surgery. The in-hospital myocardial infarction rate was 12% in patients randomized to medicine and 14% in the patients randomized to surgery. These differences were not statistically significant. There was also no significant difference in symptomatic status or return to work at long-term follow-up. At the end of 2-year follow-up, 61% of the medical group and 68% of the surgical group were working full or part time. During the average follow-up period of 42 months, 45% of patients initially randomized to medicine had undergone CABG to relieve unacceptable symptoms. The conclusion of this analysis was that patients with unstable angina and transient ST-segment elevation during pain and rest did not differ significantly from patients with pain at rest associated with transient ST-segment depression or T-wave inversion.

Critique

Although attempts were made to obtain electrocardiograms (ECG) during most episodes of chest pain, only one ECG during pain was necessary to enter the patient into the randomized study. ECGs were not necessarily obtained during *every* episode of pain. If a patient manifested ST-segment elevation on any single ECG, the patient was considered in the group with ST-segment elevation, even if subsequent ECGs showed ST depression or T-wave changes. In addition, patients with pathological Q waves or old infarctions were not separated from those without Q waves. ST-segment elevation in leads with previous pathological Q waves may be very different from ST elevation in leads without Q waves. The former may merely reflect wall motion abnormalities in the area of a previous infarction, whereas ST-segment elevation in leads without pathological Q waves, such as reported in Prinzmetal's angina, appear to represent transmural ischemia. It should be emphasized that this ST-segment elevation was seen in patients who had > 70% narrowing in the coronary arteries and may be substantially different from the ST-segment elevation seen in patients with minimal coronary disease, where coronary spasm is clearly the culprit.

SUBGROUP ANALYSIS OF PATIENTS WITH LEFT ANTERIOR DESCENDING CORONARY ARTERY DISEASE

The second subgroup analysis evaluated randomized patients from the NHLBI trial who had left anterior descending (LAD) coronary artery disease (4). LAD disease was defined as 70% or greater fixed obstruction of the left anterior descending coronary artery. LAD disease was either isolated or combined with other disease (>50% narrowing of other major vessels). Patients were further analyzed as to whether the LAD narrowing was proximal (prior to the first septal perforator branch) or distal. The rationale for this subgroup analysis was that many clinicians believed that patients with unstable angina and obstructive disease of the left anterior descending were at particularly high risk of death or imminent myocardial infarction (particularly when the lesion was proximal). Results of this analysis follow.

Of patients with proximal LAD disease, there was one (2%) in-hospital death among 64 patients randomized to medicine, compared with five (9%) among 56 patients randomized to surgery. There were six additional deaths in the medical group and four deaths in the surgical group during the follow-up period. These differences did not reach statistical significance. Of the patients with distal LAD disease, there were one (3%) in-hospital death and three late deaths among the 38 patients randomized to medicine and one (2%) in-hospital death and three late deaths among the 44 patients randomized to surgical therapy. Again, there was no significant difference between in-hospital and late mortality. Nonfatal myocardial infarctions occurred in 9% of medically treated patients and in 23% of surgically treated patients with proximal disease, but even this difference did not reach statistical significance. The lack of a significant difference may well reflect a beta error, that is, insufficient patients included in the study to demonstrate a significant difference.

CHANGES IN MEDICAL THERAPY

Medical therapy used at the time included what was available in the early to mid-1970s. Medical therapy consisted of bed rest, sedation, nitroglycerin, and propranolol, with the goal of medical therapy to achieve a systolic blood pressure of <120 mmHg and a pulse rate equal to or less than 60 beats/min throughout the day. Other antihypertensive mediation was used as indicated. The use of heparin therapy was controversial at the time, and the decision to use heparin was at the discretion of the practicing physician.

Since this study was performed, medical therapy has improved substantially for all ischemic syndromes (7–9). Most patients in the NHLBI trial received long-acting nitrate therapy in the form of isosorbide nitrate in relatively low doses, and propranolol was also used in variable doses. Practice has evolved so that more aggressive use of nitrates and beta-blockers is now supplemented by widespread use of calcium-channel-blocking drugs and aspirin. (See Chapter 6.) How often medical therapy was less than ideal in the NHLBI trial, even by 1970 standards, has never been analyzed. With improved therapeutic options, it seems likely that mortality with medical therapy would be even lower in the 1990s than reported in the NHLBI and VA studies. The selection process, however, may have explained the low mortality seen in both the NHLBI and VA studies. It is often joked that the best way to improve prognosis of the patient is to enter that patient into a clinical trial (because, by nature, patients who enter into studies tend to be a relatively low-risk group, with the highest-risk group excluded). It needs to be explained that patients in both studies were patients for whom both medical and surgical therapy were considered options. Medical failures, older patients, patients with life-threatening medical conditions, recent myocardial infarction, left main coronary disease, poor distal vessels, and poor left ventricular function were excluded.

What percentage of all patients who presented to these participating centers does the randomized cohort represent? This key question remains unanswered. This lack of key information is one of the troubling deficiencies of the NHLBI Unstable Angina Study. At the time of initiation of this study, many practicing physicians already had substantial prejudices (often toward bypass surgery) and would not allow their patients to be randomized. Whether the patients included in this study are truly representative is unclear. Near the conclusion of this study, the reverse was true, in that tentative results were known and physicians would tend to treat their patients more conservatively, that is, were less aggressive about pursuing immediate surgical therapy. A major problem in interpretating data from this study was that during the period of the study, practicing opinion changed and various therapies evolved. Surgical techniques evolved substantially even during the study (10). A few centers reported to have superb surgical results criticized this particular study as coming from centers with less than ideal surgery. However, surgery as practiced in the participating centers was at least as good as, and, probably much better than, the "average" results across the country. This is a major problem in the interpretation for any randomized surgical trial. In applying results, the practitioner really needs to know the surgical results specifically in the center where his or her patients are referred. If the study is not performed in the center with the best results, it can be criticized for not giving surgery a fair shake. The same must be true for medical therapy. Studies should be performed comparing the best surgery with the best medicine to evaluate the potential best therapy. Results may also be beneficial if one compares average surgery with average medicine to allow the practitioner who refers to the "average" center to be able to compare results.

Comparisons of the NHLBI trial with the VA trial of unstable angina are shown in Table 3. There are remarkable similarities between the patient populations included in the two large randomized studies. Although women were included in the NHLBI study, the majority of patients in this study and all patients in the VA study were men. Clinical angiographic and early outcome characteristics of the 288 randomized patients in the NHLBI study and the 468 randomized patients in the VA study are strikingly comparable. It should be emphasized that the inclusion criteria for both studies were relatively similar [i.e., patients admitted to coronary care units with "unstable angina" (90% of whom had rest pain) with transient ECG changes required] and the exclusion criteria for both studies were relatively similar (age over 70 years, left main disease, normal coronaries or "inoperable" disease, or ejection fraction less than 30%). The VA study had the foresight to keep records on all patients initially screened as potential candidates. Of the 3159 patients screened, 2433 were excluded on clinical criteria and an additional 258 were excluded on arteriographic criteria. Thus, 468 patients, or 14.8% of the 3159 patients screened, were eventually randomized. Similar records over the length of the study were not kept for the NHLBI study. Exactly how representative this randomized patient population is in relation to the average patient with the same clinical problem remains unknown.

Therapy for acute coronary syndromes has evolved substantially since these trials were performed (7–9). Both surgical and medical therapy have advanced considerably. Surgical advances include use of internal mammary arteries as the conduit of choice, the use of cold cardioplegia and ventricular assist devices, and the use of antiplatelet agents in an attempt to maintain graft patency. Medical advances include use of aspirin and antiplatelet agents to abort unstable angina, more widespread use of calcium-channel-blocking drugs, intravenous nitroglycerin, heparin, and selective beta-blocking drugs, as well as the selective use of percutaneous intraaortic balloon counterpulsation. Although results are somewhat disappointing, the use of thrombolytic therapy continues to be evaluated as primary therapy for unstable angina. The role of coronary angioplasty in the acute setting also remains to be determined (11). The availability of these additional therapeutic modalities needs to be taken into account in the design of any future prospective randomized trials of unstable angina. Since the impact of many of these therapies is unclear with respect to mortality, morbidity, and symptomatic status of patients with unstable angina, they will need to be controlled for in any future study. Since practice patterns often vary from center to center, a consensus will have to be achieved among participating centers as to standardized therapy. Remembering the difficulties in getting a small number of centers participating in the NHLBI study to agree on such simple therapy as heparin versus no heparin, there may be difficulty in arriving at a consensus with regard to the numerous and various therapeutic modalities now available.

A future prospective trial of unstable angina may have to have numerous limbs comparing CABG, thrombolytic therapy, optimal medical therapy, and percutaneous coronary transluminal angioplasty. Stratification of patients with respect to clinical syndrome and arteriographic findings, including complexity and location of the "culprit" lesion, may also be important.

The terminology and clinical definitions remain somewhat elusive (12). Patients with new-onset or crescendo angina have been included with those with rest pain (which may be acute, subacute, de novo, superimposed on chronic stable angina, or following acute myocardial infarction). Each of these presentations may have differing pathophysiological mechanisms, prognoses, and responses to therapy. Clear-cut definitions and stratifications of various clinical subgroups are recommended in future prospective trials.

SUMMARY

In summary, the NHLBI-sponsored National Cooperative Study of Unstable Angina randomized a large number of patients from nine centers in the early to mid-1970s to urgent CABG versus medical management. The results failed to demonstrate a survival benefit for urgent surgery.

The NHLBI study has been criticized with respect to:

1. Problems with clinical definitions
2. Concern that the patient population was not representative
3. Less than ideal surgical therapy
4. Relatively short follow-up
5. Large percentage of crossover patients making interpretation of long-term results difficult.

Despite these and other limitations, this early large randomized study is a model for further prospective trials.

REFERENCES

1. Cooperative Unstable Angina Study Group. Unstable angina pectoris: National Cooperative Study Group to Compare Medical and Surgical Therapy. I. A report of protocol and patient populations. Am J Cardiol 1976; 37:896–902.
2. Cooperative Unstable Angina Study Group. Unstable angina pectoris: National Cooperative Study Group to Compare Medical and Surgical Therapy. II. In-hospital experience and initial follow-up results in patients. Am J Cardiol. 1978; 42;839–48.
3. Cooperative Unstable Angina Study Group. Unstable angina pectoris: National Cooperative Study Group to Compare Medical and Surgical Therapy. III. Results in patients with S-T segment elevation during pain. Am J Cardiol 1980; 45:819–24.
4. Cooperative Unstable Angina Study Group. Unstable angina pectoris: National Cooperative Study Group to Compare Medical and Surgical Therapy. IV. Results in patients with left anterior descending coronary artery disease. Am J Cardiol 1981; 48:517–24.
5. Luchi RJ, Scott SM, Deupree RA, and the investigators and their associates of a VA Cooperative Study. Comparison of medical and surgical treatment for unstable angina pectoris: Results of a Veterans Administration Cooperative Study. N Eng J Med 1987; 316:977–84.
6. Parisi AF, Khuri S, Deupree RH, Sharma GVRK, Scott SM, Luchi RJ. Medical compared with surgical management of unstable angina—5-year mortality and morbidity in the Veterans Administration Study. Circulation 1989; 80:1176–89.
7. Lubsen J. Medical management of unstable angina—What have we learned from the randomized trials? Circulation 1989; 82:II82–7.

8. Broadhurst P, Raftery ED. Unstable angina: Pathophysiologic concepts and therapeutic options. Int J Cardiol 1989; 24:1–7.
9. Bashour TT, Myler RK, Andrea GE, Stertzer SH, Clark DA, Ryan CJM. Current concepts in unstable myocardial ischemia. Am Heart J 1988; 115:850–61.
10. Plotnick GD. The role of coronary artery bypass graft surgery. In: Plotnick GD, ed. Unstable angina. Chapter 3. Mt. Kisco, NY: Futura, 1985:49–92.
11. Myler RK, Shaw RE, Stertzer SH, Bashour TT, Ryan C, Hecht HS, Cumberland DC. Unstable angina and coronary angioplasty. Circulation 1989; 82:II88–95.
12. Braunwald E. Unstable angina—A classification. Circulation 1989; 80:410–4.

10

The Veterans Affairs Surgical Registry
Identification of the High-Risk Surgical Patient

Frederick L. Grover

Veterans Affairs Medical Center
Denver, Colorado

BACKGROUND

Since 1971, the Department of Veterans Affairs (VA) has had a quality assurance committee for cardiac surgery, which has reviewed the volume and mortality at each of the approximately 45 VA cardiac surgery programs. This Committee, known as the VA Cardiac Surgery Consultants Committee, meets twice yearly to review each 6 months' statistics for the individual hospitals. The Committee is composed of six cardiothoracic surgeons (three primarily VA surgeons, three university surgeons) and three cardiologists, two of whom are university and one of whom is VA. The program directors of each of the cardiothoracic surgical services fill out a one-page form (Fig. 1). The mortality and volume data for each 6-month period are compiled, and hospitals that have two times or greater than the average mortality for that 6-month period or a mortality for coronary artery bypass procedures of two times or greater than the average for the 6-month period are required to submit paper audits of those deaths to the Committee. In addition, hospitals that have a mortality rate of greater than 5% for any consecutive 2-year period for primary (not reoperation) coronary bypass procedures also must submit paper audits of those deaths. Hospitals that experience two consecutive 6-month periods during which they meet the above criteria for paper audits are also site visited by two members of the Committee, one cardiologist and one cardiothoracic surgeon, to evaluate potential problems at that institution. In addition, site visits are also carried out in those instances where paper audits

VA **Veterans Administration**		**SEMI-ANNUAL REPORT OF CARDIAC SURGERY ON VETERANS** (M-2 PART 14, CHAPTER 8)			*REPORTS CONTROL SYMBOL* 10-0123

RETURN TO	DIRECTOR SURGICAL SERVICE VA CENTRAL OFFICE (112) WASHINGTON, D.C. 20420	NAME AND LOCATION OF FACILITY
		SIGNATURE AND TITLE OF REPORTING OFFICIAL

PERIOD COVERED BY THIS SEMI-ANNUAL REPORT		NUMBER OF PROCEDURES	NUMBER OF OPERATIVE OR POST OPERATIVE DEATHS (Within 30 days of operation)
FROM	TO	(1)	(2)
A. Number of Cardiac Procedures Performed on Veteran Patients Using Cardiopulmonary Bypass			
1. Aortic Valve Replacement (AVR) Alone			
2. AVR with Coronary Artery Bypass Graft (CABG)			
3. Mitral Valve Replacement Alone (MVR)			
4. MVR with CABG			
5. AVR plus MVR, Without CABG			
6. AVR plus MVR, with CABG			
7. Other Valve Operations Without CABG			
8. Other Valve Operations with CABG			
9. CABG: Single Bypass Graft			
a. # Primary_____ # Deaths_____			
b. # Redo_____ # Deaths_____			
10. CABG: Multiple Bypass Grafts			
a. # Primary_____ # Deaths_____			
b. # Redo_____ # Deaths_____			
11. Operations on Left Ventricle (LV) Alone: (Aneurysmectomy, Plication, Infarctectomy)			
12. Operations on LV with CABG			
13. Other Cardiac Operations with or without CABG **			
14. Operations on Great Vessels Requiring Extracorporeal Circulation			
TOTAL			
B. For Procedures Reported in above:			
1. Number of Procedures Performed on Veterans:			
a. By VA Surgical Teams:			
b. By University Surgical Teams:			
c. By Combined Surgical Teams:			
2. Number of Procedures Performed on Veterans in the following locations:			
a. Your VA Hospital			
b. Affiliated University Hospital:			
c. Other Facility:			
C. Number of Cardiac Procedures, not reported above by VA Surgeons on non-veterans in Affiliated Hospital:			
D. Current Backlog of Open Heart Operations: (At end of reporting period.)			
E. Estimated Volume of Open Heart Operations for Next Fiscal Year:			
F. Number of fully-trained Staff Surgeons performing Cardiac Surgery during this period (Include consultants and attendings; exclude residents)			

* This is defined as a death occurring within 30 days of surgery, or, if later, as a direct result of complication of the operative procedure.

   ** Of total cases in A., 13., above, denote # of Cardiac Transplants _____/Deaths_____

      and # of Elective Physiologic Operations (Excluding Pacemakers): _____/Deaths_____

NOTE: Original plus one copy to be sent to VACO (112).

VA FORM 10-2192	SUPERSEDES VA FORM 10 2'92. JAN 1983.

Figure 1 Semiannual report of cardiac surgery. This form is completed semiannually by each of the VA cardiac surgery program directors and is submitted to the VA Central Office for the purposes of quality assurance. Only volume and raw mortality data are collected on this form.

reveal severe enough problems to warrant earlier closer scrutiny or at the request of the local facility or region. Based on the site visit report, the Committee may place a program on probation and eventually, if significant improvement is not made, may recommend closure.

It has become increasingly apparent to the VA Cardiac Surgical Consultants Committee, however, that raw mortality statistics are an inadequate means by which to determine the quality of cardiac surgery, and in order to adequately and fairly assess the quality of cardiac surgery, the risk of the patient population and not just raw mortality data must be taken into consideration. Indeed, many studies have identified important risk factors in patients undergoing myocardial revascularization (1–7). Risk factors also change from year to year, and recently there has been an increase in the preoperative risk factors of patients undergoing myocardial revascularization. The patients now tend to be older, there are more reoperations, and their disease tends to be more diffuse (8,9). As Kouchoukas and his colleagues noted (10): "Analyses incorporating these and possibly other variables [preoperative risk variables] permit stratification and identification of subgroups of patients that are of different levels of risk for coronary artery surgery. Such analyses will also permit computation of risk models and expected operative mortality rates. Comparison of these expected or predicted operative mortality rates with observed mortality rates from different institutions will provide a more meaningful assessment of quality of care than the data provided by HCFA."

The VA Cardiac Surgical Consultants Committee agreed with the importance of preoperative risk assessment and felt that the continued use of unadjusted operative mortality data for quality of care assessment could have an adverse ethical effect on the judgment of cardiothoracic surgeons, causing them to possibly deny operative treatment for very high-risk patients whose only real chance for survival would be surgical treatment. The Committee therefore requested and was authorized by the VA to perform a risk assessment study for VA Cardiac Surgery. Results of the initial 2 years of this study, from April 1, 1987, through March 31, 1989, were published in 1990 and will be reviewed here (11).

During that 24-month period, 14,475 cardiac surgical procedures were performed at 48 hospitals and 10,480 forms were received from 47 of the 48 hospitals. A total of 8567 patients underwent coronary artery bypass grafting, with 414 (4.8%) deaths. Each VA Cardiac Surgical Center was asked to complete a single-page data form on every patient undergoing cardiac surgical or great-vessel operation who was placed on cardiopulmonary bypass (Fig. 2). Clinical data, cardiac catheterization and angiographic data, operative data, and outcome data, including death and significant morbidities, were collected.

Clinical data included: age, sex, race, height, weight, type of angina, presence of associated diseases, including chronic obstructive pulmonary disease, diabetes, peripheral vascular and cerebral vascular disease, hypertension, smok-

CARDIAC SURGERY OPERATIVE RISK ASSESSMENT

Name_____, Hosp.* _ _ _, SSN _ _ _ _ _ _ _ _ _, Surg. Date _ _ _ _ _ _
    Last   First   Mo. Day Yr.

I. CLINICAL DATA

Age _ _ yrs	Angioplasty=< 7 d of surg* Y N	Preop IABP* Y N
Sex M F	Prior Heart Surgery* Y N	NYHA F. C.* I II III IV
Height ___cm, ___in	History of CHF Y N	Hypertension* Y N
Weight ___kg, ___lbs	I. V. NTG Preoperatively* Y N	Pulmonary Rales Y N
Exertional Angina*Y N	Current Diuretic Use* Y N	Resting ST Depression*Y N
Unstable Angina Y N	Current Dig Use* Y N	ECG LVH* Y N
COPD* Y N	Current Beta Blocker Use* Y N	Cardiomegaly (x-ray)* Y N
Current Smoker Y N	Current Ca++ Blocker Use* Y N	Pleural Effusion Y N
Ever Smoker Y N	Peripheral Vasc. Dis.* Y N	Creatinine _ . _ mg/dl
Active Endo-	Cerebral Vasc. Dis.* Y N	Pa02 (room air) _ _ mm Hg
carditis* Y N	Old MI (>30 d.)* Y N	PaCO2 (room air) _ _ mm Hg
Diabetes Y N	Recent MI (=<30 d.)* Y N	FEV1 (L) _ . _ L

Race: __Caucasian, __Black, __Other   General Medical Condition:* __Good, __Fair, __Poor

II. CARDIAC CATHETERIZATION AND ANGIOGRAPHIC DATA

L.V. Systolic Pressure	_ _ _ mmHg	Right Atrial Pressure (mean) _ _ mmHg
Aortic Systolic Pressure	_ _ _ mmHg	LVEDP _ _ mmHg
Pulmonary Artery Systolic Pressure	_ _ _ mmHg	Cardiac Index _ . _ L/min/M
Mean Pulmonary Artery Wedge Pressure	_ _ mmHg	LV EF (cath. or radionuclide) 0._ _
		LV End-diastolic Vol. _ _ _ ml

Coronary Arteriogram (record most severe % diameter reduction; code distal disease as 0 - none, 1 - moderate, 2 - severe)

LV Contraction Score from Contrast or Radionuclide Angiogram (NL - normal, MH - moderate hypokinesia, SH - severe hypokinesia, AK- akinesia, DY - dyskinesia, AN - aneurysmal; check one per segment):

	% Stenosis	Distal Disease
Left Main	_ _ _	
LAD	_ _ _	_
Right (include PDA)	_ _ _	_
Circ (include major marginals)	_ _ _	_

Segment (RAO)	NL	MH	SH	AK	DY	AN
Prox Ant	_	_	_	_	_	_
Mid Ant	_	_	_	_	_	_
Apical	_	_	_	_	_	_
Mid Inf	_	_	_	_	_	_
Prox Inf	_	_	_	_	_	_

Preoperative Estimate of Operative Mortality _ _ %

Priority of Surgery: EL UR EM
(EL-elective, UR-urgent, EM-emergent)

III. OPERATIVE DATA

A. Procedure(s)

CABG Distal Anastomoses:		
number with Vein	_ _	Mitral Valve Replacement Y N
number with IMA	_ _	Aortic Valve Replacement Y N
Great Vessel Repair Requiring		Tricuspid Valve Replacement Y N
Cardiopulmonary Bypass	Y N	Valve Repair Y N
Cardiac Transplant	Y N	LV Aneurysectomy or Plication Y N
		Other_____

B. Technique

Total Cross Clamp Time	_ _ _ min	Intra-op IABP Y N
Lowest Myocardial Temp	_ _ C	Post-op IABP Y N

C. Operative Death*   Y N

Date of Operative Death _ _ _ _ _ _
                     Mo. Day Yr.

D. Postoperative (30 day) Complications

Perioperative MI (new Q waves)	Y N	Reoperation for Bleeding Y N
Endocarditis	Y N	Repeat Cardiopulmonary Bypass Y N
Renal Failure Requiring Dialysis	Y N	On Ventilator => 48 Hr Y N
Low Cardiac Output State =>6 Hr	Y N	Coma => 24 Hr Y N
Mediastinitis	Y N	Stroke Y N

Figure 2 Cardiac surgery operative risk assessment data collection form. This single-page data form is filled out on every patient undergoing cardiac surgery or an operation on the great vessels requiring cardiopulmonary bypass and is submitted after the 30th postoperative day for entry of data into the risk assessment study.

ing history, prior heart surgery, angioplasty, history of congestive heart failure, cardiac drugs, myocardial infarction history, preoperative intra-aortic balloon pump, New York Heart Association functional class, electrocardiographic (EKG) and chest x-ray findings, creatinine, arterial blood gases, and FEV_1. Also included were the physician's estimate of the general medical condition, preoperative estimate of operative mortality, and whether the surgery was elective, urgent, or emergent. Invasive data collected included: right- and left-sided cardiac pressures, cardiac index, left ventricular ejection fraction, coronary angiographic data, and left ventricular contraction score. Operative data collected included the number of coronary anastomoses, the type of conduit, other cardiac procedures, ischemic time, myocardial temperature, and whether or not intraoperative or postoperative intra-aortic balloon pumping was necessary. Outcome data included operative mortality defined as death within 30 days of the procedure or complication resulting from the operative procedure. The following 30-day postoperative complications were recorded: perioperative myocardial infarction, endocarditis, renal failure requiring dialysis, low cardiac output, mediastinitis, reoperation for bleeding, repeat cardiopulmonary bypass, ventilator therapy greater than 48 hr, coma for longer than 24 hr, and stroke.

These data were collected twice yearly prior to each semiannual Cardiac Surgery Consultants Committee meeting. They were analyzed in such a fashion as to access the performance of each VA Cardiac Surgical Center and to identify the variables predictive of operative mortality. The prognostic variables were identified separately for coronary artery bypass grafting patients and for valve operation patients and for those undergoing other cardiac surgical procedures with or without coronary artery bypass grafting.

METHODS OF DATA ANALYSIS

The analyses were performed in two stages, the first a univariate screening process followed by a multivariate, stepwise logistic regression analysis. Continuous variables were measured for the difference between means and discrete variable for the distribution for operative survivors and deaths. These were tested with students t test for paired data and X^2 statistic, respectively. Variables that had a value of less than 0.2 were then entered into the logistic regression analysis for which the dependent variable was operative death. Variables with a p value of less than 0.05 were considered to be statistically significant for the logistic regression analysis.

RESULTS

Results for the purpose of this review will be confined to those concerning coronary artery bypass grafting procedures. During the 2-year period from April 1, 1987, through March 31, 1989, 8569 patients underwent coronary artery

Table 1 Variables Found to Be Significant by Univariate Analysis

Variable	Survivors			Nonsurvivors			p value
	No.	Mean	± SD	No.	Mean	± SD	
Age	8,136	61.0	8.0	412	63.2	7.8	0.002
Weight (kg)	7,877	82.67	14.04	390	80.64	15.17	0.009
BSA (m^2)	7,856	1.96	0.2	389	1.94	0.18	0.007
Creatinine	6,925	112.27	70.72	339	123.76	44.2	0.023
[μmol/L (mg/dL)]		(1.27)	(0.8)		(1.4)	(0.5)	
PaO$_2$ (mm Hg)	2,943	79.2	11.9	154	77.2	13.0	0.042
FEV$_1$	2,481	2.7	0.7	104	2.4	0.7	0.001
Height (cm)	7,859	172.5	7.75	389	171.75	7.25	0.084
PaCO$_2$	2,994	37.1	6.0	158	36.6	5.0	0.252
LV systolic pressure (mmHg)	5,247	131.1	23.4	245	135.8	25.9	0.003
Aortic systolic pressure (mmHg)	5,317	130.6	23.6	256	135.6	26.1	0.001
PA systolic pressure (mmHg)	1,789	30.1	11.0	101	32.4	11.4	0.047
PA wedge pressure (mmHg)	1,804	13.1	6.5	107	14.9	7.6	0.005

						p
Cardiac index (L/min/m²)	1,787	2.9	1.0	100	2.6	0.7	0.001
LV ejection fraction	6,525	0.54	0.14	337	0.50	0.15	0.001
Left main stenosis (%)	5,626	23.1	32.1	289	36.4	37.9	0.001
LAD stenosis (%)	7,424	82.7	21.0	362	86.0	19.9	0.008
Right (with PDA) stenosis (%)	7,241	82.3	27.2	361	86.9	22.8	0.006
Circumflex (with marginals) stenosis (%)	7,063	75.5	29.0	352	79.3	26.2	0.017
MD's estimate of operative mortality (%)	6,315	4.9	4.8	322	10.0	11.6	0.001
Distal disease score	4,615	1.8	1.8	231	2.3	1.9	0.001
LV contraction score	6,322	8.3	3.6	290	9.5	4.1	0.002
LVEDP (mm Hg)	5,152	15.9	7.8	240	17.0	8.6	0.051
Right atrial pressure (mm Hg)	1,629	6.5	4.1	93	6.6	4.2	0.722
LVEDV (mL)	1,633	144.3	58.5	69	148.1	64.1	0.596

[a] During the 2-year period of this study, 8569 patients underwent coronary artery bypass grafting; 414 (4.8%) died.
BSA = body surface area; FEV_1 = forced expiratory volume in 1 sec; LAD = left anterior descending coronary artery; LV = left ventricular; LVEDP = left ventricular end-diastolic pressure; LVEDV = left ventricular end-diastolic volume; MD = surgeon or cardiologist; PA = pulmonary artery; $PaCO_2$ = arterial carbon dioxide tension; PaO_2 = arterial oxygen tension; PDA = posterior descending coronary artery; SD = standard deviation.

bypass grafting, with an operative mortality of 4.8%. Data were collected on 72% of patients who underwent operation. Those continuous variables that were found to be significant ($p < 0.05$) by univariate analysis are listed in Table 1. Variables with a p value of less than 0.01 are greater age, lower body weight, lower body surface area, lower FEV_1, higher left ventricular (LV) systolic pressure, higher aortic systolic pressure, higher pulmonary artery wedge pressure, lower cardiac index, lower ejection fraction, the presence of left main stenosis, the presence of LAD stenosis, the presence of right with PDA stenosis, the physician's estimate of operative mortality being higher, more severe distal disease, and decreased LV function as determined by the LV contraction score. Those that were significant with a p value of less than 0.05 but greater than 0.01 were increased creatinine, decreased PAO_2, increased PA systolic pressure, and the presence of circumflex stenosis.

The effects of age, weight, FEV_1, LV ejection fraction, and LV contraction score are shown in Figures 3–7. Of interest is the fact that an age of greater than 80 years carries an operative mortality of 11.4% versus a 4.8% mortality in patients under 80 years (Fig. 3). A patient weighing less than 130 lb (58.5 kg) has an operative mortality of 9.6%, compared to a patient who weighs more than 130 lb, whose operative mortality is 4.6% (Fig. 4). A patient whose forced expiratory volume in 1 sec is less than 1.25 liters has an operative mortality of

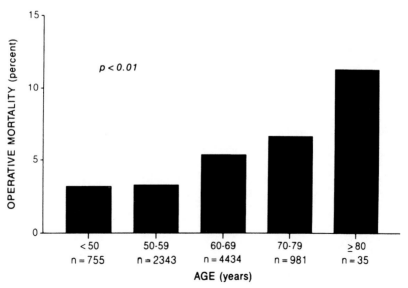

Figure 3 Coronary artery bypass surgery—effect of age on operative mortality. A marked increase in operative mortality for patients 80 years of age or older (11.4%) versus younger patients (4.8%) is noted.

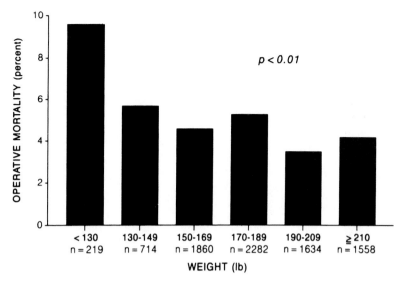

Figure 4 Coronary artery bypass surgery—effect of weight on operative mortality. Low weight, less than 58.5 kg (130 lb), was associated with a greater operative mortality than greater weight and obesity.

11.7%, compared to an operative mortality of 3.8% for those with an FEV_1 of greater than 1.25 liters (Fig. 5). Patients whose ejection fraction is less than 20% have an operative mortality of 13.8% versus an operative mortality of 4.9% if the LV ejection fraction is greater than 20% (Fig. 6). Those with a contraction score of less than 15 have an operative mortality of 4%, compared to an operative mortality of 8.3% if the contraction score is equal to or greater than 15 (Fig. 7).

Discrete variables that were predictive of operative mortality are listed in Table 2. Twenty of these variables were significant predictors of operative mortality by univariate analysis. The most significant ones, i.e., those that demonstrated a twofold or greater increase in operative mortality, are patients in whom intravenous nitroglycerin was given preoperatively (9.4% versus 3.8% operative mortality), those who had a previous cardiac operation (12.5% versus 3.9%), those patients who had pulmonary rales (12.0% versus 4.3%), those in whom an intra-aortic balloon pump was inserted preoperatively (15.8% versus 4.5%), those patients who are a New York Heart Classification IV versus I, II, or III (8.0% versus 3.3%), those whose operation was emergent instead of urgent or elective (12.6% versus 4.2%), patients who had a pleural effusion (16.7% versus 5.2%), and those whose general medical condition was felt to be poor rather than fair or good (18.8% versus 3.8%).

Table 3 lists the discrete variables that were not predictive of operative mortality by univariate analysis. Of this group, it is noteworthy that diabetes,

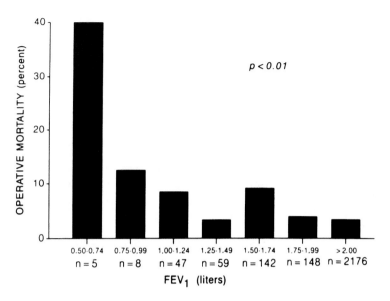

Figure 5 Coronary artery bypass surgery—effect of forced expiratory volume in 1 sec (FEV₁) on operative mortality. Operative mortality on patients with a FEV₁ of less than 1.25 liters/sec was 11.7%, compared to 3.8% for those who had a FEV₁ of greater than 1.25 liters/sec.

smoking history, and the presence of LV hypertrophy of EKG were almost of statistical significance.

Those variables with a *p* value of less than 0.2 by univariate analysis and with less than 20% of data missing were entered into a stepwise logistic regression analysis as shown in Figures 8 and 9. Figure 8 shows a combination of univariate and logistic regression analysis of noninvasive variables reflecting both the chronic and acute status of patients undergoing coronary artery bypass surgery. Those with a univariate analysis of significance of less than 0.2 are shown in the upper two boxes, reflecting chronic status on the left and acute status on the right. Those variables which were significant with a *p* value of less than 0.05 after the multivariate analysis are listed in the second two boxes. These variables were combined and a third logistic regression analysis was performed to get the final noninvasive model as depicted in the lowest box. Variables are listed in the order of significance in all boxes. Those noninvasive variables which were found to be statistically significant are prior heart surgery, priority of surgery, New York Heart Association Functional Class, presence of peripheral vascular disease, increased age, presence of pulmonary rales, and current diuretic use. Figure 9 illustrates the model used for analyzing both noninvasive and invasive variables. Four invasive variables that had less than 20% missing data were

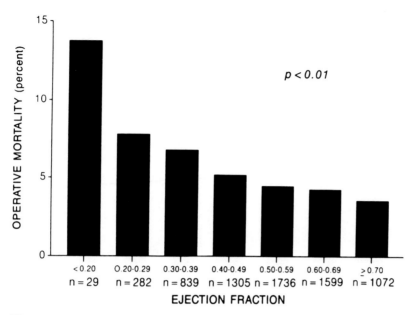

Figure 6 Coronary artery bypass surgery—effect of ejection fraction on operative mortality. A progressive increase of operative mortality was correlated with a decrease in ejection fraction, with a 13.8% operative mortality occurring in patients with an ejection fraction of less than 0.20.

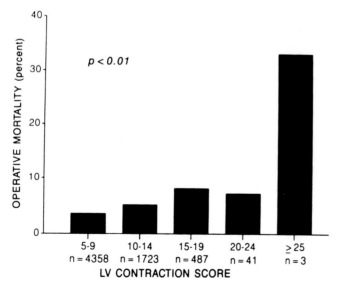

Figure 7 Coronary artery bypass surgery—effect of LV contraction score on operative mortality. Higher contraction scores correlated with increased operative mortality, with those patients having a score of 15 or greater having an operative mortality of 8.3%, compared to 4% for those whose score was less than 15.

167

Table 2 Discrete Variables That Were Predictive of Operative Mortality

Variable	Variable absent			Variable present			
	No. of patients	Operative deaths	%	No. of patients	Operative deaths	%	p value
COPD	6,048	262	4.3	2,092	134	6.4	0.001
IV nitroglycerin preoperatively	6,546	247	3.8	1,477	139	9.4	0.001
Prior cardiac operation	7,645	299	3.9	888	111	12.5	0.001
History of CHF	7,092	304	4.3	1,176	97	8.2	0.001
Current diuretic use	5,958	234	3.9	2,063	146	7.1	0.001
Peripheral vascular disease	6,128	240	3.9	1,889	144	7.6	0.001
Cerebrovascular disease	6,850	293	4.3	1,165	91	7.8	0.001
Pulmonary rales	7,465	323	4.3	523	63	12.0	0.001
Resting ST depression	6,496	271	4.2	1,394	109	7.8	0.001
Preop IABP	8,028	363	4.5	279	44	15.8	0.001
Cardiomegaly (roentgenogram)	6,850	290	4.2	1,163	97	8.3	0.001
Old MI (> 30 days)	3,606	135	3.7	4,482	249	5.6	0.001
Recent MI (< 30 days)	6,657	284	4.3	1,499	111	7.4	0.001
Rest angina	3,500	120	3.4	4,404	267	6.1	0.001
Exertional angina	622	18	2.9	7,425	364	4.9	0.024

NYHA functional class							
I				251	2	0.8	
II				1,555	36	2.3	
III				3,417	132	3.9	
IV				2,523	201	8.0	0.001[a]
Priority of operation							
Elective				5,229	183	3.5	
Urgent				2,149	127	5.9	
Emergent				634	80	12.6	0.001[b]
No. of stenotic vessels							
0				26	0	0	
1				448	10	2.2	
2				1,862	64	3.4	
3				4,443	255	5.7	0.001
Left main stenosis ≥ 50%	4,210	163	3.9	1,705	126	7.4	0.001
Pleural effusion	2,892	150	5.2	42	7	16.7	0.006
General medical condition							
Good				1,488	38	2.6	
Fair				1,826	87	4.8	
Poor				319	60	18.8	0.001[c]

[a] Significance: $p < 0.001$ for class IV versus classes I, II, and III.
[b] Significance: $p < 0.001$ for emergent priority versus urgent and elective priorities.
[c] Significance: $p < 0.001$ for poor general condition versus good and fair general condition.
CHF = congestive heart failure; COPD = chronic obstructive pulmonary disease; IABP = intraaortic balloon pump; IV = intravenous; MI = myocardial infarction; NYHA = New York Heart Association.

Table 3 Discrete Variables That Were Not Predictive of Operative Mortality by Univariate Analysis

Variable	Variable absent			Variable present			
	No. of patients	Operative deaths	%	No. of patients	Operative deaths	%	p value
Race							
White	—	—	—	7,410	345	4.7	0.104
Black	—	—	—	552	36	6.5	
Other	—	—	—	334	13	3.9	
Sex							
Male	—	—	—	8,477	408	4.8	0.726
Female	—	—	—	70	4	5.7	
Diabetes	6,065	275	4.5	1,994	111	5.6	0.061
Current smoking	4,686	208	4.4	3,379	174	5.1	0.138
Ever smoked	972	36	3.7	7,003	346	4.9	0.091
Active endocarditis	8,036	389	4.8	25	0	0	0.259
Operation within 7 days of angioplasty	8,119	390	4.8	240	15	6.3	0.304
Current digitalis use	7,089	324	4.6	939	53	5.6	0.144
Current β blocker use	3,633	168	4.6	4,361	212	4.9	0.620
Current Ca^{2+} blocker use	1,495	62	4.1	6,523	318	4.9	0.232
LV hypertrophy (ECG)	6,804	316	4.6	1,030	61	5.9	0.074
Hypertension	3,345	156	4.7	4,652	232	5.0	0.507

ECG = electrocardiogram; LV = left ventricular.

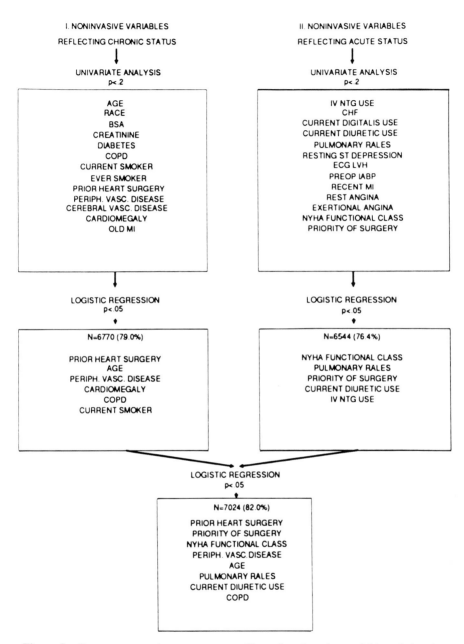

Figure 8 Coronary artery bypass surgery—effect of noninvasive variables of chronic and acute status on operative mortality. The lowest box lists the variables in order of significance after univariate and multivariate regression analysis (BSA = body surface area; CHF = congestive heart failure; COPD = chronic obstructive pulmonary disease; ECG = electrocardiographic; IABP = intraaortic balloon pump; IV = intravenous; LVH = left ventricular hypertrophy; MI = myocardial infarction; NTG = nitroglycerin; NYHA = New York Heart Association.

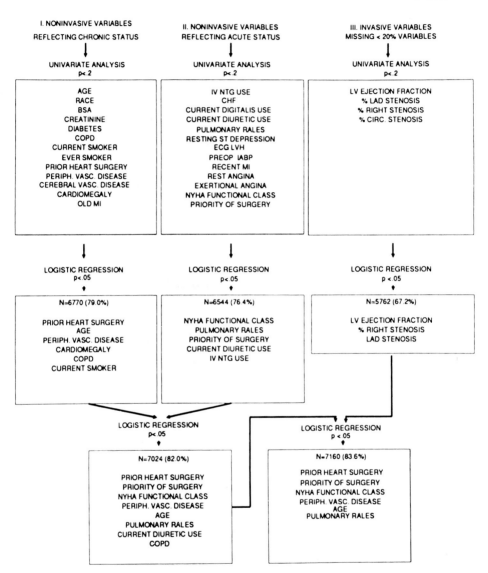

Figure 9 Coronary artery bypass surgery—effect of noninvasive and invasive variables of chronic and acute status on operative mortality using univariate and multivariate logistic regression analysis. The lower right box lists the variables in the order of their significance after the above analysis. LAD = left anterior descending coronary artery; LV = left ventricular; other abbreviations are the same as in Figure 8.

VA CARDIAC SURGERY RISK ASSESSMENT PROGRAM
A RESPONSE MUST BE PROVIDED FOR ALL DATA ITEMS
(For use beginning 9-1-90)

I. IDENTIFYING DATA   Surgery Date: Mo _ _ Day _ _ Yr _ _

Name_____, _____   Hosp Num _ _ _ SSN _ _ _ _ _ _ _ _ _ _
  Last   First

II. CLINICAL DATA

		PTCA:	None recent 12 hr - 72 hr < 12 hr of surg.
Sex	M F	Prior MI: None ≤ 7 days of surg. > 7 days of surg.	
Age	_ _ years	Prior heart surgery	Y N
COPD	Y N	Peripheral vascular disease	Y N
Cardiomegaly (x-ray)	Y N	NYHA functional class	I II III IV
Pulmonary rales	Y N	Current diuretic use	Y N
Current smoker	Y N	Current digoxin use	Y N
Creatinine	_._ mg/dl	IV NTG within 48 hr of surgery	Y N
Rest angina	Y N	Preoperative use of IABP	Y N

III. CARDIAC CATHETERIZATION AND ANGIOGRAPHIC DATA (Write NS for no study)

LVEDP   _ _ mm Hg LV Contraction Grade (from contrast or radionuclide
Aortic systolic pressure   _ _ _ mm Hg angiogram or 2D echo) CIRCLE APPROPRIATE GRADE
*PA systolic pressure   _ _ mm Hg
*PAW mean pressure   _ _ mm Hg
*patients having right heart cath.

Grade	Ejection Fraction Range	Definition
I	≥ 0.55	Normal
II	0.45-0.54	Mild dysfunction
III	0.35-0.44	Moderate dysfunction
IV	0.25-0.34	Severe dysfunction
V	< 0.25	Very severe dysfunction
?	unknown	No LV study

Left main stenosis   _ _ _%
Number of major coronaries
  with stenosis(es) ≥ 50%
  (left main, LAD, circ.,
  right) CIRCLE ONE   0 1 2 3

IV. OPERATIVE RISK SUMMARY DATA (MUST BE COMPLETED PREOPERATIVELY)

Physician's preoperative   General medical condition: good, fair, poor
estimate of operative mortality _ _%
DO NOT USE CALCULATED ESTIMATE   Surgical priority: elective, urgent, emergent

---

V. OPERATIVE DATA

A. Procedure(s)

CABG distal anastomoses:		Valve repair	Y N
number with vein	_	LV aneurysmectomy	Y N
number with IMA	_	Great vessel repair requiring	
Aortic valve replacement	Y N	cardiopulmonary bypass	Y N
Mitral valve replacement	Y N	Cardiac transplant	Y N
Tricuspid valve replacement	Y N	Electrophysiologic procedure	Y N

Miscellaneous cardiac procedures requiring cardiopulmonary bypass: (CIRCLE)
  ASD repair   Myxoma resection   Myectomy for IHSS   Other tumor resection
  VSD repair   Foreign body removal Pericardiectomy   Other procedure(s)

B. Operative Death   Y N   Date of death   _ _ _ _ _ _
                                                            Mo Day Yr

C. Perioperative (30 day) Complications

Perioperative MI	Y N	Reoperation for bleeding	Y N
Endocarditis	Y N	On ventilator ≥ 48 hr	Y N
Renal failure requiring		Repeat cardiopulmonary	
dialysis	Y N	bypass	Y N
Low cardiac output ≥ 6 hr	Y N	Coma ≥ 24 hr	Y N
Mediastinitis	Y N	Stroke	Y N

Figure 10   The simplified VA cardiac surgery risk assessment data form. This form is a simplified version of the original data form (Fig. 2). Many data items have been eliminated as a result of the initial analysis showing that these items were not significant predictors of operative mortality or morbidity.

significant by univariate analysis. These were, in the order of significance: LV ejection fraction, the presence of LAD stenosis, right stenosis, and circumflex stenosis. After logistic regression analysis, LV ejection fraction, right stenosis, and LAD stenosis were still significant. When entered into the final multivariant logistic regression analysis with the noninvasive variables, none of these were powerful enough to be predictors; i.e., they did not contribute additional prognostic information to those variables from the noninvasive model. From these data, estimated mortality by patient and by hospital can be calculated using the logit equation.

Based on the results of this study, many data items not found to be significant were deleted from the data form, thus simplifying it considerably. It is hoped that this simplified form will enhance the submission of data from each of the member hospitals. The revised data form is shown in Figure 10.

COMPARISON WITH RESULTS OF OTHER STUDIES

The above VA study is the largest and most contemporary database available on risk for the coronary artery bypass grafting procedure. In 1974, Hammermeister and Kennedy(1) examined preoperative exercise and hemodynamic and quantitative angiocardiographic variables as predictors of operative mortality in 160 patients. They found that operative mortality was significantly elevated in those patients who had an end-diastolic volume of greater than or equal to 103 ml/m^2, in those whose ejection fraction was less than or equal to 33%, and in those patients who had a LV end-diastolic pressure greater than or equal to 18 mmHg. Loop and his colleagues(2) in 1975 compared 60 patients who died following coronary artery bypass grafting procedures performed from 1967 to 1973 to 1188 patients who survived this operation in 1973. Twenty-six clinical, angiographic, and operative variables were analyzed by discriminate analysis to ascertain preoperative risk factors. Those factors found to be highly significant predictors of increased risk were marked cardiomegaly, uncompensated congestive heart failure, triple-vessel coronary artery disease, obstruction of the left main coronary artery, generalized impairment of left ventricular function, contraction or segmental wall motion abnormalities, and elevated left ventricular end-diastolic pressure. The most significant of these factors was congestive heart failure.

Kennedy and his colleagues(4) in 1980 reported on a review of 6176 patients from the CASS study who underwent coronary artery bypass grafting between August 1975 and December 1978 with an operative mortality of 2.3%. The authors performed a multivariate discriminate analysis of numerous clinical and angiographic variables after they had been analyzed in a univariate fashion. They found that the clinical variables most predictive of operative death were increased age, female sex, cardiomegaly, and congestive heart failure. Significant angiographic variables were left ventricular wall motion abnormalities and the presence of left main coronary disease. In addition, the priority of operation, i.e., elective versus urgent versus emergent, was also a significant predictor of operative mortality, with an increased mortality in the emergent/urgent group as opposed to the elective group. Using a discriminate analysis, the authors, found in descending order of importance, the following variables: increased age, left main coronary stenosis greater than or equal to 90%, female sex, ventricular wall motion abnormalities, an elevated LV end-diastolic pressure, and rales. In addition, the authors calculated the estimated mortality for individual patients based on clinical and angiographic characteristics and also did the same for each of the participating hospitals.

In 1981, in a further analysis of the CASS study mortality, Kennedy and his coauthors(3) noted an overall operative mortality of 2.3%. They found that mortality increased with age, going from 0 in the 20- to 29-year-old age group to 7.9% in the 70-year-old and older age group. Operative mortality was higher in women for each age group. Congestive heart failure was associated with an increased operative mortality, as was multivessel disease, with the mortality being 1.4% for one-vessel, 2.1% for two-vessel, and 2.8% for three-vessel disease. In the left main coronary artery stenotic subgroup, the operative mortality ranged from 1.6% for patients who had mild left main stenosis and a right dominant system to 25% in patients with severe left main stenosis. In addition, the authors noted that ejection fraction had a profound effect on operative mortality, with the mortality being 1.9% in those patients with an ejection fraction greater than or equal to 50%, but 6.7% in those whose ejection fraction was less than 19%. Operative mortality ranged from 1.7% for those patients who had the least abnormal LV wall motion score to 9.1% for those with the most abnormal score. Operative mortality was 1.7% for elective bypass versus 3.5% for urgent and 10.8% for emergent.

Fisher and his colleagues (12) in 1982 examined the effects of sex and physical size on operative mortality for coronary artery bypass surgery from the CASS data bank. They noted that following multivariate analysis, the physical size of the patient, including the coronary artery diameter, was predictive of operative mortality, after adjusting for differences in risk predicted by the basic variable and gender. They therefore concluded that a possible explanation for the increased risk of coronary artery bypass surgery in females was the fact that they are smaller and have smaller-diameter coronary arteries.

In 1983, Miller and his Stanford colleagues (13) compared patients who underwent coronary artery bypass grafting during the years 1971–1975 to those who were grafted from 1977 to 1979. Multiple variables were analyzed using univariate and multivariate logistic regression analysis. They found that emergency operation, left main coronary artery disease, congestive heart failure, hypertension, and mitral regurgitation were related to operative mortality in the first group, whereas only emergency operation and congestive heart failure were

independent determinants of operative mortality in the later group. They opti-
mistically felt at that time that in spite of the fact that the later group had higher
potential risks than the earlier group, the operative mortality had declined from
8.7% to 4.6%, thus indicating that the adverse effects of patient-related disease
variables had been neutralized by improvements in patient management. Similarly, in 1984 Cosgrove and his Cleveland Clinic colleagues (14) reported on
24,672 patients who underwent isolated coronary artery bypass grafting from
1970 to 1982. They divided this large group into four groups: group 1—patients
operated on from 1970 to 1973, group 2—from 1974 to 1976, group 3—from
1977 to 1979, and group 4—from 1980 to 1982. Their overall operative mortality was 1.2%, with an operative mortality of 1.2%, 1.4%, 1.6%, and 0.8% for
groups 1–4, respectively. Group 4's mortality was significantly lower in spite of
increased risk factors. Those factors which were significant predictors of operative mortality were: emergency operation, congestive heart failure, left main
disease, female sex, increased age, normothermic arrest, increased number of
grafts, poor LV function, and incomplete revascularization. Congestive heart
failure replaced emergency operation as a principal risk factor, and left main
disease, the number of grafts, and poor ventricular function were neutralized as
risk factors. Thus Cosgrove and his colleagues were also optimistic that despite
increased risk factors, the quality of care was more than keeping up and operative
mortality was decreasing.

McCormick and his colleagues reviewed the CASS experience in patients
who underwent coronary artery bypass surgery for unstable angina (6). They
analyzed data from 3311 patients who were operated on for unstable angina and
who had an overall operative mortality of 3.9%. There was no difference in the
various subsets of unstable angina patients for operative mortality between the
coronary insufficiency group, new-onset angina group, rest angina, or those who
had changing patterns of angina. The logistic regression analysis demonstrated
that age, LV score, and the presence of left main stenosis with a left dominant
circulation were indicators of increased operative mortality. They also noted that
the operative mortality of patients who underwent coronary artery bypass grafting during their initial hospitalization with unstable angina was similar to that of
those who were discharged and readmitted at a later date.

Kouchoukos and his colleagues (15) compared operative mortality in patients
undergoing coronary artery bypass surgery from 1970 to 1973 to those undergoing it from 1974 to 1977. The operative mortality in the first period was 2.7%,
compared to 1.2% in the second period. The incidence of probable myocardial
perioperative myocardial infarction decreased from 11.4% to 2.4%. At the same
time, however, the incidence of three-vessel disease increased from 42% to 54%
and the mean number of vessels grafted per patient increased from 1.9% to
2.9%. The percentage of patients with unstable angina, congestive heart failure,
left main coronary artery disease, and angiographic evidence of LV dysfunction

was similar for the two time periods. Kouchoukos et al. also concluded that improved quality of care of patients, including anesthesia, surgical techniques, intraoperative myocardial preservation, as well as preoperative stabilization of patients with unstable angina, counterbalanced the risk factors.

In 1987, Wright el al. (7) reviewed the Loyola experience. Fifty clinical and angiographic variables were analyzed initially univariately and 22 were then subjected to multivariate discriminate analysis. It was found that in patients undergoing elective coronary artery bypass surgery, the variables predictive of operative mortality were: age greater than 70, severe stenosis of more than six vessels, diffuse disease, positive family history, and increasing number of coronaries bypassed.

In 1988, Naunheim and his colleagues at St. Louis University (8) reported on a reversal of the improved survival that the Cleveland Clinic, Kouchoukos, and others had reported in the late 1970s and early 1980s. Naunheim's group compared the first 100 consecutive patients undergoing coronary artery bypass surgery in 1975 to an identically selected group from 1985 and found that there was a significant worsening of the preoperative condition in that time interval. The patients were older, there was a higher incidence of congestive heart failure and LV dysfunction, a greater severity of coronary artery disease, and a higher incidence of emergency operation. In addition, more patients in their 1985 group had associated medical problems such as diabetes and chronic lung disease, and there was an increase in vascular diseases, including hypertension, renal dysfunction, and peripheral vascular and cerebral vascular disease. The operative mortality increased from 1% in 1975 to 8% in 1985. The significant increase in operative mortality was mainly due to an increased incidence of emergency operations. The operative mortality for elective coronary artery bypass surgery was similar in both time periods.

In 1989, Naunheim et al. (16) reviewed the pertinent risk factors involved in the subgroup of patients undergoing emergency coronary artery bypass grafting for failed angioplasty. They found that the angioplasty group had a lower risk profile shown by a lower mean age, less diseased vessels, better ventricular function, fewer left main stenosis, and few patients with acute ischemia requiring an intravenous administration of nitroglycerin. However, in spite of this relatively good risk group, they had a higher operative mortality rate of 11% versus 1%, as well as a higher incidence of perioperative infarction. A multivariate analysis, however, demonstrated that LV function score, the need for ionotropic support after the angioplasty failure but prior to surgery, and increasing age were independent predictors of operative mortality in the group with failed angioplasty who required surgery.

In 1988, Conner and his colleagues (17) at the Mayo Clinic reviewed the operative risks of coronary artery bypass grafting after failed angioplasty procedures. They found that in those patients requiring coronary artery bypass grafting within 24 hr of an unsuccessful percutaneous coronary artery angioplasty, the operative mortality was 2.7% and that the risk was significantly increased among those patients who were hemodynamically unstable or had a new occlusion or further narrowing of the dilated vessel (3.8% versus 0%).

In 1989, Naunheim et al. (18) reviewed the preoperative risk factors in patients with unstable angina who had to undergo coronary artery bypass grafting. In this group of patients the operative mortality was 6.2%. Univariate analyses revealed that age, cross-clamp time, and cardiopulmonary bypass time were significant factors predictive of death. But after multivariate analyses, only age remained a predicting factor.

Ottino's group from Turin, Italy (19), analyzed risk factors for operative mortality and aortocoronary bypass surgical patients in 1990, including 437 consecutive patients, and found that significant risk factors of operative mortality were age and cross-clamp time after stepwise logistic regression. In addition, a decrease in LV ejection fraction was very close to statistical significance (p = 0.06). Mattila and colleagues from Helsinki (20) in 1990 reviewed 202 consecutive patients with coronary bypass grafting and found that by univariate analysis, patients with critical left main coronary stenosis and an LV ejection fraction of less than 30% were at greater risk for operative death. In addition, these factors remained significant after multivariate analysis, with a 2.6- and 2.8-fold increase in mortality, respectively. Huysmans and van Ark from The Netherlands (21) found, in a study of 220 patients greater than 70 years of age, that mortality was related to preoperative hypertension, prior myocardial infarction, and the severity of coronary artery disease.

In 1990, Hannan et al. (22) reported data from the New York State new cardiac surgery reporting system. Although this study analyzes the risk factors in terms of all cardiac surgical procedures, not just coronary artery bypass procedures, the coronary bypass procedure group comprised about 75% of the total group. Significant risk factors for operative mortality noted were: increased age, female gender, decreased ejection fraction, previous myocardial infarction, increasing number of previous open heart operations, diabetes requiring medication, dialysis, renal failure, cardiogenic shock, unstable angina, intractable congestive heart failure, and greater than 90% left main stenosis.

The results of the VA study confirm many of the risk factors noted in the above studies. Increased age was noted by the VA study as a significant predictor of mortality. Decreased weight and body surface area were also found to be significant predictors, as reported before. The VA study, however, documented that the presence of chronic obstructive pulmonary disease and a decreased forced expiratory volume in 1 sec was associated with a higher operative mortality. Hypertension was also noted to be a predictor of operative mortality, as was a decreased ejection fraction, as many other studies have also reported.

The same is true for the presence of left main coronary disease and an abnormal LV contraction score. Other very significant factors were the preoperative use of intravenous nitroglycerin and reoperation, which was found to increase the operative mortality by a factor of 3.2. A history of congestive heart failure was associated with an increased operative mortality, as other studies have shown. Also of interest in this particular study was the fact that both peripheral vascular disease and cerebral vascular disease were noted to cause a 1.9- and 1.8-fold increase in operative mortality, respectively. These factors have not been identified in most other studies. The use of an intra-aortic balloon pump preoperatively was associated with a 3.5-fold increase in operative mortality and rest angina, with a 1.8 times increase in mortality. New York Heart Association class IV patients had a 2.1 times greater operative mortality than those in class III, those having an emergent operation had a 3.6 times operative mortality compared to those with elective procedures, and patients undergoing urgent operation were 1.7 times more likely to die than those having elective procedures.

A logistic regression analysis of the VA patients revealed that a prior operation and the priority of the operation, i.e., elective versus emergent versus urgent, were the two leading prognostic indicators. This is of particular importance at present because of the increasing incidence of patients requiring reoperation and those being operated on for unstable angina or in the process of acute events such as involving myocardial infarctions.

Since patients who are unstable, who require reoperation, who are on i.v. nitroglycerin, and/or an intra-aortic balloon pump, and those with severe LV dysfunction are at highest risk, it is reasonable to consider whether another mode of therapy exists that could either allow postponement of surgery or render surgery unnecessary. It is this particular subset of patients who may benefit from a percutaneous coronary angioplasty to convert them from an unstable to stable state to salvage myocardium. Such patients who are very unstable may be candidates for angioplasty in conjunction with femoral artery-vein bypass. As noted by Rankin and Sabiston (23), successful dilatation rates per stenosis for percutaneous transluminal coronary angioplasty now exceed 90% and the rate of major complications for elective angioplasty has decreased to approximately 4%, with procedure-related myocardial infarction death being uncommon. Of major concern, however, is the long-term stability of angioplasty revascularization, with significant restenosis occurring within the first year in up to 40% of lesions. He notes that the goal of the cardiothoracic surgeons and cardiologists "should be conversion of currently competing therapies into complementary ones through scientific assessment." It may be that cooperative investigation of the use of angioplasty in those patients who are at very high risk for surgery attempting to either eliminate the need for surgery or convert them into a more stable condition prior to surgery would be a cooperative investigation well worthwhile.

REFERENCES

1. Hammermeister KE, Kennedy JW. Predictors of surgical mortality in patients undergoing direct myocardial revascularization. Circulation 1974; (Suppl II) 49&50:II-112–II-115.
2. Loop FD, Berrettoni JN, Pichard A, Siegel W, Razavi M, Effler DB. Selection of the candidate for myocardial revascularization: A profile of high risk based on multivariate analysis. Thorac Cardiovasc Surg 1975; 69:40–51.
3. Kennedy JW, Kaiser GC, Fisher LD, Fritz JK, Myers W, Mudd JG, Ryan TJ. Clinical and angiographic predictors of operative mortality from the collaborative study in coronary artery surgery (CASS). Circulation 1981; 63(4):793–802.
4. Kennedy JW, Kaiser GC, Fisher LD, Maynard C, Fritz JK, Myers W, Mudd JG, Ryan TJ, Coggin J. Multivariate discriminant analysis of the clinical and angiographic predictors of operative mortality from the Collaborative Study in Coronary Artery Surgery (CASS). J Thorac Cardiovasc Surg 1980; 80:876–87.
5. Fisher L, Kennedy JW. Operative mortality in coronary bypass grafting. Letters to the Editor. J Thorac Cardiovasc Surg 1983; 85:146–51.
6. McCormick JR, Schick EC, McCabe CH, Kronmal RA, Ryan TJ. Determinants of operative mortality and long-term survival in patients with unstable angina: The CASS experience. J Thorac Cardiovasc Surg 1985; 89:683–8.
7. Wright JG, Pifarre R, Sullivan HJ, Montoya A, Bakhos M, Grieco J, Jones R, Foy B, Gunnar RM, Bieniewski CL, Scanlon PJ. Multivariate discriminant analysis of risk factors for operative mortality following isolated coronary artery bypass graft: Loyola University Medical Center experience, 1970 to 1984. Chest 1987; 91:394–9.
8. Naunheim KS, Fiore AC, Wadley JJ, McBride LR, Kanter KR, Pennington DG, Barner HB, Kaiser GC, Willman VL. The changing profile of the patient undergoing coronary artery bypass surgery. J Am Coll Cardiol 1988; 11(3):494–8.
9. Rich MW, Keller AJ, Schechtman KB, Marshall WG, Kouchoukos NT. Morbidity and mortality of coronary bypass surgery in patients 75 years of age or older. Ann of Thorac Surg 1988; 46:638–44.
10. Konchoukos NT, Ebert PA, Grover FL, Lindesmith GG. Report of the ad hoc committee on risk factors for coronary artery bypass surgery. Ann Thorac Surg 1988; 45:348–9.
11. Grover FL, Hammermeister KE, Burchfiel C, and cardiac surgeons of the Department of Veterans Affairs. Initial report of the Veterans Administration preoperative risk assessment study for cardiac surgery. Ann Thorac Surg 1990; 50:12–28.
12. Fisher LD, Kennedy JW, Davis KB, Maynard C, Fritz JK, Kaiser G, Myers WO, and the participating CASS clinics. Association of sex, physical size, and operative mortality after coronary artery bypass in the Coronary Artery Surgery Study (CASS). J Thorac Cardiovasc Surg 1982; 84:334–41.
13. Miller DC, Stinson EB, Oyer PE, Jamieson SW, Mitchell RS, Reitz BA, Baumgartner WA, Shumway NE. Discriminant analysis of the changing risks of coronary artery operations: 1971–1979. J Thorac Cardiovasc Surg 1983; 85:197–213.
14. Cosgrove DM, Loop FD, Lytle BW, Baillot R, Gill CC, Golding LAR, Taylor PC, Goormastic M. Primary myocardial revascularization: Trends in surgical mortality. J Thorac Cardiovasc Surg 1984; 88:673–84.

15. Kouchoukos NT, Oberman A, Kirklin JW, Russell RO, Karp RB, Pacifico AD, Zorn GL. Coronary bypass surgery: Analysis of factors affecting hospital mortality. Circulation 1980; 62 (Suppl I):I84–9.

16. Naunheim KS, Fiore AC, Fagan DC, McBride LR, Barner HB, Pennington DG, Willman VL, Kern MJ, Deligonul U, Vandormael MC, Kaiser GC. Emergency coronary artery bypass grafting for failed angioplasty: Risk factors and outcome. Ann Thorac Surg 1989; 47:816–23.

17. Conner AR, Vlietstra RE, Schaff HV, Ilstrup DM, Orszulak TA. Early and late results of coronary artery bypass after failed angioplasty. Actuarial analysis of late cardiac events and comparison with initially successful angioplasty. J Thorac Cardiovasc Surg 1988; 96:191–7.

18. Naunheim KS, Fiore AC, Arango DC, Pennington DG, Barner HB, McBride LR, Harris HH, Willman VL, Kaiser GC. Coronary artery bypass grafting for unstable angina pectoris: Risk analysis. Ann Thorac Surg 1989; 47:569–74.

19. Ottino G, Bergerone S, Di Leo M, Trucano G, Sacchetti C, De Paulis R, Vuolo A, Golzio PG, Brusca A, Morea M. Aortocoronary bypass results: A discriminant multivariate analysis of risk factors of operative mortality. J Cardiovasc Surg 1990; 31:20–5.

20. Mattila P, Vento A, Rist, Kan Kare M, Mattila S. Multivariate analysis of operative mortality and late outcome after coronary bypass surgery. J Cardiovasc Surg (Torino) 1990; 31:220–4.

21. Huysmans HA, van Ark E. Predictors of perioperative mortality, morbidity and late quality of life in coronary bypass surgery. Eur Heart J 1989; 10 (Suppl H):10–12.

22. Hannan EL, Kilburn H, O'Donnell JF, Lukacik G, Shields EP. Adult open heart surgery in New York State: An analysis of risk factors and hospital mortality rates. JAMA 1990; 264(21):2768–74.

23. Rankin JS. Relative roles of PTCA and CABG in the treatment of stable and unstable angina.

11

Surgery for Unstable Angina Pectoris

Karl E. Hammermeister

Department of Veterans Affairs Medical Center and
University of Colorado School of Medicine
Denver, Colorado

SYNOPSIS

Aortocoronary artery bypass surgery, introduced in 1967, was the first clinically successful revascularization procedure for ischemic heart disease and continues to have an important role in the treatment of ischemic heart disease, including unstable angina. Despite similar symptom relief and improvement in exercise tolerance with coronary bypass surgery for unstable angina patients as for stable angina, it is clear that the risk of operative death is higher in patients with evidence of unstable ischemia. Aspirin and heparin have been shown in randomized trials to produce dramatic reductions in the risk of myocardial infarction and death in patients with unstable angina, compared to no therapy, but have not been compared against coronary revascularization by surgery or percutaneous transluminal coronary angioplasty (PTCA). Similarly, contemporary randomized trials assessing the effects of surgery or PTCA against medical therapy or each other are lacking. Thus, the selection of therapy for patients with unstable angina poses several dilemmas: (a) How frequently is resting chest pain in patients with coronary artery disease due to myocardial ischemia? (b) How do we interpret randomized trial data now nearly a decade old? (c) Are there subgroups of patients with unstable angina in whom nonoperative forms of therapy should be considered?

In patients with stable exertional angina, the characteristics of the chest pain—particularly the precipitation by factors that increase myocardial oxygen demand and relief by rest or nitroglycerin—are highly reliable indicators that obstructive coronary artery disease and resultant myocardial ischemia are the causes of the pain. However, for unstable angina patients these specific predictive characteristics are lacking by definition. In many unstable angina patients, transient ST-segment changes on the resting electrocardiogram and/or the visceral character and location of the pain make causation by myocardial ischemia likely. However, there are many patients with resting chest pain, the character of which is atypical, and who do not have transient electrocardiographic changes. In such patients, even though they have documented coronary artery disease, alternative causes of pain, such as skeletal muscle or esophageal spasm, should be considered.

Large randomized trials conducted in patients with stable angina have shown that surgical revascularization is more effective than medical therapy in relieving angina and improving exercise tolerance for at least several years; however, survival was improved by surgical therapy only in limited high-risk subgroups. The decreased operative mortality plus better graft patency rates of the last decade imply that survival following coronary artery bypass may be improved in a broader spectrum of coronary disease patients than is documented in the randomized trials. The trials of medical versus surgical therapy in unstable angina patients, although smaller and less detailed, suggest similar outcomes. The development of atherosclerosis in the vein grafts plus progression of disease in the native vessels results in a return of angina in a substantial proportion of patients 5–10 years after the procedure.

Overall, patients with unstable angina have a risk of operative death at coronary bypass surgery approximately 1.5–2 times that of patients with stable ischemic heart disease. Based on contemporary data from the Department of Veterans Affairs Cardiac Surgery Risk Assessment Program, we have identified subsets of unstable angina patients with particularly high operative mortality: those with prior heart surgery, cardiomegaly, evidence of congestive heart failure, on intravenous nitroglycerin, severe other organ system disease, and severe left ventricular dysfunction. The relative efficacy of medical therapy, surgical revascularization, or PTCA can only be determined by a large-scale randomized trial. In the absence of this much-needed randomized trial data, we have proposed an algorithm for evaluation and treatment of such patients based on currently available evidence.

INTRODUCTION

Chest pain at rest suggestive of myocardial ischemia occurs frequently both in patients with manifest coronary artery disease and in those without. Such patients account for a substantial proportion of admissions to coronary care units, as well as of patients undergoing coronary artery bypass grafting and percutaneous transluminal coronary angioplasty. At the Denver Department of Veterans Affairs (DVA) Medical Center in the past 2 years approximately 90% of patients undergoing PTCA had chest pain at rest in their presenting history. For all cardiac surgical centers in the DVA medical care system, 53% (6752/12,712) of patients undergoing coronary artery bypass grafting reported having had unstable angina at the admission for their surgery. In such patients the operative mortality was almost twice that of those who did not report unstable angina (6.1% versus 3.4%) (1). Furthermore, older studies suggest that unstable angina patients experience a high incidence of recurrent rest angina, myocardial infarction, and death on long-term follow-up (2,3). Despite strong evidence that this poor outcome can be dramatically altered by aspirin (4–6), the perception of poor long-term prognosis and need for revascularization persists.

The evaluation and treatment of patients with rest angina pose a number of dilemmas. The most important of these is which form of therapy is most likely to produce the best short- and long-term results. A central thesis of this monograph is the need for contemporary, well-controlled studies to study this issue. This chapter will review and discuss the limitations of the existing data comparing medical and surgical therapy; at this time (early 1991) there are no randomized trial data comparing medical therapy versus angioplasty or surgical therapy versus angioplasty in these patients.

Other important related dilemmas include the distinction between chest pain due to ongoing myocardial ischemia and noncardiac causes of chest pain in patients with known coronary artery disease, but no diagnostic electrocardiographic (ECG) changes; and what to do with the subgroups of rest angina patients who have a poor short-term outcome with surgical therapy. This chapter will also discuss these two topics and suggest clinical research to resolve these issues.

Regardless of the significant limitations in our knowledge base, decisions for diagnosis and treatment of unstable angina must be made. This chapter will conclude with an algorithm for clinical decision making in patients with rest angina.

HISTORICAL

Surgical procedures to relieve angina have included several techniques to stimulate collateral flow from the pericardium to the heart (7), internal mammary artery ligation (8,9), and internal mammary artery implantation into the myocardium (10). While initial reports suggested that most patients had symptomatic relief, two randomized trials showed that internal mammary ligation was no better than a sham operation (8,9). Subsequently, the volume of additional blood flow to the heart through the implanted internal mammary artery was demonstrated to be small (11). Thus, all these procedures have been abandoned.

In 1967 Favaloro and colleagues at the Cleveland Clinic initiated the use of aortocoronary saphenous vein bypass grafting performed with the aid of cardiopulmonary bypass (12). Blood flow through these bypass grafts measured at the time of surgery represented a substantial proportion of total coronary artery blood flow. The operative mortality was acceptable, and most patients appeared to have relief of angina and improved exercise tolerance. Although applied initially to stable patients, patients with rest angina were soon undergoing coronary artery bypass grafting. The relatively low operative mortality and excellent symptomatic results resulted in great enthusiasm for this procedure as a therapy for both stable, exertional angina and rest angina. However, this enthusiasm has been tempered by randomized trials showing survival benefit only in limited subgroups for surgical therapy compared to medical therapy in both stable and unstable angina patients, and by the rapid development of atherosclerosis in vein grafts and progression of atherosclerosis in native vessels resulting in recurrent angina in many patients after 5–10 years. Thus it becomes important to consider whether alternative treatment strategies, such as PTCA or PTCA combined with surgical therapy, would be as or more effective than surgical therapy alone in some subsets of unstable angina patients.

THE FIRST DILEMMA: IS THE CHEST PAIN DUE TO MYOCARDIAL ISCHEMIA?

Significance of the Problem

For patients presenting with resting chest pain or discomfort, one of the first diagnostic tasks is to determine whether there is objective evidence of coronary artery disease, such as diagnostic ECG changes, history of myocardial infarction, previous positive stress testing, or coronary obstruction demonstrated by coronary ateriography. If such data are not available, then coronary arteriography is often appropriate to establish whether there is obstructive coronary artery disease. If there is no obstructive coronary artery disease, then the chest pain can be attributed to noncardiac causes or relatively rare other causes of myocardial ischemia, such as syndrome X; in either case, the prognosis is generally good.

However, there is a real diagnostic dilemma when patients with known coronary artery disease present with resting chest pain without transient ECG changes. Is the chest pain always due to myocardial ischemia, or are there noncardiac causes? The distinction is absolutely vital, as frequently the decision to undertake potentially hazardous invasive diagnostic or interventional procedures is based on whether there is ongoing myocardial ischemia.

Relation Between Angina and Myocardial Ischemia

Angina is commonly, but incorrectly, felt to be synonymous with myocardial ischemia. Angina is a clinical syndrome based largely on historical findings with no obligatory relationship to myocardial ischemia. A common definition is chest, arm, or neck discomfort of a visceral nature precipitated by exercise or emotion and relieved by rest or nitroglycerin. In its classic form in men, exertional angina is highly predictive of obstructive coronary artery disease (13). Furthermore, the objective, transient, physiological abnormalities that accompany stress-induced angina (e.g., ST-segment depression, perfusion deficits on radionuclide scintigraphy, and left ventricular wall motion abnormalities) indicate that this syndrome is indeed a reflection of myocardial ischemia in 80 or 90% of patients. It is likely that the two key components in this definition of angina that result in its high degree of specificity for myocardial ischemia are the precipitating factors and the relief by rest or nitroglycerin. It is more than ironic that these two key components are obligatorily missing from the definition of unstable angina, suggesting that rest angina may be less specific for myocardial ischemia than exertional angina. Secondary chest skeletal muscle spasm and pain of esophageal origin undoubtedly confound the picture, but to what extent is uncertain.

Characteristics of Resting Myocardial Ischemic Pain

History and Physical Examination
Most types of noncardiac chest pain are relatively easily distinguished from the pain or discomfort of myocardial ischemia. Table 1 lists several historical and physical examination characteristics that this author has found useful in distinguishing the pain or discomfort of myocardial ischemia from nonischemic pain. Important characteristics of rest myocardial ischemic pain are its vague, deep-seated nature, poor or diffuse localization, location between diaphragm and mandible, associated dyspnea and/or diaphoresis, and absence of pleuritic character. Although the specificity and sensitivity of these findings for identification of active myocardial ischemia have not been rigorously tested, most clinicians are comfortable diagnosing noncardiac chest pain in a patient whose pain is clearly pleuritic or reproducible by pressure over a costochondral junction.

The Electrocardiogram
ST-segment and/or T-wave changes on the electrocardiogram have been the mainstay for the diagnosis of myocardial ischemia for over 50 years. Although it is well known that about two-thirds of patients with obstructive coronary artery disease will develop ST-segment depression with exertion or other types of stress, the frequency with which transient ECG changes occur with resting myocardial ischemia is unknown. While few doubt that transient ST-segment depression accompanying rest angina is highly specific for myocardial ischemia, there is no information to indicate the frequency with which resting myocardial ischemia occurs in the absence of electrocardiographic changes.

Noncardiac Chest Pain Simulating Angina

It seems likely that most types of noncardiac resting chest pain can be correctly diagnosed using the characteristics given in Table 1. However, two important

Table 1 Characteristics of Resting Chest Pain Useful in Distinguishing Nonischemic Causes from Myocardial Ischemia

Characteristic	Consistent with myocardial ischemia	Possibly myocardial ischemia	Inconsistent with myocardial ischemia
Location	Confined between diaphragm and mandible	Includes, but overlaps, outside of region between diaphragm and mandible	Confined outside of region between diaphragm and mandible
Localization	Diffuse, described with flat of hand	Somewhat localized	Discretely localized; described with end of tip of finger(s)
Nature of pain	Vague, discomfort not pain, tightness, burning	Some sharpness or mild changes with respiration	Sharp, pleuritic
Associated findings	Diaphoresis, dyspnea	Dyspnea, anxiety	No diaphoresis or dyspnea
Physical examination	S_3 gallop or wall motion abnormality with pain	No findings	Chest pain reproduced by chest palpation or arm or shoulder motion

causes of chest pain or discomfort are not easily distinguishable from myocardial ischemia: secondary skeletal muscle spasm and esophageal pain.

Secondary Skeletal Muscle Spasm

It is the author's belief that ischemic myocardial pain may serve as a trigger for secondary skeletal muscle spasm involving the pectoral and intercostal muscles; this is analogous to paravertebral muscle spasm accompanying and magnifying a variety of thoracic, lumbar, and sacral spine disorders. Neuronal pathways facilitating such reflex pain have been described (14). The evidence supporting this belief is sketchy, but includes the frequent observation of high-frequency artifact in leads I, II, and aVL of the resting ECG recorded during pain probably due to involuntary muscle spasm, limited documentation of pectoral muscle spasm by electromyography, tender pectoral muscles in many coronary artery disease patients, and symptomatic response to biofeedback and/or skeletal muscle relaxants. Such secondary skeletal muscle spasm could easily explain the very long-lasting (many hours or days), often low-grade left chest discomfort frequently reported by patients with coronary artery disease. Unfortunately, the characteristics of secondary skeletal muscle spasm do not easily distinguish it from pain or discomfort due to myocardial ischemia (Table 1).

Esophageal Pain

The pain and associated findings of typical reflux esophagitis are usually easily distinguished from those of myocardial ischemia. Useful findings are the ascending nature of the discomfort, relief with antacids, relationship to gravity, and the taste of acid in the mouth. However, the pain of esophageal spasm and variants of reflux is easily confused with that of myocardial ischemia. The report that the pain of esophageal spasm may be relieved by nitroglycerin (rare in the author's experience) raises the question as to whether myocardial ischemia may serve as a trigger for spasm of esophageal muscle, as postulated above for skeletal muscle.

Summary

The definition of angina is based on historical findings that are not clearly linked to myocardial ischemia. The precipitation of angina by a stress increasing myocardial oxygen demand and its relief by rest or nitroglycerin appear to provide a specific link to myocardial ischemia. However, medically refractory rest angina by definition lacks these criteria. Coronary arteriography is a very useful tool for identifying those patients whose anginal symptoms are not due to obstructive coronary artery disease, and who therefore have a favorable prognosis. Unfortunately, it seems likely that patients with obstructive coronary artery disease frequently have symptoms due to both myocardial ischemia and noncardiac causes of pain, such as skeletal muscle spasm or esophageal pain. In the absence of transient ECG changes, the distinction between ischemic and nonischemic pain is difficult. Because lifesaving diagnostic and therapeutic decisions often depend on this distinction, this would be an area of fruitful research.

THE SECOND DILEMMA: HOW DO WE INTERPRET THE RANDOMIZED TRIAL DATA?

Two moderate-sized randomized trials comparing medical and surgical therapy of unstable angina have been conducted. The National Cooperative Study Group, representing nine university hospitals in the United States, randomized 288 patients between 1972 and 1976 (15–17). The Veterans Administration Cooperative Study randomized 468 patients between 1976 and 1982 at 12 VA medical centers (18). Eligibility requirements were similar in both studies: age < 70 years, either progressive or rest angina associated with ST-segment or T-wave changes, and no recent myocardial infarction; the VA study excluded women. In both studies the interpretation of long-term results is complicated by the rapid rate of crossover to surgical therapy of medically assigned patients: 36% at 30 months in the National Cooperative Study and 34% at 2 years in the VA Cooperative Study.

Results: Effects of Coronary Bypass Surgery on Nonfatal End-Points

Short-Term Effects on Symptoms

The rate of symptom relief following revascularization for unstable angina appears to be similar to that for stable patients. Much of the randomized trial data comparing symptomatic and functional outcomes between medically and surgically treated patients with coronary artery disease come from studies in stable angina patients (19–23).

There is a broad consensus that coronary artery bypass grafting is initially effective in relieving angina and improving exercise tolerance. This consensus exists even though it has not been possible to account for the placebo effect of surgery and observer bias in assessing the outcome by blinding patient and physician to type of treatment in the randomized trials comparing medical to surgical therapy. While subjective assessment of outcome, such as functional class, could be significantly affected by placebo effect and observer bias, the persistence of symptomatic benefit for at least several years, plus improvement in a multitude of objective exercise parameters, indicates that much of the benefit reported by the patient is the result of improved myocardial blood supply eliminating ischemia.

The National Cooperative Study Group reported that only 14% of surgically treated patients with multivessel disease had significant symptoms (New York Heart Association functional class III or IV) at 1 year after surgery, compared to

40% of those assigned to medical therapy (15). In general, 70–80% of patients undergoing coronary artery bypass grafting for angina pectoris are markedly improved or completely free of angina 1 year after surgery; similar patients assigned to medical therapy may show some improvement in symptoms, but most continue to have angina (19–21).

Long-Term Effects on Symptoms

All three of the major randomized trials in patients with stable angina show a modest deterioration in the proportion of surgically treated patients free of angina or markedly improved compared to preoperatively between 1 and 5 years following surgery; the magnitude of this deterioration has been approximately 10%, falling from 70–80% improved in the first year to 60–70% at year 5 (21–23).

Longer follow-up has shown continued deterioration in symptomatic status, such that 50% or more of patients undergoing saphenous vein bypass grafting have significant angina 10 years after surgery (24). In the VA Cooperative Study on stable angina, only 52% of surgically treated patients were reported as improved 10 years postoperatively compared to 46% of medically treated patients (25). The symptomatic deterioration with time following coronary artery bypass surgery is the result of both de novo development of atherosclerosis in vein grafts and progression of atherosclerosis in the native coronary arteries. Only 40% of vein grafts studied 10–12 years after surgery by the Montreal Heart Institute group revealed satisfactory patency; 37% had occluded, while 24% had significant (≥50%) stenoses (24). Similarly, significant progression of atherosclerotic obstruction was observed in 47% of ungrafted native coronary arteries over the same time period.

Mechanisms for Relief of Angina

It is generally agreed that the primary mechanism for relief of angina is restoration of normal blood flow to previously ischemic myocardium. However, alternative mechanisms may play a role, including placebo effect of surgery, perioperative myocardial infarction, and possibly an alteration in the perception of cardiac pain (26). The relationship between graft patency and relief of angina has been inconsistent. While Campeau and colleagues reported a significantly greater rate of relief of angina in patients with one or more patent grafts (89%) than in those with all grafts closed (57.5%), the most striking observation is that over half those with no revascularization were symptomatically improved after surgery, suggesting a powerful placebo effect (24). Similarly, the VA Cooperative Study found a poor relationship between graft patency and angina relief at 5 years (22).

Effects on Exercise Tolerance

Nearly all the information available on the comparative effects of coronary artery bypass grafting versus medical therapy on exercise capacity comes from the three large randomized trials in patients with stable angina or no angina (20,21,23).

All three of these trials reported significantly greater improvement in exercise tolerance in surgically treated patients than medically treated patients. Both the European Coronary Artery Survey Study and CASS showed modest deterioration in exercise performance between 1 and 5 years (20,23).

The mechanisms for improved exercise performance have been evaluated in a careful, detailed study of exercise hemodynamics in 70 patients before and after coronary artery bypass grafting by Hossack and colleagues (27). There was marked improvement in maximal oxygen consumption, cardiac index, and maximal pressure-rate product and a fall in pulmonary arterial pressure at the postoperative study in patients with complete revascularization. The increase in maximal cardiac index was largely due to being able to achieve a higher exercise heart rate, although patients with complete revascularization also experienced a significant increase in stroke volume index at maximal exercise. In contrast, patients with incomplete revascularization had no significant improvement in exercise oxygen consumption, cardiac index, heart rate, or stroke volume from pre- to postoperatively. These data provide strong evidence that the major mechanism for the beneficial effects of coronary artery bypass surgery is improved myocardial blood supply.

Effects on Myocardial Infarction

Neither of the major randomized trials comparing medical versus surgical therapy for unstable angina showed protection from myocardial infarction with surgical revascularization (15,18). In the National Cooperative Study, at a median follow-up of 30 months, 19% of medically treated patients experienced a nonfatal acute myocardial infarction compared to 30% of surgically treated patients. Most of this difference was due to the high rate of perioperative infarction (17%) in surgically treated patients, as the rates of late infarction were essentially identical in the two treatment groups. The rates of nonfatal myocardial infarction were lower in the VA Cooperative Study, but still similar in the medically and surgically treated patients: 12% in each treatment group at 2 years after randomization (18).

Effects on Left Ventricular Function

Most available evidence indicates that left ventricular function is not improved by revascularization in patients with stable angina pectoris; the implication is that the dysfunction is due to irreversible myocardial damage. In contrast to stable angina patients, patients with an acute myocardial ischemic syndrome, such as unstable angina or cardiogenic shock, might be expected to have reversible left ventricular dysfunction. Improved left ventricular performance after coronary artery bypass grafting in such patients has been suggested by several uncontrolled series (28–30).

Results: Effects on Survival

Although neither of the two major randomized trials designed to test the hypothesis that surgical revascularization improves survival of unstable angina patients confirmed this hypothesis, there remains a widespread consensus that coronary bypass grafting is lifesaving in many of these patients. What are the data to support this belief?

Summary of Major Randomized Trials

In the National Cooperative Study, in-hospital mortality was only 3% for those randomized to medical therapy and 5% for those randomized to surgical therapy (difference not significant) (15). Survival at a median of 30 months after randomization was also similar between those randomized to medical or surgical therapy. Subgroup analyses from this study failed to show any survival benefit with surgical therapy for patients with ST-segment changes with their chest pain (16) or with obstruction of the proximal left anterior descending coronary artery (17).

In the VA Cooperative Study, survival at 2 years was identical for all patients assigned to medical or surgical therapy, as well as subgroups defined by type of angina or number of diseased vessels (18). However, a post hoc multivariate analysis showed a striking effect of ejection fraction on survival of medically treated patients, but little effect on survival of surgically treated patients. When survivals in the subset with ejection fraction = 0.30–0.59 were compared, the surgically treated patients had significantly better survival (31).

Nonrandomized Observational Data Analyses

The Coronary Artery Surgery Study (CASS) reported that preoperative left ventricular function, congestive heart failure, other noncardiac illness, extent of coronary artery disease, and cardiomegaly were significant predictors of survival on multivariate analysis of 3311 patients undergoing coronary artery bypass for unstable angina (32). However, no comparison with similar medically treated patients was reported.

The Impact of Changes in Medical and Surgical Therapy

Nearly a decade has passed since the last patient in the VA Cooperative Unstable Angina Study (the most recent randomized trial) was operated on; patients were operated on in the other major randomized trials up to nearly 20 years ago. Major changes in the medical and surgical therapy of coronary artery disease have occurred during this period, including intraoperative myocardial protection with cold potassium cardioplegia, widespread use of the internal mammary artery as a conduit, the use of thrombolytic agents and beta-blocking agents in the treatment of myocardial infarction, and the use of aspirin in the prevention of myocardial infarction and death in patients with unstable angina (4–6). Although randomized trial and observational data analyses indicate better outcome of patients treated with these medical and surgical innovations than those without, the relative impact on the comparison of outcome with medical versus surgical therapy is unknown. It seems unlikely that a randomized trial to compare outcome following medical versus surgical therapy will be repeated for patients with stable angina, because short-term symptomatic results of both coronary artery bypass grafting and PTCA are good. As reviewed elsewhere in this book, a number of randomized trials are underway to compare the results of PCTA with coronary artery bypass grafting. The only trial to compare outcome of medical therapy to PTCA is confined to patients with relatively mild coronary disease.

However, some clinically relevant insights have been obtained from observational data analyses of patients entered into the registry of all patients undergoing coronary arteriography at Duke University Medical Center. Analyses by Califf and colleagues suggest that the absolute survival difference after 5 years between medically and surgically treated patients increases with increasing operative risk (33). Furthermore, survival after surgery has improved with operations done in more recent years, even though the best evidence is that the risk for operative death has gone up (34). These analyses suggest that a broader spectrum of patients may experience survival benefit with revascularization than heretofore considered, based on randomized trial data.

THE THIRD DILEMMA: SHOULD NONOPERATIVE THERAPY BE CONSIDERED IN PATIENTS IN WHOM CORONARY ARTERY BYPASS SURGERY IS NOT LOW RISK?

Operative mortalities for patients undergoing coronary artery bypass grafting are commonly reported in the range of 1–4%, but are highly dependent on patient risk factors (35–38). Urgency of surgery, reoperation, age, angina severity, congestive heart failure, and severity of left main coronary artery stenosis have been consistently reported as risk factors for operative mortality. Women have about twice the operative mortality as men (38). However, most of these reports are based on patients operated on a decade or more ago and do not separate stable angina patients from unstable angina patients.

The Department of Veterans Affairs Cardiac Surgery Risk Assessment Program

Study Design

We have analyzed data from patients in the DVA Cardiac Surgery Risk Assessment Program reported as having unstable angina at their admission for coronary artery bypass grafting between April 1987 and March 1990. This program, which collects data on 54 preoperative risk factors, the operative procedure, and short-term operative outcomes on all patients undergoing cardiac surgery at DVA medical centers, has four major goals:

1. To develop multivariate models for prediction of operative death and complications from prospectively collected preoperative risk data
2. To provide risk-adjusted operative mortality to the DVA Cardiac Surgery Consultants Committee to aid it in its quality assurance role
3. To provide these risk data and predictive models to DVA cardiology-cardiac surgery teams to aid them in their clinical decision making and internal quality assurance
4. To determine risk factors relevant to operative mortality and morbidity in the present era (1,39)

In its first 3 years, this program has collected data on 12,712 patients undergoing coronary artery bypass grafting as the primary procedure, of whom 6752 (53%) had unstable angina, although not necessarily "medically refractory angina," as defined for this book. A single page data form is completed by a member of the cardiac surgical team. The preoperative risk data are analyzed by a series of univariate and multivariate analyses to develop models for prediction of operative mortality (1) or one or more perioperative complications (39). The individual patients' estimated operative mortalities can be summed to give an estimated operative mortality (E) for a cardiac surgical center. The comparison between observed operative mortality (O) and estimated operative mortality in the form of an O/E ratio may be an indicator of quality of care.

To identify unstable angina patients who may be at particularly high risk for operative death at coronary artery bypass grafting (and thus candidates for alternative forms of therapy, such as PTCA), we have analyzed the preoperative risk factors and constructed a risk model for prediction of operative mortality specifically for unstable angina patients.

Results of Univariate Analyses

Table 2 shows the preoperative variables reflecting chronic status significantly predictive of operative mortality, while Table 3 shows the preoperative variables reflecting acute status at the time of surgery that are significantly predictive of operative death. Operative mortality for unstable angina patients was 5.6% (376/6752). Some of the more important preoperative variables relevant to operative death are also illustrated in Figures 1–9.

As other studies have shown (32,35,36,38), age is a potent predictor of operative mortality; as Figure 1 illustrates, patients with unstable angina over age 70 have more than twice the risk of operative death of patients under age 60. We also confirmed the deleterious effect of smaller body size, as previously reported by Fisher and colleagues (40).

Figure 2 shows that variables reflecting the extent and previous therapy of

Table 2 Preoperative Variables Significantly Predictive of Operative Death in 6752 Patients with Unstable Angina Undergoing Coronary Artery Bypass Grafting Between April 1987 and March 1990: Variables Reflecting Chronic Status

	Variable absent		Variable present			
Variable	Number patients	Operative mortality	Number patients	Incidence (%)	Operative mortality	p
Age (years)						
<50			566	(8.4)	3.5%	0.000
50–59			1745	(25.9)	3.8%	
60–69			3510	(52.0)	6.0%	
≥70			927	(13.7)	8.5%	
Body surface area (M²)						
<1.96			3295	(49.4)	6.2%	0.011
≥ 1.96			3374	(50.6)	4.8%	
Prior MI (>30 days)	2873	4.1%	3721	(56.4)	6.5%	0.000
Prior heart surgery	5911	4.3%	837	(12.4)	12.3%	0.000
COPD	4723	5.2%	1897	(28.7)	6.9%	0.005
Peripheral vascular disease	4967	4.6%	1603	(24.4)	8.4%	0.000
Cerebral vascular disease	5519	5.0%	1031	(15.7)	8.4%	0.000
Cardiomegaly	5546	4.9%	1057	(16.0)	9.3%	0.000
Creatinine (mg/100 ml)						
≤1.4			4923	(81.5)	4.6%	0.000
1.5–2.0			914	(15.1)	7.7%	
>2.0			206	(3.4)	12.1%	

Table 3 Preoperative Variables Significantly Predictive of Operative Death in 6752 Patients with Rest Angina Undergoing Coronary Artery Bypass Grafting Between April 1987 and March 1990: Variables Reflecting Acute Status

Variable	Variable absent		Variable present			p
	Number patients	Operative mortality	Number patients	Incidence (%)	Operative mortality	
History of CHF	5592	4.8%	1116	(16.6)	9.7%	0.000
Recent MI (≤30 days)	5190	4.7%	1484	(22.2)	8.5%	0.000
Current dig. use	5703	5.2%	853	(13.0)	7.4%	0.007
Current diur. use	4773	4.6%	1791	(27.3)	8.0%	0.000
i.v. NTG preop.	4591	3.8%	1978	(30.1)	9.7%	0.000
Preop. IABP	6369	5.1%	314	(4.7)	15.6%	0.000
Pulmonary rales	6020	4.8%	537	(8.2)	14.0%	0.000
Resting ST dep.	4931	4.8%	1542	(23.8)	8.2%	0.000
ECG LVH	5525	5.2%	916	(14.2)	7.5%	0.005
FEV_1 (L)						
<1.0			17	(0.8)	17.6%	0.002
1.0–1.5			141	(6.5)	8.5%	
1.6–2.0			307	(14.2)	4.6%	
>2.0			1692	(78.4)	3.7%	
NYHA functional class						
I			122	(1.9)	2.5%	0.000
II			861	(13.2)	2.3%	
III			2419	(37.2)	3.8%	
IV			3109	(47.7)	7.8%	
General medical condition						
Good			1598	(36.9)	2.9%	0.000
Fair			2280	(52.7)	4.8%	
Poor			450	(10.4)	17.3%	

Table 3 (*Continued*)

Variable	Variable absent		Variable present			p
	Number patients	Operative mortality	Number patients	Incidence (%)	Operative mortality	
Left ventricular systolic pressure (mmHg)						
<120			1649	(38.2)	4.9%	
121–130			723	(16.8)	4.4%	0.004
131–140			734	(17.0)	3.5%	
>140			1207	(28.0)	7.0%	
Aortic systolic pressure (mmHg)						
<120			1668	(38.8)	5.2%	
121–130			734	(17.1)	4.2%	0.034
131–140			706	(16.4)	3.8%	
>140			1188	(27.7)	6.6%	
Left ventricular end-diastolic pressure (mmHg)						
<10			1145	(26.6)	3.9%	
11–16			1341	(31.1)	4.8%	0.000
17–20			790	(18.3)	4.8%	
>20			1032	(24.0)	8.0%	
Number of stenotic vessels (≥50%)						
0			13	0.2	0.0	
1			339	4.1	2.6	0.000
2			1491	17.9	3.8	
3			3730	44.7	6.6	

	n	(%)		p
Left main stenosis				
≤30%	3279	(66.8)	4.6%	0.000
31–50%	474	(9.7)	6.5%	
51–70%	458	(9.3)	5.5%	
71–90%	513	(10.5)	8.4%	
>90%	183	(3.7%)	14.8%	
Left ventricular ejection fraction				
<0.20	251	(4.6)	9.2%	0.008
0.21–0.30	692	(12.7)	7.8%	
0.31–0.40	1130	(20.7)	6.0%	
0.41–0.50	1437	(26.3)	5.5%	
0.51–0.60	1196	(21.9)	4.7%	
>0.60	750	(13.7)	4.5%	
Left ventricular wall motion score				
I (normal)	2428	(39.0)	4.7%	0.003
II (mild dysfunction)	2053	(32.9)	5.1%	
III (moderate dysfunction)	1317	(21.1)	6.6%	
IV (dyskinesis)	354	(5.7%)	8.5%	
V (severe dysfunction)	81	(1.3%)	9.9%	
Priority of surgery				
Elective	3580	(54.9)	3.7%	0.000
Urgent	2228	(34.2)	6.5%	
Emergent	714	(10.9)	12.5%	

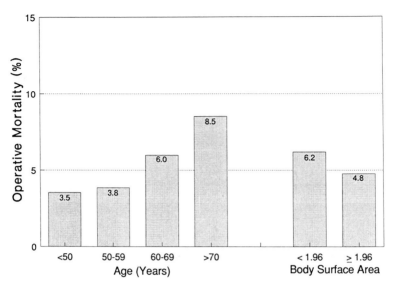

Figure 1 Effect of the demographic variables age and body surface area on operative mortality in patients with rest angina.

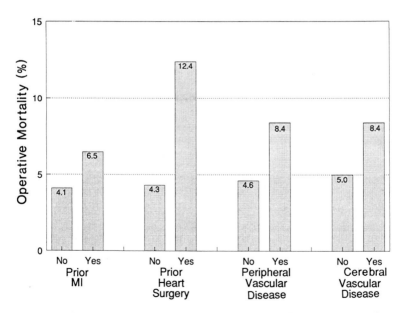

Figure 2 Effect of measures of severity of atherosclerotic vascular disease, prior myocardial infarction (MI), prior heart surgery, peripheral vascular disease, and cerebral vascular disease on operative mortality in patients with rest angina.

atherosclerotic disease are significant predictors of operative death. The most potent of these is prior heart surgery (nearly always previous coronary artery bypass graft surgery), which increases operative mortality threefold.

Not surprisingly, risk factors reflecting the presence of congestive heart failure are significantly related to operative death, as shown in Figure 3. The most powerful of these is pulmonary rales, present in 8% of our patients, which triple the risk of perioperative death; a past history of congestive heart failure (present in 17% of patients) and cardiomegaly (present in 16% of patients) each doubles the operative mortality.

Figure 4 illustrates the effect on operative mortality of variables reflecting acute or recent ischemia/infarction. ST-segment depression on the resting electrocardiogram, a myocardial infarction within 30 days, and the use of intravenous nitroglycerin preoperatively all approximately double the operative risk.

Comorbidity, disease in other organ systems, also significantly affects operative mortality (Fig. 5). There are progressive increases in operative mortality with greater severity of renal dysfunction as measured by serum creatine and pulmonary disease reflected by the force expiratory volume in 1 sec (FEV_1). While statistically significant, a simple diagnosis of chronic obstructive pulmonary disease (defined as chronic use of bronchodilators or hospitalization for

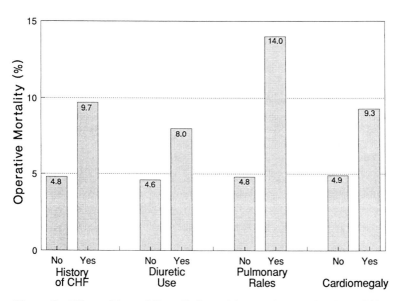

Figure 3 Effect of heart failure findings, history of congestive heart failure (CHF), diuretic use, pulmonary rales, and cardiomegaly on operative mortality in patients with rest angina.

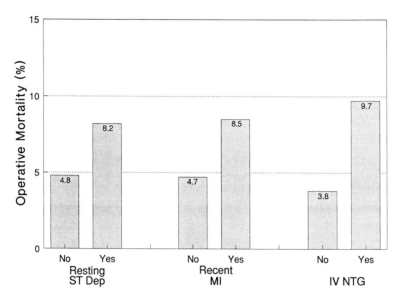

Figure 4 Effect of findings of acute ischemia, ST-segment depression on the resting ECG (Resting ST Dep), myocardial infarction (MI) within 30 days, and intravenous nitroglycerin (IV NTG) use within 48 hr on operative mortality in patients with rest angina.

chronic pulmonary disease) is not nearly as powerful or precise a predictor as the FEV_1.

Although all patients were diagnosed as having unstable angina, their physicians also noted gradations in severity of symptoms that had prognostic significance, as reflected in the New York Heart Association functional class (Fig. 6). The 48% of the patients listed as being in class IV had 2–3 times the operative mortality of the remainder in classes I–III. One of the most powerful predictors in our analyses is general medical condition; each patient is to be classified into good, fair, or poor general medical condition based on overall functional, mental, and nutritional status. The 10% of patients classified as having poor general medical condition had 6 times the operative mortality as the 37% whose condition was classified as good. However, this variable has not been included in out multivariate models, because we began collecting these data about halfway through the present reporting period.

Figure 7 shows the effects of left ventricular systolic and end-diastolic pressures on operative mortality. There is a ''U-shaped'' relationship between both aortic and left ventricular systolic pressure, with patients with the lowest and highest pressures having the greatest risk of operative death. Left ventricular

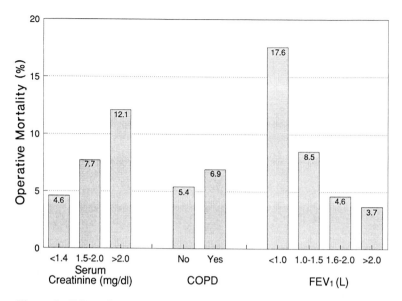

Figure 5 Effect of evidence of other organ system disease, serum creatinine, history of chronic obstructive pulmonary disease (COPD), and forced expiratory volume in 1 sec (FEV$_1$) on operative mortality in patients with rest angina.

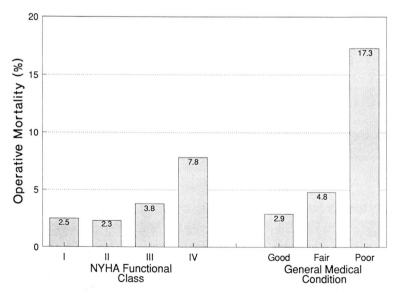

Figure 6 Influence of New York Heart Association (NYHA) functional class and general medical condition on operative mortality in patients with rest angina.

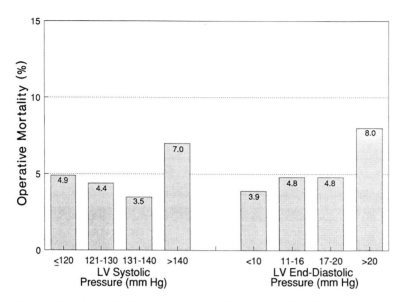

Figure 7   Effect of left ventricular systolic and end-diastolic pressures on operative mortality in patients with rest angina.

end-diastolic pressure is predictive of operative death only when it is very high, e.g., >20 mmHg.

The angiographic severity of the coronary artery disease is predictive of operative risk, as shown in Figure 8. The small subgroup (4%) of patients with very severe left main stenosis (>90%) had a very high operative mortality of 15%.

Operative risk progressively increases with decrements in left ventricular ejection fraction below 0.50 (Fig. 9). However, patients with moderate degrees of left ventricular dysfunction (ejection fraction between 0.30 and 0.50) can be successfully operated on at only a modestly increased risk (5.5–6.0% compared to 4.6% for patients with normal ejection fraction). Even with an ejection fraction of 0.20 or below, the operative mortality is only 9%. The urgency of surgery is highly predictive of operative death, with an approximate doubling of risk going from elective to urgent surgery and from urgent to emergent surgery.

Multivariate Predictive Model

Figure 10 illustrates the development of the multivariate predictive model. All preoperative patient-related risk variables are analyzed univariately, as summarized in Tables 2 and 3. Noninvasive variable reflecting the chronic status and acute status of the patient and invasive variables with $p < 0.2$ are entered into separate logistic regression analyses. The significant ($p < 0.05$) variables in

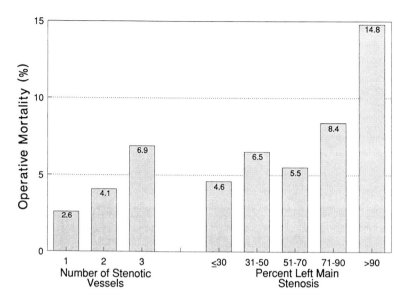

Figure 8 Influence of the extent of severity of coronary artery disease [number of vessels with stenosis(es) ≥ 50% and severity of left main coronary artery stenosis] on operative mortality in patients with rest angina.

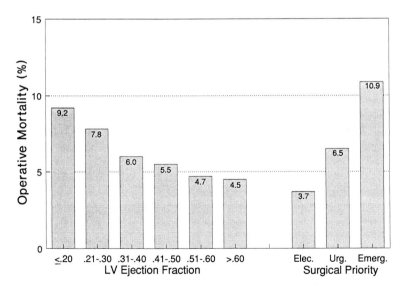

Figure 9 Influence of left ventricular ejection fraction and surgical priority on operative mortality in patients with rest angina.

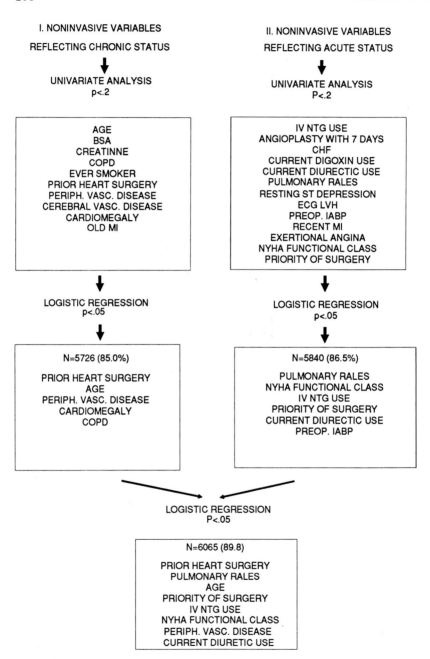

Figure 10 Development of a multivariate model to predict operative death in 6752 patients with rest angina using a series of univariate and multivariate analyses.

these analyses are then entered into a final logistic regression model. Since the invasive variables (including left ventricular ejection fraction, left ventricular wall motion score, and number of stenotic vessels) add minimal additional predictive power to the model, only the model constructed with noninvasive variables is shown.

Table 4 shows the variables in the final predictive model listed in order of their statistical significance. The odds ratio reflects increase in operative mortality for that variable after adjusting for all other variables in the model. For example, the odds of perioperative death for a patient with prior cardiac surgery is 3.2 times that of a patient without prior surgery.

Previous Studies

By comparison, the Coronary Artery Surgery Study reported a 4.3% operative mortality for 2559 patients with rest angina (32). Multivariate predictors of operative death were age, congestive heart failure score, left ventricular contraction score, and stenosis of the left main coronary artery in a left dominant circulation. Stuart et al. reported a 5.3% operative mortality for 225 patients with unstable portinfarction angina; independent predictors of operative mortality were transmural anterior myocardial infarction and need for intra-aortic balloon pumping for angina or congestive heart failure (41). Naunheim and colleagues reported an operative mortality of 6.2% in 129 patients on intravenous nitroglycerin for unstable angina; age was the only preoperative variable predictive of increased operative mortality (42).

Summary of Operative Risk

The risk of operative death for unstable angina patients undergoing coronary artery bypass grafting is significantly higher than that of patients with stable

Table 4 Multivariate Predictive Model for Identification of Patients with Rest Angina at High Risk (Operative Mortality $\geq$ 10%) for Operative Death

Variable	Beta	p	Odds ratio
Prior heart surgery	1.201	0.000	3.24
Pulmonary rales	0.731	0.000	2.08
Age	0.032	0.000	1.38[a]
Priority of surgery	0.354	0.000	1.42
i.v. nitroglycerin	0.475	0.000	1.61
NYHA functional class	0.334	0.000	1.40
Peripheral vascular disease	0.403	0.001	1.50
Current diuretic use	0.270	0.032	1.31

[a]Odds ratio computed for 10-year age increment.
NYHA = New York Heart Association; i.v. = intravenous.

angina, averaging between 4 and 6%. However, within the broad category of unstable angina, there are marked variations in operative risk, depending on preoperative patient-related risk factors. The most important of these are previous cardiac surgery, variables reflecting congestive heart failure, age, the urgency of the surgery, variables reflecting acute or recent ischemia or infarction, and comorbid conditions.

Summary: Clinical Implications and Indications for Coronary Bypass Surgery

Patients who continue to have unstable angina despite intensive in-hospital medical therapy are, obviously, candidates for revascularization. If they have single-vessel disease (not involving the left main coronary artery), coronary artery angioplasty is usually the therapy of choice. If they have multivessel disease, coronary artery bypass surgery is generally performed. However, such patients are at significantly increased risk for operative death—particularly if they have had previous bypass surgery and/or a recent myocardial infarction. The relative risks and efficacy of surgery versus angioplasty in these patients need further study in a randomized trial.

Most patients presenting with unstable angina can have their symptoms controlled with medical therapy consisting of bed rest, oxygen, heparin and/or aspirin, nitrates, calcium-channel blocking agents, and beta-adrenergic-blocking agents. The question is then whether these patients should be continued on medical therapy or considered for revascularization. Even though the two randomized trials of initial medical versus prompt surgical therapy showed no overall survival benefit for surgery (15,18), there is a consensus that patients who are otherwise acceptable operative risks should undergo coronary ateriography. The reason for this is the high rate of crossover from medical to surgical therapy because of recurrent ischemia in these two randomized trials. Although not specifically studied, it is generally accepted that preoperative characteristics indicating improved survival with surgery in stable angina patients also apply to unstable angina patients. Patients with left main coronary artery stenosis, three-vessel disease, and left ventricular dysfunction, and probably patients with three-vessel disease with normal left ventricular function and patients with two-vessel disease with left anterior descending coronary artery involvement are likely to experience improved survival with coronary bypass surgery.

AN ALGORITHM FOR CLINICAL DECISION MAKING AND PLANNING CLINICAL TRIALS

Both heparin and aspirin (separately and in combination) have been demonstrated to reduce mortality and/or risk of myocardial infarction compared to placebo in patients with unstable angina (4–6). However, aspirin clearly increases the risk of postoperative bleeding in those patients who will subsequently undergo coronary artery bypass grafting (43). Figure 11 illustrates our algorithm for the preoperative care and diagnostic evaluation of unstable angina patients. The first step is to initiate anti-ischemic and antithrombotic therapy with short-acting agents: intravenous nitroglycerin and heparin. The next step is to make a quick estimate of risk of coronary artery bypass surgery based on age, general medical condition, comorbid conditions, congestive heart failure, and left ventricular function. Then, most patients who are an acceptable surgical risk should undergo coronary arteriography. Until a decision is made based on the coronary arteriogram regarding the need for surgical revascularization, these patients should be maintained on intravenous nitroglycerin and heparin with electrocardiographic monitoring in an intensive care setting. Patients recommended for surgery will generally have this procedure during the same hospitalization while being maintained on heparin until shortly before the procedure. Patients who are felt to be at high risk or otherwise not suitable for surgical therapy may be switched to oral antianginal therapy plus aspirin and gradually ambulated. Those who have persistent angina due to myocardial ischemia will likely require

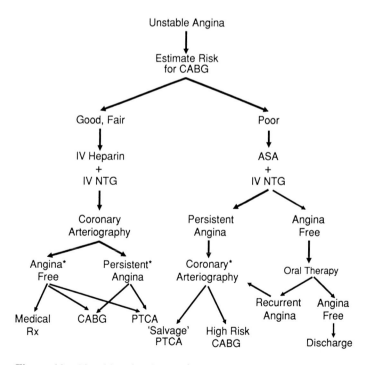

Figure 11 Algorithm for the preoperative care, evaluation, and treatment of patients with rest angina. *Subsets of patients for randomized trial.

coronary arteriography and a difficult decision whether to recommend "salvage" PTCA or high-risk coronary artery bypass surgery. Because controlled clinical trial data regarding the most efficacious therapy for many of these subsets are lacking, such patients would be appropriate for a randomized trial.

ACKNOWLEDGMENT

Data reported from the Department of Veterans Affairs (DVA) Cardiac Surgery Risk Assessment Program are based on research supported by the DVA Health Services Research and Development Service.

REFERENCES

1. Grover FL, Hammermeister KE, Burchfiel C, Cardiac Surgeons of the Department of Veterans Affairs. Initial report of the Veterans Administration preoperative risk assessment study for cardiac surgery. Ann Thorac Surg 1990; 50:12–28.
2. Gazes PC, Mobley EM, Faris HM, Duncan RC, Humphries GB. Preinfarctional (unstable angina)—A prospective study—10 year follow-up. Circulation 1973; 48:331–7.
3. Robert KB, Califf RM, Harrell FE Jr, Lee KL, Pryor DB, Rosati RA. The prognosis for patients with new-onset angina who have undergone cardiac catheterization. Circulation 1983; 68:970–8.
4. Lewis, HD Jr, Davis JW, Archibald DG, et al. Protective effects of aspirin against acute myocardial infarction and death in men with unstable angina: Results of a Veterans Administration Cooperative Study. N Engl J Med 1983; 309:396–403.
5. Cairns JA, Gent M, Singer J, et al. Aspirin, sulfinpyrazone, or both in unstable angina: Results of a Canadian multicenter trial. N Engl J Med 1985; 313:1369–75.
6. Theroux P, Ouimet H, McCans J, et al. Aspirin, heparin, or both to treat acute unstable angina. N Engl J Med 1988; 319:1105–11.
7. Beck CS. The development of a new blood supply to the heart by operation. Ann Surg 1935; 102:801–13.
8. Cobb LA, Thomas GI, Dillard DH, et al. An evaluation of internal-mammary-artery ligation by a double-blind technique. N Engl J Med 1959; 260:115–8.
9. Dimond EG, Kittle CF, Crockett JE. Comparison of internal mammary artery ligation and sham operation for angina pectoris. Am J Cardiol 1960; 5:483–6.
10. Vinberg AM, Miller WD. An experimental study of the physiological role of the anastomosis between the left coronary circulation and the left internal mammary artery implanted in the left ventricular myocardium. Surg Forum 1950; 1:294–9.
11. Dart CH Jr, Kato Y, Scott SM, et al. Internal thoracic (mammary) arteriography. A questionable index of myocardial revascularization. J Thorac Cardiovasc Surg 1970; 59:117–27.
12. Favaloro RG. Saphenous vein graft in the surgical treatment of coronary artery disease: Operative technique. J Thorac Cardiovasc Surg 1969; 58:178–85.
13. Weiner DA, Ryan TJ, McCabe CH, Kennedy JW, Schloss M, Tristani F, Chaitman BR, Fisher LD. Correlations among history of angina, ST segment response and

prevalence of coronary artery disease in the Coronary Artery Surgery Study (CASS). N Engl J Med 1979; 301:230–5.

14. Hammermeister KE, Bonica JJ. Cardiac and aortic pain. In: Bonica JJ, ed. The management of pain. 2nd ed. Philadelphia: Lea & Febiger, 1990: 1001–42.

15. Unstable angina pectoris: National Cooperative Study Group to Compare Surgical and Medical Therapy. II. In-hospital experience and initial follow-up results in patients with one, two and three vessel disease. Am J Cardiol 1978; 42:839–48.

16. Unstable angina pectoris: National Cooperative Study Group to Compare Surgical and Medical Therapy. III. Results in patients with ST segment elevation during pain. Am J Cardiol 1980, 45:819–24.

17. Unstable angina pectoris: National Cooperative Study Group to Compare Medical and Surgical Theory. IV. Results in patients with left anterior descending coronary artery disease. Am J Cardiol 1981; 48:517–24.

18. Luchi RJ, Scott SM, Deupree RH, et al. Comparison of medical and surgical treatment for unstable angina pectoris. Results of a Veterans Administration Cooperative Study. N Engl J Med 1987; 316:977–84.

19. European Coronary Surgery Study Group. Prospective randomised study of coronary artery bypass surgery in stable angina pectoris. Lancet 1980; 2:491–5.

20. CASS Principal Investigators and Their Associates. Coronary Artery Surgery Study (CASS): A randomized trial of coronary artery bypass surgery. Quality of life in patients randomly assigned to treatment groups. Circulation 1983; 68:951–60.

21. Hultgren HN, Peduzzi P, Detre K, et al. The 5 year effect of bypass surgery on relief of angina and exercise performance. Circulation 1985; 72:V-79–V-83.

22. Peduzzi P, Hultgren H, Miller C, et al. The five-year effect of coronary artery bypass surgery on relief of angina. Prog Cardiovasc Dis 1986; 28:267–72.

23. European Coronary Surgery Study Group. Long-term results of prospective randomized study of coronary artery bypass surgery in stable angina pectoris. Lancet 1982; 2:1173–80.

24. Campeau L, Enjalbert M, Lesperance J, et al. Course of angina 1 to 12 years after aortocoronary bypass surgery related to changes in grafts and native coronary arteries. Can J Surg 1985; 28:496–8.

25. Peduzzi P, Hultgren H, Thomsen J, et al. Ten-year effect of medical and surgical therapy on quality of life: Veterans Administration Cooperative Study of Coronary Artery Surgery. Am J Cardiol 1987; 59:1017–23.

26. Ribeiro P, Shea M, Deanfield JE, et al. Different mechanisms for the relief of angina after coronary bypass surgery. Physiological versus anatomical assessment. Br Heart J 1984; 52:502–9.

27. Hossack KF, Bruce RA, Ivey TD, et al. Improvement in aerobic and hemodynamic responses to exercise following aorta-coronary bypass grafting. J Thorac Cardiovasc Surg 1984; 87:901–7.

28. Chatterjee K, Swan HJC, Parmley WW, et al. Depression of left ventricular function due to acute myocardial ischemia and its reversal after aortocoronary saphenous-vein bypass. N Engl J Med 1972; 286:1117–22.

29. Kolibash AJ, Goodenow JS, Bush CA, et al. Improvement in myocardial perfusion and left ventricular function after coronary artery bypass grafting in patients with unstable angina. Circulation 1979; 59:66–74.

30. Leinbach RC, Gold HK, Dinsmore RE, et al. The role of angiography in cardiogenic shock. Circulation 1973; 48(Suppl III):95–8.
31. Scott SM, Luchi RJ, Deupree RH. Veterans Administration Cooperative Study for treatment of patients with unstable angina. Results in patients with abnormal left ventricular function. Circulation 1988; 78 (Suppl I):I-113–I-121.
32. McCormick JF, Schick EC Jr, McCabe CH, Kronmal RA, Ryan TJ. Determinants of operative mortality and long-term survival in patients with unstable angina. J Thorac Cardiovasc Surg 1985; 89:683–8.
33. Califf RM, Harrell FE, Lee KL, et al. Changing efficacy of coronary revascularization. Implications for patient selection. Circulation 1988; 78 (Suppl I):I-185–I-191).
34. Califf RM, Harrel FE, Lee KL, et al. The evolution of medical and surgical therapy for coronary artery disease. A 15-year perspective. J Am Med Soc 1989; 261:2077–86.
35. Kennedy JW, Kaiser GC, Fisher LD, et al. Multivariate discriminant analysis of the clinical and angiographic predictors of operative mortality from the Collaborative Study in Coronary Artery Surgery (CASS) J Thorac Cardiovasc Surg 1980; 80:876–87.
36. Kennedy JW, Kaiser GC, Fisher LD, et al. Clinical and angiographic predictors of operative mortality from the Collaborative Study in Coronary Artery Surgery (CASS). Circulation 1981; 63:793–802.
37. Gersh BJ, Kronmal RA, Frye RL, et al. Coronary arteriography and coronary artery bypass surgery: Morbidity and mortality in patients ages 65 and older. Circulation 1983; 67:483–91.
38. Loop FD, Golding LR, Macmillan JP, et al. Coronary artery surgery in women compared with men: Analyses of risks and long-term results. J Am Coll Cardiol 1983; 1:383–90.
39. Hammermeister KE, Burchfiel C, Johnson R, Grover FL. Identification of patients at greatest risk for developing major complications at cardiac surgery. Circulation 1990; 82 (Suppl IV):IV-380–IV-389.
40. Fisher LD, Kennedy JW, Davis KB, Maynard C, Fritz JK, Kaiser G, Myers WO. Association of sex, physical size and operative mortality after coronary artery bypass in the Coronary Artery Surgery Study (CASS). J Thorac Cardiovasc Surg 1982; 84:334–41.
41. Stuart RS, Baumgartner WA, Soule L, Borkon AM, Gardner TJ, Gott VL, Watkins L Jr, Reitz BA. Predictors of perioperative mortality in patients with unstable postinfarction angina. Circulation 1988; 78 (Suppl I):I-163–II-165.
42. Naunheim KS, Fiore C, Arango DC, Pennington DG, Barner HB, McBride LR, Harris HH, Willman VL, Kaiser GC. Coronary artery bypass grafting for unstable angina pectoris; risk analysis. Ann Thorac Surg 1989; 47:569–74.
43. Sethi GK, Copeland JG, Goldman S, and Participants in Veterans Administration Cooperative Study on antiplatelet therapy. Implications of preoperative administration of aspirin in patients undergoing coronary artery bypass grafting. J Am Coll Cardiol 1990; 15:13–20.

V
CORONARY ANGIOPLASTY
FOR UNSTABLE ANGINA

12

Percutaneous Transluminal Coronary Angioplasty in Patients with Unstable Angina
Historical Perspectives, Mayo Clinic Experience, and the BARI Study

Malcolm R. Bell

Mayo Clinic and Mayo Foundation
Rochester, Minnesota

David R. Holmes, Jr.

Mayo Medical School and Mayo Clinic
Rochester, Minnesota

INTRODUCTION

When percutaneous transluminal coronary angioplasty (PTCA) was first introduced into clinical cardiology practice in 1978 (1), its application was limited to patients with stable angina pectoris who had single-vessel disease. The target lesion was generally a single, discrete, concentric, subtotal stenosis situated in the proximal portion of the coronary vessel. Eligible patients also generally had normal left ventricular function. However, as operator experience developed, technology improved, and success rates increased, patient selection broadened to include higher-risk patients with more complicated lesions.

One important group of patients in clinical practice who had often posed a vexing problem of management were those with medically refractory unstable angina in whom the only available treatment option had been coronary artery bypass (CABG) surgery. These patients were generally considered at higher risk than those treated in the early period of PTCA because of the presence of multivessel coronary disease, eccentric or ulcerated lesions often associated with the presence of intracoronary thrombus, and the presence of impaired left ventricular function. Nevertheless, reports of the efficacy of PTCA in these patients first began to appear in 1981, and today its use continues to be invaluable in the management of selected patients with refractory unstable angina as an alternative to surgical revascularization.

This chapter will first discuss the safety and efficacy of PTCA in the management of patients with unstable angina from a historical perspective. The differences in outcome and complications following PTCA between patients with single-vessel disease and multivessel disease will be discussed. In some patients with multivessel disease, a strategy of dilating only the identifiable ''culprit'' lesion has been advocated; since this strategy results in incomplete revascularization, it is important to examine the outcome of such treated patients. A number of important randomized studies are now in progress comparing the outcome of patients, including those with unstable angina, treated with PTCA or CABG surgery. The final discussion will therefore focus on whether or not such trials, which include the National Heart, Lung, and Blood Institute (NHLBI)–sponsored Bypass Angioplasty Revascularization (BARI) study, will be able to fully address the important issue of choosing the most appropriate revascularization strategy for patients with unstable angina.

FEASIBILITY OF PTCA IN UNSTABLE ANGINA

Retrospective Series

Safety and Efficacy

The first published reports of the use of PTCA in patients with unstable angina appeared in 1981, one from North America and the other from Europe. The first of these dealt with 17 patients with unstable angina who underwent PTCA, with successful dilation achieved in 13 patients (76%) (2). All these patients had disabling angina, including angina at rest, with 10 experiencing medically refractory angina during hospitalization. Although all four failures underwent CABG surgery, only one of these was performed as an emergency. The only death occurred in a patient undergoing elective coronary surgery after the lesion could not be crossed with a guidewire. No myocardial infarctions occurred in this early series. At a mean follow-up of approximately 11 months, all patients were alive, with all but one patient asymptomatic, and none had had a myocardial infarction.

Similar results were also reported from Germany of 40 patients (3) who underwent PTCA in the setting of unstable angina with rest pain and transient ST or T-wave changes of ischemia, with a success rate of 63%. One patient required emergency bypass surgery after abrupt occlusion with the subsequent development of a myocardial infarction. Of the 14 failures, 11 underwent elective bypass surgery. No other complications or deaths were observed in this series.

These early series clearly demonstrated the feasibility of PTCA in selected patients with unstable angina, including patients with rest angina, demonstrating at least modest success rates with minimal complication rates and mortality. Since then a number of other authors (4–14) have reported their experiences with

Table 1 Use of PTCA in Patients with Unstable Angina

Author (year)	Number of patients	Mean age (years)	Included medically refractory unstable angina	Medical therapy included antiplatelet therapy	Success rate (%)	Acute complications		
						Death (%)	MI (%)	Emergency CABG (%)
Williams (1981)(2)	17	50	Yes	No	76	0	0	6
Meyer (1981)(3)	40	51	—	No	63	0	3	3
Meyer (1983)(4)	50	50	Yes	No	74	0	4	2
de Feyter (1985)(5)	60	59	Yes	No	93	0	7	7
Quigley (1986)(6)	25	53	No	No	81	4	12	12
de Feyter (1987)(7)	71	57	No	Yes	87	0	10	11
Steffenino (1987)(8)	89	55	No	Yes	90	0	5	4
Timmis (1987)(9)	56	53	No	No	70	5	7	13
Plokker (1988)(10)	469	57	Yes	Yes	88	1	5	3
Sharma (1988)(11)	40	56	Yes	Yes	88	0	0	13
de Feyter (1988)(12)	200	56	Yes	No	90	0.5	8	9
Perry (1988)(13)	105	50	Yes	Yes	87	2	9	4
Kamp (1989)(14)	334	54 (median)	—	No	87	0	9	10

MI = myocardial infarction; CABG = coronary artery bypass surgery.

therapeutic PTCA in the setting of unstable angina, with larger numbers of patients and overall success rates that have reached almost 90% (Table 1). Thus PTCA has been demonstrated to be safe and effective in patients with unstable angina who have been initially stabilized with medical therapy and has also proved to be safe and effective in patients refractory to intensive medical therapy. In the former patients, PTCA success rates have averaged 84% and in the latter group, averaged 87%.

The immediate mortality in these studies has ranged from 0% to 5.4% and acute myocardial infarction complicating the procedure has been reported to occur in 0–12% of attempted procedures (2–14). Although emergency CABG surgery has been necessary in 2–13% of cases, most of the larger series have reported rates of about 6% (10, 12–14).

Importance of Complex Lesions

Serial angiography has demonstrated that many patients with unstable angina will have rapidly progressive lesions (15) which are often complex, including lesions that may be ulcerated or contain intraluminal thrombus, as well as lesions in tandem, or lesions that have led to total occlusion (16). This probably explains the relatively high acute occlusion rates during or after PTCA with consequent procedural-related myocardial infarction, since more complex lesions are dilated in unstable angina patients (7,13) compared to patients with stable angina, in whom lower rates of myocardial infarction are generally anticipated. Although the recognition of complex lesions is very important, the stenosis severity of the lesion itself may actually be the most important predictive factor for procedural-related complications (12). The relation between the presence of intracoronary thrombus and the risk of acute complications is controversial (12,17) but may become clearer as more sensitive imaging technology is utilized in the future, which may enable improved visualization of intracoronary thrombus.

At the same time, it should be remembered that the natural history of patients with unstable angina treated with medical therapy has demonstrated that acute infarction among hospitalized patients approaches a rate that is similar to, if not higher than, those documented in the above studies (18,19). In recent years, aspirin therapy in medically treated patients has dramatically altered the immediate outcome of patients with unstable angina with respect to acute myocardial infarction and mortality (20,21). Antiplatelet therapy begun 24 hr prior to PTCA also reduces the acute complication rate associated with this procedure (22), but the effect of longer preprocedural administration in patients with unstable angina is unknown. It is important to emphasize that of the reported series of patients undergoing PTCA, only five studies (Table 1) included patients who had been receiving aspirin as part of their antianginal medical therapy (7,8,10,11,13), but there appears to have been little decrease in the overall abrupt occlusion rates when these latter studies are compared to the earlier studies. The majority of patients currently treated with PTCA in the setting of unstable angina are likely to have received antiplatelet and/or anticoagulant therapy during their initial hospitalization. It is possible that preprocedural heparin therapy (>24 hr) may increase success rates and decrease complications during PTCA (23). Whether this relates to the fact that patients who are more unstable cannot be managed conservatively on heparin for more than 24 hr, and require more urgent dilation with increased complications, is not certain. This will be a particularly interesting and important area for future research.

What is certain is that these patients represent a high-risk group who should be vigorously treated pharmacologically, and if PTCA is employed, vigilant awareness of potential acute vessel closure should be maintained while continuing adequate anticoagulant and antiplatelet therapy. If acute closure does occur, either in or out of the catheterization laboratory, immediate recatheterization and redilation, if appropriate, should be performed. The concomitant use of thrombolytic therapy in these emergency situations has been advocated by some, usually with intracoronary administration. It must be kept in mind that as many of these abrupt in-laboratory closures represent severe dissection rather than thrombus formation alone, thrombolytic therapy will probably only be effective when recurrent thrombus formation is evident as the cause of occlusion. If these maneuvers fail, then emergency CABG surgery should be considered in all suitable patients.

Early Outcome After Successful PTCA

Successful dilation of obstructive coronary lesions in these patients with unstable angina will result in relief of angina in the majority and improvement in objective functional testing (2,9,11). This is presumably due to sustained improvement in the vessel patency, with increased coronary blood flow, decreased coronary vascular resistance, and preservation of aerobic metabolism (2). Patients experiencing unstable angina will often have impaired ventricular function due to recurrent acute ischemia, which may improve after successful PTCA. Improvement in segmental and global wall motion, (24–26) and improvement in diastolic dysfunction (27), a sensitive indicator of myocardial ischemia, have all been observed after successful PTCA in these patients.

Follow-up Results

Long-term follow-up evaluation of these patients (mean duration ranging from 6 to 26 months) has documented that improvement in anginal symptoms can be maintained in the majority of patients, with most remaining asymptomatic (Table 2) (2–12,14). Functional improvement during follow-up has been confirmed with exercise testing, often combined with radioisotope imaging (2,5,7–9,11,12).

It appears that during the first few months or years following PTCA, the incidence of death and/or myocardial infarction is very low in successfully treated patients. Angiographic restenosis occurs in about 30% of cases restudied for recurrence of symptoms. Although these rates appear similar to those after PTCA in patients with stable angina, recent evidence suggests that restenosis

220

Table 2 Follow-up Data for Patients with Unstable Angina Undergoing Successful PTCA

Author (year)	Duration of follow-up (mean; months)	Asymptomatic or class I or II angina (%)	Objective functional testing data	Death (%)	MI (%)	CABG (%)	Angiographic restenosis (%)
				Follow-up events			
Williams (1981)(2)	11	92	Yes	0	0	0	—
Meyer (1982)(3)	5	59	No	0	0	0	29
Meyer (1983)(4)	5	64	No	0	0	0	25
de Feyter (1985)(5)	9	88	Yes	2	0	7	28
Quigley (1986)(6)	14	—	No	0	0	5	32
de Feyter (1987)(7)	12	92	Yes	2	2	5	25
Steffenino (1987)(8)	10	73	Yes	0	1	5	37
Timmis (1987)(9)	6	93	Yes	3	3	0	100[a]
Plokker (1988)(10)[b]	19	—	No	—	—	—	28
Sharma (1988)(11)	11	86	Yes	0	0	6	57
de Feyter (1988)(12)	>24	97	Yes	3	12	15	32
Kamp (1989)(14)	25	—	No	5	14	21	—

[a]Only the six patients (21%) with recurrent angina underwent repeat angiography—all had restenosis.
[b]Actuarial follow-up data revealed that after 5 years, 78.8% of patients had remained event-free (recurrence of angina, myocardial infarction, re-PTCA, coronary artery bypass grafting, or death).
Abbreviations as for Table 1.

rates may be higher among patients with unstable angina versus stable angina, reflecting a more "active" lesion at the time of dilation (28). Factors that may increase the risk of restenosis in these patients include the present of lesions in the left anterior descending coronary artery, presence of collateral vessels, ST-segment depression, multivessel disease, recent onset of pain, multiple luminal irregularities and poor distal flow (12,29). Many of these patients with restenosis can be satisfactorily managed with repeat angioplasty, but surgical revascularization may be necessary in some patients, particularly if multivessel disease is present, although the need for late CABG surgery appears to be low (approximately 1–5%).

Additional Indications for PTCA in Unstable Angina
The vast majority of these early and late series of patients have dealt with relatively younger patients (average age approximately 50–55 years), yet many patients admitted to hospital with unstable angina are much older and continue to present vexing problems with regard to the most appropriate choice of therapy, especially if they are refractory to intensive pharmacological management. Little is known about the outcome of elderly patients following attempted PTCA in unstable angina. In a series of patients reported from the Mayo Clinic (30), the immediate and long-term outcomes of 54 patients aged 70 years or older undergoing PTCA for unstable angina were examined. The success rate of attempted dilation was 80% in this patient population and was achieved with no mortality and minimum morbidity. The incidence of late ischemic events appeared to be acceptably low for this aged population, with over 70% of patients remaining asymptomatic during late follow-up.

Another important consideration for PTCA is in the management of the increasing number of patients with previous CABG surgery who present with medically refractory unstable angina. These patients present a clinical challenge since the results of repeat CABG surgery in patients with stable effort angina are generally not as good as those achieved with the first operation and may be associated with a higher complication rate. In addition, the cause of the deterioration in anginal symptoms may represent not only progression of ungrafted native vessel disease but also occlusion of one or more of the bypass grafts. Morrison (31) has shown that PTCA may be a feasible therapeutic option in patients presenting with refractory unstable angina who have had prior surgery. Although only a small group of 34 patients was studied, a PTCA success rate of 94% was achieved with no deaths or infarctions. In this series, almost half the dilated lesions were located in the bypass grafts.

Included in the spectrum of patients with unstable angina are also those who experience refractory angina, usually at rest, during the early recovery phase of an acute myocardial infarction. Although these are high-risk patients, with the potential for reinfarction and progressive myocardial necrosis, PTCA can be successfully performed with success rates similar to those associated with other types of unstable angina, as discussed above (32–35).

NHLBI PTCA Registry

In addition to the series of patients discussed above, which were all retrospectively analyzed, data from the initial NHLBI PTCA registry (1979–1982) also support the view that PTCA can be performed safely and successfully in patients with unstable angina (36). This registry cohort included 1939 patients with single–lesion–single–vessel disease, 66% of whom had unstable angina. The success rates for patients with stable and unstable angina were almost identical, 65.6% versus 64.6%, respectively, with no difference observed in the incidence of acute complications or need for emergency CABG surgery. Follow-up of about one-half the patients revealed that symptomatic improvement and event rates were similar between the two groups of patients; however, patients who initially had unstable angina had a higher rate of late CABG surgery.

While the outcome of PTCA in patients with unstable angina and single-vessel disease appeared favorable, the question then arose as to the overall outcome of patients when those with multivessel disease were included. The initial registry experience was confined to patients with single-vessel disease, but toward the end of the registry enrollment period, a substantial number of patients with multivessel disease were also added (total of 768 of 3079 patients). Analysis of the entire registry cohort revealed that success rates were only slightly lower among patients with multivessel disease compared to single-vessel disease, 63% and 68%, respectively (37). As with the single-vessel disease cohort alone, the success rate of PTCA in patients with unstable angina (67%) was also similar to the rate in those with stable angina (66%).

Subsequent to these reports, preliminary data from the 1985 NLBI PTCA registry, which included patients with multivessel disease, poor left ventricular function, and prior CABG surgery, have shown that success rates have continued to improve (38). Indeed, the success rate for 350 unstable angina patients was 82.3% versus 72.5% of 260 patients with stable angina, although major nonfatal complications (coronary occlusion or myocardial infarction) were slightly more common in the unstable angina patients (7.7% versus 5.0%).

Prospective Series

The high success rates and relatively low complication rates, as well as the favorable long-term clinical outcome, found in retrospective studies have also been confirmed in prospective analyses (29,39). These studies thus emphasize the feasibility of the use of PTCA in patients with unstable angina. Furthermore, such prospective analyses have enabled identification of patients who have multiple luminal irregularities and thrombolysis-in-myocardial-infarction flow grade less than 3 as being at high risk of restenosis (29).

PTCA IN PATIENTS WITH MULTIVESSEL DISEASE AND UNSTABLE ANGINA

Among the reported series of patients undergoing PTCA with unstable angina, the vast majority of treated patients had single-vessel disease (2–10,12,13,37). Nevertheless, patients with multivessel disease have also had PTCA performed in this situation with primary success rates and complication rates similar to those with single-vessel disease (9–12,39). The presence of multivessel disease and total coronary occlusions appear to represent important risk factors for late coronary events (myocardial infarction, recurrent angina, or death) during follow-up (12).

While most of the PTCA experience in patients with unstable angina and multivessel disease has involved single-lesion dilation, multilesion PTCA in these patients has also been performed without appearing to affect the primary success rate, the incidence of acute complications, or long-term follow-up results, including the incidence of angiographic restenosis. Whether this experience can be generalized is uncertain, but there are a number of reasons why multilesion angioplasty has not been widely embraced for the management of patients with unstable angina. PTCA of each lesion carries with it the risk of acute occlusion; therefore, dilation of additional lesions, even if less complex, will expose the patient to some increased risk (40). Any hemodynamic deterioration associated with vessel occlusion will also adversely affect coronary blood flow through the area of additionally dilated segments with the risk of acute closure. Many patients will have impaired ventricular function from previous infarctions or because of stunned myocardium related to the ischemia-causing vessel. It should be obvious that in the unstable patient with already limited contractile reserve, multiple balloon dilations in multiple vessels will further compromise left ventricular function acutely and multiple occlusions will certainly not be well tolerated.

Dilation of the "Culprit" Lesion

The issue in multivessel disease patients of single versus multilesion angioplasty is very relevant since many of those undergoing single-lesion PTCA remain incompletely revascularized, although many of these will continue to experience long-term symptomatic improvement similar to those after successful dilation of single-vessel disease (8,10,11).

The systematic approach to dilating only the ischemia-causing vessel (the "culprit" lesion) has been studied and advocated in the management of patients with multivessel disease who have refractory unstable angina (41,42). Identification of the culprit lesion is possible in many patients using angiographic (severity of stenosis, presence of thrombus, or ulcerated plaque) and electrocardiographic evidence. The primary success rates with this approach are generally excellent, with subsequent resolution of symptoms in most patients. Improvement in left ventricular function can be expected in many patients after successful dilation (26). Myocardial infarction again occurs with a frequency of about 9% but is generally confined to the failed PTCAs and can be managed with emergency CABG surgery (42).

While long-term follow-up of successfully treated patients using this strategy reveals that many patients will remain clinically improved (41,42), the results of exercise testing and radionuclide scintigraphy suggest that a significant number of patients will have residual ischemia. This is presumably because of incomplete revascularization in most and restenosis of the dilated lesion in others. Consistent with this observation is the higher recurrence rate of angina compared to similarly treated patients with single-vessel disease (completely revascularized) (42). Careful clinical follow-up of patients with multivessel disease should be maintained as those with incomplete revascularization may potentially continue to have myocardial ischemia as documented by electrocardiography and perfusion scintigraphy during exercise (7).

Prospective studies, preferably randomized, will be required to confirm the overall efficacy and safety of culprit lesion angioplasty versus multilesion angioplasty in patients with unstable angina and multivessel disease. Extended follow-up of these patients will also be necessary to determine the recurrence rates of angina, as well as survival and incidence of late myocardial infarction. Not all institutions have had good experiences with this strategy (43), and as increasing numbers of patients with more extensive coronary disease are referred for PTCA with unstable angina, the need for more data is crucial. Meanwhile, it does appear that in selected patients, PTCA remains a worthwhile alternative to surgery. However, in some patients PTCA should only be considered as an initial therapy since further revascularization, with either PTCA or surgery at a later date may be required. Therefore, careful clinical follow-up of these patients with incomplete revascularization is essential.

THE MAYO CLINIC EXPERIENCE: PTCA FOR REST PAIN

At the Mayo Clinic the current strategy employed for patients who have been hospitalized with unstable angina is to attempt initially to treat the ischemia with intensive medical therapy (aspirin, intravenous heparin, nitrates, beta-blockers, and calcium-channel antagonists). Patients who fail to respond adequately to this medical regimen are generally referred directly for diagnostic angiography and patients with suitable coronary anatomy are considered for immediate PTCA. We currently attempt to dilate only the culprit lesion in patients with multivessel disease, particularly if this lesion is complex and is associated with thrombus, or if the other lesions appear to be high-risk lesions. In some cases it is not always possible to accurately assess the severity of other lesions at the time of angiography, but future application of on-line digital quantitative angiographic techniques may overcome this limitation. Patients who have responded to medical therapy and who are then referred for catheterization will usually be considered for complete revascularization if possible.

A review through a computerized data bank of all patients undergoing PTCA at the Mayo Clinic since 1979 reveals that 1296 patients (average age of 64 years) with unstable angina had experienced rest angina immediately prior to their procedure. Of these patients, 431 (33%) had single-vessel disease and 865 patients (67%) had multivessel disease (55% two- and 45% three-vessel disease). The baseline features of these patients are listed in Table 3. More patients with multivessel disease had undergone prior CABG surgery and had a history of prior myocardial infarction compared to patients with single-vessel disease; left ventricular ejection fraction was also slightly lower in the former group. Despite these baseline differences, the overall success rate of PTCA (improvement in luminal diameter of >40% with no in-hospital coronary artery surgery) in this setting was very similar (86% for single-vessel disease and 87% for multivessel disease) (Table 4). Angiographic evidence of intracoronary thrombus at the site of the lesion to be dilated was present in approximately 5% of patients.

We have found that this success rate has been achieved with a relatively low rate of acute complications, considering that all patients had rest pain (Table 4).

Table 3 Baseline Characteristics of 1296 Patients at the Mayo Clinic Undergoing PTCA for Rest Pain and Unstable Angina

Characteristic	Single-vessel disease ($n = 431$) n (%)	Multivessel disease ($n = 865$) n (%)
Age, years (mean ± SD)	61 ± 11	66 ± 11
Males	277(64)	553(64)
Prior coronary artery bypass surgery	53(12)	164(19)*
History of myocardial infarction	186(43)	479(55)*
Current smoker	118(28)	176(20)*
Diabetes	44(10)	164(19)*
Hypertension	172(40)	480(56)*
Vessels diseased		
Two	—	478(55)
Three	—	387(45)
Left ventricular ejection fraction, %	63 ± 11 (in 315 patients)	60 ± 14 (in 613 patients)
Vessel diameter stenosis, % (mean ± SD)	89 ± 11	87 ± 11

*$p < 0.05$ single- versus multivessel disease.

Table 4 Immediate Outcome of PTCA in Patients with Rest Angina

Number of vessels diseased	Success (%)	Acute complications			Angiographic restenosis (%)
		In-hospital mortality (%)	Acute MI (%)	Emergency CABG (%)	
Single-vessel disease	86	0.9	3.7	4.6	50
Multivessel disease					
All patients	87	3.6*	3.8	3.6	56
Single-lesion PTCA	83	2.8	3.5	3.7	57
Multilesion PTCA	93	5.0	4.4	3.4	55

*$p < 0.05$ compared to single-vessel disease.

PTCA = percutaneous transluminal coronary angioplasty; other abbreviations as for Table 1.

In-hospital mortality was 0.9% among patients with single-vessel disease but significantly higher among patients with multivessel disease (3.6%). A total of 51 patients (3.9%) required emergency CABG surgery following complications of the procedure, with no major difference noted between patients with single- versus multivessel disease. Compared to the studies discussed earlier, the incidence of myocardial infarction has been low in both groups, 3.7% and 3.8%, respectively. Corresponding to this is an in-lab abrupt occlusion rate of about 6% among all patients. Overall symptomatic improvement in hospital survivors has been excellent, with 97% of single-vessel disease patients and 94% of multivessel disease patients experiencing improvement in anginal class.

During an average of 2.8 years of follow-up, the cumulative 5-year survival for hospital survivors has been 88%. Five-year event-free survival (freedom from Canadian Cardiovascular Society class III or IV angina, myocardial infarction, or CABG) has been lower (47%). Not surprisingly, patients with multivessel disease consistently have higher predicted event rates compared to patients with single-vessel disease, although this is mainly in terms of mortality and occurrence of myocardial infarction.

Follow-up angiography is not routine at our institution and is generally requested only if there is a suspicion of restenosis or residual ischemia. Among 181 patients with successfully dilated single-vessel disease returning for angiography, angiographic restenosis has been documented in 50% of dilated lesions. The restenosis rate has been 56% (p = NS) among 316 patients with multivessel disease. These relatively high rates undoubtedly reflect a selection bias in referral patterns for repeat angiography. The overall restenosis rates would be lower if all successfully dilated patients were included in the denominator.

Multivessel Disease: Single- Versus Multilesion PTCA

Sixty-six percent of the 865 patients with multivessel disease underwent only single-lesion angioplasty; the remaining 34% had multilesion dilation performed. There has been a trend toward a higher number of patients with three-vessel disease undergoing multilesion angioplasty (49%) versus single-lesion angioplasty (42%). Success has been achieved in 83% of single-lesion angioplasty and in 93% of multilesion angioplasty patients (at least one segment successfully dilated). Again, no significant difference was observed in the need for emergency bypass surgery, which was required in 3.5% overall. We have observed an in-hospital mortality of 2.8% and 5% for single and multilesion angioplasty, respectively. Occlusions in the catheterization laboratory have occurred in 8% of single-lesion and 10% of multilesion patients, and acute myocardial infarction complicated the course in 4% of patients in each group. At the time of hospital dismissal, 94% of patients had experienced symptomatic improvement.

During extended follow-up, no significant differences in either survival or event-free survival (vida supra) have been found between patients in whom single-lesion versus multilesion angioplasty had been initially performed. In those patients who have been studied with follow-up angiography, restenosis has been documented in 57% of lesions after single-lesion angioplasty and 55% of lesions after multilesion angioplasty (p = NS). These figures correspond to restenosis rates per patient of 57% and 71%, respectively. It therefore appears that despite incomplete angiographic follow-up, restenosis rates per patient increase after multilesion angioplasty, but this is probably due to the presence of more lesions at risk rather than any inexplicable aggressive pathophysiological process.

PTCA VERSUS CABG SURGERY IN UNSTABLE ANGINA

Whether the outcome of suitable patients with unstable angina differs between patients treated with PTCA versus CABG surgery can probably only be satisfactorily answered with a prospective randomized trial. Until the results of such ongoing studies become available, we are left with the notion that PTCA appears to be an acceptable treatment option in selected patients, yet we remain unsure as to whether it has the same efficacy and safety as surgery.

Analysis of the outcome of patients from the initial NHLBI PTCA registry with unstable angina, who had single-vessel disease and underwent PTCA, showed that outcome compared favorably with single-vessel-disease patients from the Coronary Artery Surgery Study (CASS) registry who underwent CABG surgery for unstable angina (Table 5) (44). The latter patients underwent surgical revascularization with an in-hospital mortality rate (0.9%) similar to those treated with PTCA, and after accounting for the baseline differences between the

Table 5 Comparison of Use of PTCA in Patients from NHLBI PTCA Registry with Unstable Angina Versus Stable Angina Versus Patients with Unstable Angina Treated Surgically in the CASS registry

Group (angina)	Number of patients	Mean age (years)	Success rate (%)	In-hospital mortality (%)	No angina or class I or II at 12 months (%)	Follow-up events (18 months)	
						Deaths (%)	MI (%)
PTCA (unstable)	442	53.6	61	0.9	90	2.6	9.5
PTCA (stable)	214	51.7	64	0.4	—	1.4	8
Surgical (unstable)	330	53.3	—	0.9	80	2.7	7

Abbreviations as for Tables 1 and 4.
Source: Faxon et al. (44).

two groups, no difference was found in the combined mortality plus myocardial infarction rate after 18 months. The only evident difference was in the functional status of the patients after 1 year of follow-up. Ninety percent of the PTCA group were in Canadian Cardiovascular Society class I or II or were asymptomatic, compared to 80% of the surgical group, with 82% of the patients treated with PTCA remaining asymptomatic versus only 63% of the surgical patients. Most of the immediate ischemic problems were confined to those patients in whom PTCA had been unsuccessful, and e majority of patients with failed PTCA underwent CABG surgery prior to hospital dismissal.

Although these data from the initial NHLBI registry (44) are encouraging, a number of important caveats should be emphasized. First, these patients represent a select population—all had single-vessel disease, a condition well known to be associated with an excellent long-term prognosis, and so major differences in outcome would be unlikely. Second, the PTCA registry data pertain to the "learning curve" period of angioplasty at a time when steerable guidewire systems were not yet available. Finally, the two studies were performed a few years apart, during which time a number of advances in the medical management of angina were made. For instance, aspirin was probably not employed in the medical management of patients prior to either PTCA or CABG surgery being performed. Whether it would have influenced the immediate outcome is not clear, but we have since learned that antiplatelet therapy at the time of CABG surgery does improve the early and late (1-year) patency rates of saphenous vein grafts (45,46). The lack of antiplatelet therapy could well have influenced the late follow-up results in the surgical group in this analysis.

These caveats should cause the reader to interpret these results cautiously, since improvements in medical therapy, technical developments, and improved operator expertise with PTCA, and refinements in surgical technique, suggest that extrapolation of these results to today may be fraught with error.

One prospective, but nonrandomized, study comparing the use of PTCA and surgery in unstable angina has been reported (39) dealing with 104 consecutive patients who were hospitalized with unstable angina (Table 6). In comparison to the NHLBI registry and CASS reports, more than half these patients had multivessel disease. The total in-hospital mortality for these patients was 4%, while 8% suffered acute myocardial infarction, which again emphasizes the serious nature of unstable angina. Forty-four percent were refractory to intensive pharmacological therapy, which included aspirin or heparin, or both. During hospitalization, only 13% of patients were continued on medical therapy alone, whereas 46% were referred for CABG surgery and 41% for PTCA. PTCA was successful in 88% of patients referred for this procedure, with four of the failed patients requiring CABG surgery (two emergency). There were no in-hospital deaths after attempted angioplasty, compared to a surgical mortality rate of 9% (4 of 45 patients). The majority of deaths and acute myocardial infarctions occurred in patients who had initially been unresponsive to medical therapy.

Long-term follow-up in this study revealed that the mortality in the PTCA group was extremely low, and no cases of myocardial infarction occurred. Although more patients in the medically responsive group treated with PTCA were free of angina than surgically treated patients, the reverse was true for patients who were refractory to medical treatment. Despite the fact that this study was not randomized and that surgically treated patients tended to have more extensive coronary disease than PTCA-treated patients, it does support the role of PTCA as a viable alternative to surgery in selected patients with unstable angina, particularly if symptoms are unresponsive to medical therapy.

Patients with unsuitable coronary anatomy, such as significant (> 50% diameter stenosis) left main coronary artery disease or technically complex lesions present in a vessel supplying a large amount of viable myocardium in

Table 6 Early and Late Outcome of Patients with Unstable Angina Assigned to PTCA or CABG Surgery

Group	Number of patients	Mean number of diseased vessels	Success rate (%)	In-hospital complications Death (%)	MI (%)	Emergency CABG (%)	Follow-up status (mean 16.7 months) Number of patients	Death (%)	MI (%)	CABG (%)	Free of angina (%)
PTCA	41	1.7	88	0	12	5	36	3	0	0	61
Surgical	45	2.9	—	9	2	—	39	8	10	3	69

Abbreviations as for Tables 1 and 4.
Source: Leeman et al. (39).

patients with severely impaired left ventricular function, should probably be considered for surgery rather than PTCA at the outset. Patients with severe three-vessel disease, even with depressed left ventricular function, may still be considered for PTCA if there is suitable anatomy, but at present it is not clear whether this is as effective as surgical revascularization.

Prospective, Randomized Trials of PTCA Versus CABG Surgery in Unstable Angina

Since its introduction, there has been explosive growth in the numbers of patients undergoing PTCA. It is estimated that 300,000–400,000 patients had this procedure in 1990, surpassing the number of coronary surgical revascularization procedures during the same time period. Well-controlled cooperative studies have been carried out to define the role of CABG surgery in varying subsets of patients with coronary artery disease. Such trials have been notably lacking in the field of interventional cardiology dealing with PTCA. This is being remedied by five trials that are currently enrolling patients or have finished enrollment.

The BARI Study

The Bypass Angioplasty Revascularization Investigation study (BARI) will be the largest American study. It includes both a randomized group of 2400 patients randomly assigned to either PTCA or CABG surgery as well as a registry group of patients who could have been randomized, but were not, for reasons ranging from patient to physician preference. This study is a comparative study of PTCA versus CABG surgery in patients who have multivessel coronary artery disease and severe angina or ischemia and who are suitable for either revascularization procedure. The trial was constructed to test the hypothesis that in those patients who could receive either treatment, an initial strategy of PTCA does not compromise clinical outcome during a 5-year follow-up period. The major end-point is mortality, with secondary end-points being infarction, repeat revascularization, and recurrent ischemia.

Patient Selection

The intent was to study patients currently being treated with either PTCA or CABG surgery for multivessel disease and severe angina pectoris or ischemia. As such, eligible patients must (a) have clinically severe angina or ischemia requiring a revascularization procedure, (b) have angiographically documented multivessel coronary artery disease, (c) be suitable for either PTCA and CABG after review by both an angiographer and a cardiovascular surgeon, and (d) be able to give informed consent. Patients with primary valvular heart disease, prior PTCA or CABG surgery, single-vessel disease, or advanced age greater than 80 years were excluded.

Other criteria include suitability for CABG surgery or PTCA. For the latter, the lesions to be dilated must have anatomical characteristics associated with a reasonable likelihood of successful dilatation. While not all arteries were required to be dilated (i.e., complete revascularization was not necessary by protocol), the major stenoses felt to be responsible for the clinical ischemia must be amenable to dilatation. Angiographic exclusions included lesions unlikely to be successfully dilated because of excessive tortuosity, angulation, length, chronic old total occlusion, or excessive lesion calcification. Other exclusion criteria included lesions of such importance that abrupt closure would result in cardiogenic shock or lesions with a major side branch that could not be adequately protected. Suitability for CABG surgery included assessment as to presence of vessels of adequate size (>1 mm) in the vessels to be grafted, satisfactory distal runoff, absence of severe diffuse involvement or extreme aortic calcification, and finally, enough disease to warrant surgery.

Completeness of Revascularization

Complete revascularization is not a requirement for patient entry. As has been documented, complete revascularization is more readily achieved with CABG. In patients undergoing PTCA in the BARI trial, lesions to be dilated are prospectively coded as essential (culprit lesions) or significant (revascularization indicated). This is particularly important in patients with unstable angina and multivessel disease. In these patients, as has been emphasized, PTCA of culprit lesions may result in a satisfactory clinical outcome. In the BARI trial, the majority of randomized patients have unstable angina. This trial should therefore allow objective assessment of the strategy of dilating the culprit lesion in patients with multivessel disease and unstable angina.

Quality Control and End-Points

Quality control and comparable procedures among the participating institutions are essential in a multicenter study such as this. Core laboratories include quantitative angiography, left ventricular angiography, electrocardiographic reading, and assessment of exercise tests, as well as lipid analysis. Prospective criteria for qualifications of angiographers and cardiovascular surgeons were set up and monitored so that quality was maintained throughout. Follow-up patient visit schedules were outlined with appropriate follow-up data forms. Finally, a central data registry was designed.

As has been mentioned, the primary aim was to test the hypothesis that an initial strategy of PTCA in patients eligible for either PTCA or CABG does not compromise clinical outcome. Nine major end-points are being assessed: mortality, myocardial infarction, angina/chest pain, myocardial ischemia, subsequent revascularization, resource utilization, quality of life, angiographic characteristics at 5 years, and left ventricular function at 5 years.

Potential Limitations of Study

Design of a long-term study such as BARI has many potential problems. Designing any study to have applicability when it is finished in 7 years (2 years of recruitment, 5 years of follow-up) is problematic given the rapid evolution of medical care that has occurred over the past 10 years and continues to occur. To an extent that new devices will play a major role in solving the problems of PTCA, this potentially could have a major impact on results. Given that the technology of CABG surgery is more mature and stable compared to interventional cardiology, any change in technology may impact more on PTCA than surgery. The BARI trial by design does not include new devices such as atherectomy, laser, or stents as primary treatment options, although these new devices can be used to treat complications of the initial PTCA procedure or to treat restenosis that occurs during follow-up after the initial dilatation. If a new technology is developed with a device, drugs, or a combination that eliminates restenosis, that will also have major implications for analysis of the trial. At present, such a breakthrough in restenosis seems unlikely in the next few years. Development of a new device that effectively allows treatment of diffuse disease and/or old total occlusions will also have a major impact, although at present such a new device either does not exist or is not widely available. It is anticipated that for the next decade or so, PTCA will remain the mainstay of interventional cardiology, so these concerns may not cause significant problems in translating the conclusions reached from BARI to other comparable patient groups.

A second potential group of problems with any large study is patient selection and applicability of results. During design of such a study, consideration must be given to the patient population available, recruitment goals, funding, and the biases of the investigators. Some of these biases became apparent during design of the BARI study with an exclusion of patients with single-vessel proximal left anterior descending coronary stenoses as well as exclusion of very elderly patients (> 80 years). The BARI study is not all-inclusive. One of the most important patient exclusions is prior PTCA or CABG surgery. Given the high incidence of patients who have had PTCA in the past, a large group is thereby excluded. Patients with single-vessel disease are also excluded. Each of these exclusion criteria was extensively debated during formulation of the BARI study. An additional factor is the increased number of patients who are randomizable, but are not randomized because of either their own desires or those of the primary cardiologist. To the extent that this introduces biases into the randomized group, it may affect results. Randomizable patients who are not randomized will be enrolled in a registry and followed similarly to that seen in the CASS trial. In the latter study, conclusions from the randomized portion were translatable to the larger registry group.

In the BARI study, as is true with all other studies, conclusions are relevant to the patient population studied. In this case conclusions will be relevant to the patients with multivessel disease, many of whom have unstable angina, without prior procedures who could undergo revascularization with either PTCA or CABG surgery. In this group there will be a wealth of data with which to assess these techniques and put them into perspective.

SUMMARY

Questions remain in approaching the patient with unstable angina, whether it is responsive or refractory to medical therapy. Although a considerable body of data exists regarding mechanisms, pathophysiology, and outcome of patients with unstable angina, for any specific patient, questions remain. Revascularization is usually required, although, if possible, medical therapy to stabilize the patient is optimal. The decision as to whether to proceed with PTCA or surgery depends on the clinical setting, the specific anatomical features of the lesions involved, the extent of coronary disease, and the status of left ventricular function. PTCA is increasingly used to treat culprit lesions in this setting with often excellent results. If complete revascularization can be achieved, the results may be even better. Limitations exist with acute closure, restenosis, and inability to access some lesions. Solutions to these problems will increase the number of patients in whom a catheterization-based approach may be used. The ultimate role of PTCA in these patients will depend on these solutions as well as the information gained from the randomized trials of PTCA versus CABG surgery.

REFERENCES

1. Grüntzig A. Transluminal dilatation of coronary artery stenosis (letter). Lancet 1978; 1:263.
2. Williams DO, Riley RS, Singh AK, Gewirtz H, Most AS. Evaluation of the role of coronary angioplasty in patients with unstable angina pectoris. Am Heart J 1981; 102:1–9.
3. Meyer J, Schmitz H, Erbel R, et al. Treatment of unstable angina pectoris with percutaneous transluminal coronary angioplasty (PTCA). Cathet Cardiovasc Diagn 1981; 7:361–71.
4. Meyer J, Schmitz HJ, Kiesslich T, et al. Percutaneous transluminal coronary angioplasty in patients with stable and unstable angina pectoris: analysis of early and late results. Am Heart J 1983; 106:973–80.
5. de Feyter PJ, Serruys PW, van den Brand M, et al. Emergency coronary angioplasty in refractory unstable angina. N Engl J Med 1985; 313:342–6.
6. Quigley PJ, Erwin J, Maurer BJ, Walsh MJ, Gearty GF. Percutaneous transluminal coronary angioplasty in unstable angina: comparison with stable angina. Br Heart J 1986; 55:227–30.
7. de Feyter PJ, Serruys PW, Suryapranata H, Beatt K, van den Brand M. Coronary angioplasty early after diagnosis of unstable angina. Am Heart J 1987; 114:48–54.

8. Steffenino G, Meier B, Finci L, Rutishauser W. Follow up results of treatment of unstable angina by coronary angioplasty. Br Heart J 1987; 57:416–9.

9. Timmis AD, Griffin B, Crick JC, Sowton E. Early percutaneous transluminal coronary angioplasty in the management of unstable angina. Int J Cardiol 1987; 14:25–31.

10. Plokker THW, Ernst SM, Bal ET, et al. Percutaneous transluminal coronary angioplasty in patients with unstable angina pectoris refractory to medical therapy: Long-term clinical and angiographic results. Cathet Cardiovasc Diagn 1988; 14: 15–8.

11. Sharma B, Wyeth RP, Kolath GS, Gimenez HJ, Franciosa JA. Percutaneous transluminal coronary angioplasty of one vessel for refractory unstable angina pectoris: Efficacy in single and multivessel disease. Br Heart J 1988; 59:280–6.

12. de Feyter PJ, Suryapranata H, Serruys PW, et al. Coronary angioplasty for unstable angina: immediate and late results in 200 consecutive patients with identification of risk factors for unfavorable early and late outcome. J Am Coll Cardiol 1988; 12:324–33.

13. Perry RA, Seth A, Hunt A, Shiu MF. Coronary angioplasty in unstable angina and stable angina: A comparison of success and complications. Br Heart J 1988; 60:367–72.

14. Kamp O, Beatt KJ, de Feyter PJ, et al. Short-, medium-, and long-term follow-up after percutaneous transluminal coronary angioplasty for stable and unstable angina pectoris. Am Heart J 1989; 117:991–6.

15. Kimbiris D, Iskandrian A, Saras H, et al. Rapid progression of coronary stenosis in patients with unstable angina pectoris selected for coronary angioplasty. Cathet Cardiovasc Diagn 1984; 10:101–14.

16. Gambhir DS, Nair M, Prasad R, Sethi KK, Khanna SK, Khalilullah M. Coronary angioplasty of 'complex lesions' in patients with unstable angina. Indian Heart J 1989; 41:233–9.

17. Mabin TA, Holmes DR, Smith HC, et al. Intracoronary thrombus: role in coronary occlusion complicating percutaneous transluminal coronary angioplasty. J. Am Coll Cardiol 1985; 5:198–202.

18. Cairns JA, Fantus IG, Klassen GA. Unstable angina pectoris. Am Heart J 1976; 92:373–86.

19. Russell RO, Moraski RE, Kouchoukos N, et al. Unstable angina pectoris: National Cooperative Study Group to Compare Surgical and Medical Therapy II. In-hospital experience and initial follow-up results in patients with one, two and three vessel disease. Am J Cardiol 1987; 42:839–48.

20. Cairns JA, Gent M, Singer J, et al. Aspirin, sulfinpyrazone, or both in unstable angina. Results of a Canadian multicenter trial. N Engl J Med 1985; 313:1369–75.

21. Lewis HDJ, Davis JW, Archibald DG, et al. Protective effects of aspirin against acute myocardial infarction and death in men with unstable angina. Results of a Veterans Administration Cooperative Study. N Engl J Med 1983; 309:396–403.

22. Schwartz L, Bourassa MG, Lesperance J, et al. Aspirin and dipyridamole in the prevention of restenosis after percutaneous transluminal coronary angioplasty. N Engl J Med 1988; 318:1714–9.

23. Laskey MA, Deutsch E, Barnathan E, Laskey WK. Influence of heparin therapy on

percutaneous transluminal coronary angioplasty outcome in unstable angina pectoris. Am J Cardiol 1990; 65:1425–9.

24. Carlson EB, Cowley MJ, Wolfgang TC, Vetrovec GW. Acute changes in global and regional rest left ventricular function after successful coronary angioplasty: Comparative results in stable and unstable angina. J Am Coll Cardiol 1989; 13:1262–9.

25. Renkin J, Wijns W, Ladha Z, Col J. Reversal of segmental hypokinesis by coronary angioplasty in patients with unstable angina, persistent T wave inversion, and left anterior descending coronary artery stenosis. Additional evidence for myocardial stunning in humans. Circulation 1990; 82:913–21.

26. de Feyter PJ, Suryapranata H, Serruys PW, Beatt K, van den Brand M, Hugenholtz PG. Effects of successful percutaneous transluminal coronary angioplasty on global and regional left ventricular function in unstable angina pectoris. Am J. Cardiol 1987; 60:993–7.

27. Snow FR, Gorcsan J III., Lewis SA, Cowley MJ, Vetrovec GW, Nixon JV. Doppler echocardiographic evaluation of left ventricular diastolic function after percutaneous transluminal coronary angioplasty for unstable angina pectoris or acute myocardial infarction. Am J Cardiol 1990; 65:840–4.

28. Foley JB, Chisolm RJ, Armstrong PW. Restenosis after PTCA for unstable angina has a different natural history. Circulation 1990; 82(Suppl III):III–338 (Abstract).

29. Halon DA, Merdler A, Shefer A, Flugelman MY, Lewis BS. Identifying patients at high risk for restenosis after percutaneous transluminal coronary angioplasty for unstable angina pectoris. Am J Cardiol 1989; 64:289–93.

30. Holt GW, Sugrue DD, Bresnahan JF, et al. Results of percutaneous transluminal coronary angioplasty for unstable angina pectoris in patients 70 years of age and older. Am J Cardiol 1988; 61:994–7.

31. Morrison DA. Coronary angioplasty for medically refractory unstable angina in patients with prior coronary bypass surgery. Cathet Cardiovasc Diagn 1990; 20:174–81.

32. Morrison DA. Coronary angioplasty for medically refractory unstable angina within 30 days of acute myocardial infarction. Am Heart J 1990; 120:256–61.

33. Gottlieb SO, Walford GD, Ouyang P, et al. Initial and late results of coronary angioplasty for early postinfarction unstable angina. Cathet Cardiovasc Diagn 1987; 13:93–9.

34. de Feyter PJ, Serruys PW, Soward A, van den Brand M, Bos E, Hugenholtz PG. Coronary angioplasty for early postinfarction unstable angina. Circulation 1986; 74:1365–70.

35. Safian RD, Snyder LD, Snyder BA, et al. Usefulness of percutaneous transluminal coronary angioplasty for unstable angina pectoris after non-Q-wave acute myocardial infarction. Am J Cardiol 1987; 59:263–6.

36. Bentivoglio LG, van Raden J, Kelsey SF, Detre KM. Percutaneous transluminal coronary angioplasty (PTCA) in patients with relative contraindications: Results of the National, Heart, Lung, and Blood Institute PTCA registry. Am J. Cardiol 1984; 53:82C–88C.

37. Detre KM, Myler RK, Kelsey SF, van Raden M, To T, Mitchell H. Baseline characteristics of patients in the National, Heart, Lung, and Blood Institute per-

cutaneous transluminal coronary angioplasty registry. Am J Cardiol 1984; 54:7C–11C.

38. Bentivoglio LG, Kelsey SF, Cowley MJ, Myler RK, Williams DO, Detre MK. Outcome of PTCA in stable and unstable angina pectoris. NHLBI PTCA registry. Circulation 1986; 74(Suppl II):II–123 (Abstract).

39. Leeman DE, McCabe CH, Faxon DP, et al. Use of percutaneous transluminal coronary angioplasty and bypass surgery despite improved medical therapy for unstable angina pectoris. Am J Cardiol 1988; 61:38G–44G.

40. Gaul G, Hollman J, Simpfendorfer C, Franco I. Acute occlusion in multiple lesion coronary angioplasty: frequency and management. J Am Coll Cardiol 1989; 13:283–8.

41. Wohlgelernter D, Cleman M, Highman HA, Zaret BL. Percutaneous transluminal coronary angioplasty of the "culprit lesion" for management of unstable angina pectoris in patients with multivessel coronary artery disease. Am J Cardiol 1986; 58:460–4.

42. de Feyter PJ, Serruys PW, Arnold A, et al. Coronary angioplasty of the unstable angina related vessel in patients with multivessel disease. Eur Heart J 1986; 7: 460–7.

43. DiMarco RF, McKeating JA, Pellegrini RV, et al. Contraindications for percutaneous transluminal coronary angioplasty in treatment of unstable angina pectoris. Texas Heart Inst J 1988; 15:152–4.

44. Faxon DP, Detre KM, McCabe CH, et al. Role of percutaneous transluminal coronary angioplasty in the treatment of unstable angina. Report from the National Heart, Lung, and Blood Institute Percutaneous Transluminal Coronary Angioplasty and Coronary Artery Surgery Study Registries. Am J Cardiol 1983; 53:131C–135C.

45. Chesebro JH, Clements IP, Fuster V, et al. A platelet-inhibitor-drug trial in coronary-artery bypass operations: benefit of perioperative dipyridamole and aspirin therapy on early postoperative vein-graft patency. N Engl J Med 1982; 307:73–8.

46. Chesebro JH, Fuster V, Elveback LR, et al. Effect of dipyridamole and aspirin on late vein-graft patency after coronary bypass operations. N Engl J Med 1984; 310:209–14.

13

Coronary Angioplasty for Unstable Angina

Pim J. de Feyter and Harry Suryapranata

University Hospital Rotterdam-Dijkzigt and
Erasmus University
Rotterdam, The Netherlands

Patrick W. Serruys

Interuniversity Cardiological Institute
of The Netherlands and
Erasmus University
Rotterdam, The Netherlands

INTRODUCTION

Since the introduction of coronary angioplasty, the scope of the technique has been broadened to include various subgroups of patients with unstable angina of varying severity (1–14). The primary success rate is high, but acute major complications seem to be more common in patients with unstable angina. The higher major complication rate is related to the underlying pathophysiology of the unstable plaque. The initiating event is the development of a rupture or fissuring of an atheromatous plaque, which leads to a cascade of pathophysiological and biochemical events, including platelet activation, fibrin deposition, thrombus formation, and the release of thromboxane A2 (15–17). The exact etiology of plaque fissuring is not known, but associated factors include shear forces of blood on the lesion (18,19), different plaque configuration (20), weakening of the plaque cap (13,21), and biochemical and structural properties of the cap components (13).

The cascade of events leads to rapid encroachment on the arterial lumen, with a significant reduction in cross-sectional area that results in a marked decrease in coronary blood flow. Widening of the remaining lumen with balloon dilatation in case of failure of pharmacological therapy appears a logical step in the management of patients with unstable angina.

This paper reviews recent developments of coronary angioplasty for unstable angina, and guidelines are proposed for the management of unstable angina, including the roles of coronary angioplasty, intensive medical treatment, and bypass surgery.

Classification of patients with unstable angina pectoris

Unstable angina was classically defined by Paul Wood as follows: ''The onset of acute coronary insufficiency is sudden; a state of normal health or of relatively mild angina of effort, with or without a history of cardiac infarction changing abruptly to one of almost total incapacity. Although the pain is usually provoked by all the familiar triggers (exertion) it may also occur spontaneously, when the patient is sitting quietly in a chair reading the paper, or may wake him repeatedly from sleep. The diagnosis of acute coronary insufficiency denies evidence of coronary infarction'' (22). He believed that coronary insufficiency was a warning sign of impending myocardial infarction. Gazes et al. (23) were the first to point out that the natural history of all patients with unstable angina was not uniform. They identified a high-risk subgroup for myocardial infarction and death. High-risk patients have frequent, repeated attacks of angina, accompanied by electrocardiographic ST-T changes and little or no response to treatment.

   Due to the fact that unstable angina is a single term used to encompass a number of clinical and physiological syndromes, we believe that, to evaluate the natural history and the impact of different therapeutic modalities, it is imperative to stratify patients according to clinical subgroups. There appear to be distinct subgroups of patients who have a different prognosis and who require different plans for management:

1. Progressive angina: Patients with (a) new-onset angina of a progressive nature or with (b) chronic angina who experience a change in their anginal pattern, which has now increased in frequency or severity. These patients do not experience angina at rest. This subgroup of patients with unstable angina appears to have a more benign clinical course and may require only pharmacological intervention (including antiplatelet agents) to treat recurrent ischemia or to prevent progression to myocardial infarction and cardiac death (24–30). If the symptoms do not respond sufficiently to pharmacological treatment or even progress in severity, revascularization (PTCA or CABG) is necessary.
2. Angina at rest: Patients with (repeated periods of) angina at rest with ST-segment or T-wave changes on a baseline electrocardiogram. These patients appear to have a worse prognosis, with a high incidence of acute myocardial infarction and mortality that requires more aggressive interventions (31–35). A subgroup of these patients who have angina at rest while hospitalized or who are refractory to pharmacological treatment appears to have a worse prognosis, which dictates urgent aggressive intervention.

The above classification is also helpful in terms of the expected difference of the frequency of complications of PTCA in these subgroups. Patients with angina at rest, especially those refractory to treatment, are at increased risk of procedural complications, whereas patients with progressive angina appear to have a lower risk of procedural complications, similar to the risk of patients with stable angina pectoris who undergo coronary angioplasty (36). In this context it is also important to note that angioplasty performed in patients more than 2 weeks after onset of angina (not refractory) is associated with a complication rate similar to the rate obtained in patients with stable angina pectoris (37).

CORONARY ANGIOPLASTY FOR PROGRESSIVE ANGINA PECTORIS

Patients with progressive angina pectoris should initially be managed with pharmacological treatment and be referred for revascularization if the symptoms cannot be controlled adequately. However, when the symptoms abate after an initial trial with medical treatment, these patients should no longer be considered "unstable," and when they undergo PTCA, they are classified as having "stable angina," although with severe symptoms. There appears to be a similar initial success rate and major complication rate among patients with stable angina who have moderate or severe angina (36–39).

CORONARY ANGIOPLASTY FOR ANGINA AT REST: INITIALLY STABILIZED WITH OR REFRACTORY TO PHARMACOLOGICAL TREATMENT

Patients with chest pain at rest accompanied by significant ST-T changes in the electrocardiogram (ECG) carry an increased risk of mortality and morbidity. Although in most of these patients the clinical symptoms can be stabilized with pharmacological treatment, including nitrates, beta-blockers, Ca antagonists and heparin, further treatment of the underlying coronary lesion, by either PTCA or coronary bypass surgery, is indicated in the majority of patients. Patients refractory to pharmacological treatment should undergo urgent revascularization.

The advantages of coronary angioplasty over coronary artery bypass surgery in these critically ill patients include the avoidance of intrinsic risks of major surgery and anesthesia, the ease and speed of implementation, and a reduction of hospital stay and costs. A major drawback of coronary angioplasty is the restenosis rate.

Earlier reports have shown that coronary angioplasty is relatively safe and effective in patients with unstable angina (37–39). The initial success rate, the major complication rate, and the occurrence of coronary events after successful PTCA are shown for PTCA performed early (semielective) after initial stabilization (Table 1) (40–42) or performed acutely in patients refractory to optimal pharmacological treatment (Table 2) (43–46). The reported initial success rate of 79–90% achieved in patients with unstable angina appears to be somewhat lower than the success rate of >90% achieved now in patients with stable angina pectoris (Table 3) (36,47–51). This is primarily a result of the higher complication rate in patients with unstable angina who undergo coronary angioplasty. The procedure-related mortality is reported from 0% to 4% (Tables 1,2). A myocardial infarction (MI), which results from a complication during the angioplasty procedure, is reported between 0% and 120%, of patients; the need for emergency surgery ranges from 3% to 12% (Tables 1,2). The occurrence of major complications is definitely higher in patients with unstable angina than in patients with stable angina. These major complications are mainly associated with a higher occurrence of abrupt closure, presumably because of the more likely formation of an occlusive thrombus after PTCA in these clinically unstable patients. The prognosis is excellent, after initial successful coronary angioplasty, with a low incidence of late mortality and a low occurrence of late nonfatal MI. Finally, the angiographic restenosis rate and recurrence of angina after an initial successful coronary angioplasty appear to be comparable to those of patients with stable angina.

CORONARY ANGIOPLASTY OF THE CULPRIT LESION IN UNSTABLE ANGINA AND MULTIVESSEL DISEASE

The majority of patients with unstable angina have multivessel disease. Successful multiple dilatations in one angioplasty procedure have been performed with acceptable complication rates in patients with stable angina (52). However, there is less acceptance of and less experience with multivessel dilatation in patients with (refractory) unstable angina because multiple dilatations in these clinically unstable patients may increase the risk of major complications and because of the established efficacy of bypass surgery in this population.

Regional left ventricular wall function is often impaired in these patients as a result of chronic ischemia (hibernating myocardium) or prolonged postischemic dysfunction (stunned myocardium) and additional dilatations jeopardize additional myocardium, which may result in fatal left ventricular dysfunction (53–55). There also is the risk of performing unnecessary dilatations because of the difficulty in assessing the significance of any additional stenosis in the acute setting. To expand the potential use of coronary angioplasty as an alternative to bypass surgery in patients with unstable angina and multivessel disease, dilatation of only the "'culprit'" lesion has been recommended as an initial approach to stabilize the patient's condition (56,57). This strategy is successful in the majority of the patients; however, it is associated, not unexpectedly, with a higher occurrence of angina pectoris after the procedure, which may necessitate later

Table 1 Coronary Angioplasty for Initially Stabilized Unstable Angina Pectoris

Author	Year	No PT	Success rate (%)	Major complication rate			Coronary events after successful angioplasty			F/U (mo, mean)
				Death (%)	MI (%)	Acute surgery (%)	Death (%)	MI (%)	AP (%)	
Quigley (40)	1986	25	81	4	12	12	0	0	32	14
de Feyter (41)	1987	71	87	0	10	12	2	2	23	12
Steffenino (42)	1987	89	90	0	5	5	0	1.5	23	10
Myler (37)	1990	220	85	0	6.6	6.1	1	2.5	29	37

Definition of unstable angina: Quigley: New-onset angina, coronary insufficiency, changing pattern of preexisting angina, angina at rest, or variant angina. de Feyter: Chest pain at rest accompanied with ST-T changes. Steffenino: Worsening in the frequency or severity of chest pain or severe episodes of prolonged pain at rest. Myler: Onset 1–2 weeks before PTCA.

241

Table 2 Coronary Angioplasty for Refractory Unstable Angina Pectoris

Author	Year	No PT	Success rate (%)	Major complication rate			Coronary events after successful angioplasty			
				Death (%)	MI (%)	Acute surgery (%)	Death (%)	MI (%)	AP (%)	F/U (mo, mean)
de Feyter (43)	1988	200	89.5	0.5	8	9	2.5	4	25	24
Plokker (44)	1988	469	88	1	4.9	3	1.5	0.1	21	19.3
Sharma (45)	1988	40	88	0	0	12	0	0	34	11
Perry (46)	1988	105	87	2	9	4	—	—	—	—
Myler (37)[a]	1990	310	79	0.3	6.5	9.4	5.8	6.3	33	37

[a]UAP: onset < 1 week before PTCA.

Table 3 Coronary Angioplasty for Stable Angina Pectoris

Author	Year	No. of patients	Success rate (%)	Major complication rate		
				Death (%)	MI (%)	Acute surgery (%)
Bredlau ('83–'84) (47)	1985	1167	92	±0.2	±2.5	±2.7
Hartzler ('80–'85) (48)	1986	3986	91	1.2	0.9	1.8
NHLBl-PTCA (49)						
Registry ('85–'86)	1988	839[a]	91	0.2	3.5	1.8
Tuzcu ('80–'87) (38)	1988	2677	93	0.3	1.1	3.6
de Feyter ('86–'87) (50)	1988	523	92	0.2	2.3	1.9
O'Keefe ('85–'86) (51)	1989	404	90	1.2	4.2	3.4

[a]Only patients with single-vessel disease.

elective coronary artery bypass surgery or elective coronary angioplasty of other vessels (43). Angioplasty of the culprit lesion in patients with unstable angina and multivessel disease should be regarded as an initial treatment strategy in patients whose symptoms do not respond adequately to pharmacological treatment. In most patients, this approach will have a long-term success, but in some patients further dilatations or even bypass surgery will be required. Thus this strategy does not provide a definitive long-term treatment in all patients. However, the subsequent interventions can be performed on a more elective basis with less risk.

PROPOSED MANAGEMENT OF PATIENTS WITH UNSTABLE ANGINA

The latest improvements in surgical technique and myocardial preservation have certainly decreased the operative mortality and the perioperative myocardial infarction rate in patients with unstable angina, which now is reported between 1.8% and 7.7% and 1% and 16.7%, respectively (Table 4) (58–65). The results obtained by acute surgery and angioplasty cannot be compared directly since patients who undergo angioplasty are a select group with predominantly one-vessel disease and preserved left ventricular function, whereas patients selected for surgery tend to have three-vessel disease, left main stem disease, and compromised left ventricular function, factors known to adversely influence prognosis.

There is a lack of recent randomized studies to establish the merits of current pharmacological treatment, current bypass surgery, and coronary angioplasty in the management of patients with unstable angina. Until further information becomes available, we propose the following practical approach (Figs. 1,2). This approach is based on (a) the classification of unstable angina, (b) the time interval between the last attack of chest pain and instituted therapy, (c) the

Table 4 Surgical Mortality and Perioperative Myocardial Infarction Rate in Unstable Angina

Study	Year	No. of patients	Perioperative mortality (%)	Perioperative MI (%)
Ahmed et al. (58)	1980	71	4.2	7.0
Brawley et al. (59)	1980	130	7.7	8.0
Rankin et al. (60)	1984	48	4.0	6.1
Rahimtoola et al. (61)	1983	1282	1.8	—
Cohn et al. (62)	1985	222	3.0	1.0
Goldman et al. (63)	1985	299	5.0	16.7
McCormick et al. (64)	1985	3311	3.9	—
Luchi et al. (65)	1987	468	4.1	10.3

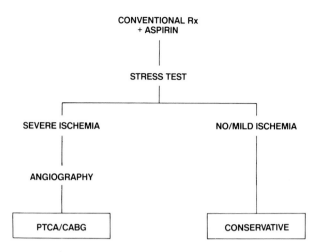

Figure 1 Triage approach to the patient with unstable angina who presents with progressive angina.

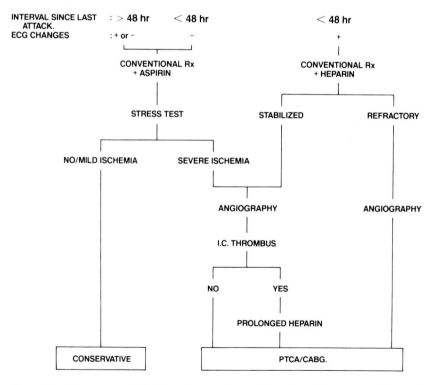

Figure 2 Triage approach to the patient with unstable angina who presents with angina at rest.

Table 5 Optimal Pharmacological Treatment for Patients with Unstable Angina

Bed rest (CCU) and sedation
Treatment of precipitating factors (anemia, hypertension, tachycardia)
Anticoagulant (heparin) or antiplatelet treatment (aspirin)
Stepwise intensification with individual tailoring of a pharmacological regimen,
   including adequate administration of beta-adrenergic blockade to achieve a resting
   pulse of <60 bpm
Calcium antagonists and nitroglycerin (long-acting or i.v.) to optimize preload
   (pulmonary capillary wedge pressure <14 mmHg) and afterload (systolic aortic
   pressure <110 mmHg)

presence of ECG changes of ST segment and T wave, (d) the response to
pharmacological treatment, and (e) the coronary anatomy and left ventricular
function. In the management of unstable angina it has now become standard
practice to initiate treatment with bed rest and sedation and optimal pharmacological treatment (Table 5) and to proceed to revascularization (PTCA or
surgery) if ischemia persists or is easily provoked by exercise testing. It appears
extremely important to "cool down" a patient with unstable angina and to
perform PTCA after a stabilization period of about 14 days, because then the
acute major complication rate has been shown to be similar to the rate observed
in patients with stable angina (Table 6). The choice of bypass surgery or
angioplasty to treat a medically nonresponsive patient is still subject to much
debate. However, it is generally agreed that surgery should be reserved for two
subsets of patients: those with life-threatening coronary anatomy (i.e., significant left main disease, significant three-vessel disease) and those with a depressed ejection fraction. Angioplasty should be reserved for patients with
suitable coronary anatomy (i.e., single-vessel disease, suitable culprit lesion in
multivessel disease) and those with preserved left ventricular function.

CONCLUSIONS

Coronary angioplasty is an effective treatment for patients with angina at rest
(either refractory to or initially stabilized with pharmacological treatment for
unstable angina). The procedure has a high initial success rate, but there is an
increased risk of major complications resulting in a higher incidence of acute
closure, which may be related to preexisting platelets, fibrin, thrombus, or
thromboxane A2 activity. Resolution of this problem may be achieved by the use
of more potent antiplatelet treatment or treatment that can be applied locally
(laser energy, atherectomy, stenting, sweating balloon).

Table 6 Initial Success and Major Complication Rate in Relation to Symptom Duration Before Angioplasty

Duration of symptoms	Unstable angina pectoris			Stable angina pectoris
	< 1 week	1–2 weeks	2–4 weeks	
Success (%)	79	85	86	88
Major complication event	11.5	10.1	4.8	4.7
Death (%)	0.3	0.0	0.3	0.2
Acute myocardial infarction (%)	6.5	6.6	1.6	2.3
Emergency CABG	9.4	6.1	4.8	3.8

CABG = coronary artery bypass grafting.
Source: Abstracted from Myler et al. (37).

241

REFERENCES

1. Williams DO, Riley RS, Singh AK, Gewirtz H, Most AS. Evaluation of the role of coronary angioplasty in patients with unstable angina pectoris. Am Heart J 1981; 102:1–9.
2. Meyer J, Schmitz HJ, Kiesslich T, et al. Percutaneous transluminal coronary angioplasty in patients with stable and unstable angina pectoris: Analysis of early and late results. Am Heart J 1983; 106:973–80.
3. Faxon DP, Detre KM, McGabe CH, et al. Role of percutaneous transluminal coronary angioplasty in the treatment of unstable angina: Report from the National Heart, Lung and Blood Institute Percutaneous Transluminal Coronary Angioplasty and Coronary Artery Surgery Study Registries. Am J Cardiol 1983; 53:131C–35C.
4. de Feyter PJ, Serruys PW, Brand van den M, Balakumaran K, Mochtar B, Soward AL, Arnold AER, Hugenholtz PG. Emergency coronary angioplasty in refractory unstable angina. N Engl J Med 1985; 313:342–7.
5. Falk E. Plaque rupture with severe pre-existing stenosis precipitating coronary thrombosis: characteristics of coronary atherosclerotic plaques underlying fatal occlusive thrombi. Br Heart J 1983; 50:127–34.
6. Davies MJ, Thomas A. Thrombosis and acute coronary artery lesions in sudden cardiac ischemic death. N Engl J Med 1984; 310:1137–40.
7. Levin DC, Fallon JT. Significance of angiographic morphology of localized coronary stenoses. Histopathologic correlations. Circulation 1982; 66:316–20.
8. Gorlin R, Fuster V, Ambrose JA. Anatomic-physiologic link between acute coronary syndromes. Circulation 1986; 74:6–9.
9. Sherman CT, Litvack F, Grundfest W, et al. Coronary angioscopy in patients with unstable angina pectoris. N Engl J Med 1986; 315:913–9.
10. Fitzgerald DG, Roy L, Catelle F, Fitzgerald GA. Platelet activation in unstable coronary disease. N Engl J Med 1986; 315:983–93.
11. Fuster V, Chesebro JH. Mechanisms of unstable angina. N Engl J Med 1986; 315:1023–5.
12. Maseri A, L'Abbate, Baroldi G, et al. Coronary vasospasm as a possible cause of myocardial infarction: A conclusion derived from the study of "preinfarction" angina. N Engl J Med 1978; 229:1271–7.
13. Davies MJ, Thomas AC. Plague fissuring—The cause of acute myocardial infarction, sudden ischemic death and crescendo angina. Br Heart J 1985; 53:363–73.
14. Falk E. Unstable angina with fatal outcome: Dynamic coronary thrombosis leading to infarction or sudden death. Circulation 1985; 71:699–708.
15. Davies MJ, Thomas AC, Knapman PA, Hangartner JR. Intramyocardial platelet aggregation in patients with unstable angina suffering sudden ischemic cardiac death. Circulation 1986; 73:418–28.
16. Epstein SE, Talbot TL. Dynamic coronary tone in precipation, exacerbation and relief of angina pectoris. Am J Cardiol 1981; 48:797–803.
17. Fuster V, Badimon L, Cohen M, Ambrose JA, Badimon JJ, Chesebro JH. Insights into the pathogenesis of acute ischemic syndromes. Circulation 1988; 77:1213–20.
18. Badimon L, Badimon JJ, Galvez, et al. Influence of arterial wall damage and wall shear rate on platelet depositions: Ex vivo study in a swine model. Arteriosclerosis 1986; 6:312–30.

19. Glagov S, Zarins C, Giddens DP, Zarins CK, Ku DN. Hemodynamics and atherosclerosis. Insights and perspectives gained form studies of human arteries. Arch Pathol Lab Med 1988; 112:1018–31.
20. Richardson PD, Davies MJ, Born GVR. Influence of plaque configuration and stress distribution on fissuring of coronary atherosclerotic plaques. Lancet 1989; 2:941–4.
21. Constantinides P. Plaques fissuring in human coronary thrombosis. J Atheroscler Res 1966; 6:1–17.
22. Wood P. Acute and subacute coronary insufficiency. Br Med J 1961; 1:1779–82.
23. Gazes PC, Mobley EM, Farris HM, Duncan RC, Humphries GB. Preinfarction (unstable) angina—A prospective study. Ten year follow-up. Circulation 1973; 48:331–8.
24. Conti CR, Brawley RK, Griffith LSC, Pitt B, Humhries JO, Gott VL, Ross RS: Unstable angina pectoris morbidity and mortality in 57 consecutive patients evaluated angiographically. Am J Cardiol 1973; 32:745–50.
25. Harris PH, Harrell FE, Lee KL, Behar VS, Rosati RA. Survival in medically treated coronary artery disease. Circulation 1979; 60:1259–69.
26. Duncan B, Fulton M, Morrison SL, Lutz W, Donald KW, Kerr F, Kirby BJ, Julian DG, Oliver MF. Prognosis of new and worsening angina pectoris. Br Med J 1976; 1:981–5.
27. Roberts KB, Califf RM, Harrell FE, Lee KL, Pryor DB, Rosati RA. The prognosis for patients with new onset angina who have undergone cardiac catheterization. Circulation 1983;68:970–8.
28. Heng MK, Norris RM, Singh BN, Partridge JB: Prognosis in unstable angina. Br Heart J 1976; 38:921–5.
29. Mulcahy R: Natural history and prognosis of unstable angina. Am Heart J 1985; 109:753–9.
30. Krauss KR, Hutter AM, de Sanctis RW: Acute coronary insufficiency: Course and follow-up. Arch Intern Med 1972; 129:808–13.
31. Gazes PC, Mobley EM, Farris HM, Duncan RC, Humphries GB. Preinfarction (unstable) angina—A prospective study. Ten year follow-up. Circulation 1973; 48:331–8.
32. Bertolasi C, Tronge J, Riccitelli M, Villamayor RM, Zuffardi E: Natural history of unstable angina with medical therapy. Chest 1976; 70:596–605.
33. Olson HG, Lyons KP, Aronow WS, Stinson RJ, Kuperus J, Waters HJ. The high-risk angina patients. Circulation 1981; 64:674–84.
34. Quyang P, Brinker JA, Mellits ED, Weisfeldt ML, Gerstenblith G. Variables predictive of successful medical therapy in patients with unstable angina pectoris: Selection by multivariate analysis from clinical, electrocardiographic and angiographic variables. Circulation 1984, 70:376–84.
35. Report of the Holland Interuniversity Nifedipine/Metoprolol Trial (HINT) Research Group. Early treatment of unstable angina in the coronary care unit: A randomised, double blind, placebo controlled comparison of recurrent ischaemia in patients treated with nifedipine or metoprolol or both. Br Heart J 1987; 56:400–13.
36. Black AJ, Brown CS, Feres F, Roubin GS, Douglas JS. Coronary angioplasty and the spectrum of unstable angina pectoris: What determines increased risk? Circulation 1988; 78:(Suppl II;11–8 (Abstract).

37. Myler RK, Shaw RE, Stertzer SH, Bashour TT, Ryan C, Hecht HS, Cumberland DC. Unstable angina and coronary angioplasty. Circulation 1990; 82(Suppl II):II:88–95.
38. Tuzcu EM, Simpfendorfer C, Badhwar K, Chambers J, Dorosti K, Franco J, Hollman J, Whitlow P. Determinants of primary success in elective PTCA for significant narrowing of a single major coronary artery. Am J Cardiol 1988; 62: 873–5.
39. Faxon DP, Detre KM, McGabe CH, et al. Role of percutaneous transluminal coronary angioplasty in the treatment of unstable angina: Report from the National Heart, Lung and Blood Institute Percutaneous Transluminal Coronary Angioplasty and Coronary Artery Surgery Study Registries. Am J Cardiol 1983; 53:131C–35C.
40. Quigley PJ, Erwin J, Maurer BJ, Walsh MJ, Gearty GF. Percutaneous transluminal coronary angioplasty in unstable angina; comparison with stable angina. Br Heart J 1986; 55:227–30.
41. de Feyter PJ, Serruys PW, Suryapranata H, Beatt K, van den Brand M. PTCA early after the diagnosis of unstable angina. Am Heart J 1987; 114:48–54.
42. Steffenino G, Meier B, Finci L, Rutishauer W. Follow-up results of treatment of unstable angina by coronary angioplasty. Br Heart J 1987; 57:416–9.
43. de Feyter PJ, Suryapranata H, Serruys PW, Beatt K, van Domburg R, van den Brand M, Tijssen JJ, Azar AJ, Hugenholtz PG. Coronary angioplasty for unstable angina: Immediate and late results in 200 consecutive patients with identification of risk factors for unfavorable early and late outcome. J Am Coll Cardiol 1988; 12:324–33.
44. Plokker HWT, Ernst SMPG, Bal ET, van den Berg ECJM, Mast GEG, Feltz TA, Ascoop CAPL. Percutaneous transluminal coronary angioplasty in patients with unstable angina pectoris refractory to medical therapy. Cathet Cardiovasc Diagn 1988; 14:15–8.
45. Sharma B, Wyeth RP, Kolath GS, Gimenez HJ, Franciosa JA. Percutaneous transluminal coronary angioplasty of one vessel for refractory unstable angina pectoris: efficacy in single and multivessel disease. Br Heart J 1988; 59:280–6.
46. Perry RA, Seth A, Hunt A, Shiu MF. Coronary angioplasty in unstable angina and stable angina: A comparison of success and complications. Br Heart J 1988; 60:367–72.
47. Bredlau CE, Roubin GS, Leimgruber PP, Douglas JS, King SB, Gruentzig AR. In-hospital morbidity and mortality in patients undergoing elective coronary angioplasty. Circulation 1985; 72:1044–52.
48. Hartzler G. Complex coronary angioplasty: multivessel/ multilesion dilatation. In: Ischinger T, ed. Practice of coronary angioplasty. New York: Springer-Verlag, 1986:250–67.
49. Holmes DR, Holubkov R, Vlietstra RE. Comparison of complications during PTCA from 1977 to 1981 and from 1985 to 1986: The NHLBI-PTCA Registry. J Am Coll Cardiol 1988; 12:1149–55.
50. de Feyter PJ, van den Brand M, Serruys PW, Suryapranata H, Beatt K, Zijlstra F, van Domburg R, Patijn M. Increase of initial success and safety of single-vessel PTCA in 1371 patients: A seven-years experience. J Interven Cardiol 1988; 1:1–9.
51. O'Keefe J, Reeder GS, Miller GA, Bailey KR, Holmes R. Safety and efficacy of

PTCA performed at time of diagnostic catheterization compared with that performed at other times. Am J Cardiol 1989; 63:27–9.

52. Myler RK, Topol EJ, Shaw RE, Stertzer SH, Clark DA. Multiple vessel coronary angioplasty: Classification, results and patterns of restenosis in 494 consecutive patients. Cathet Cardiovasc Diagn 1987; 13:1–14.

53. Braunwald E, Rutherford JD. Reversible ischemic left ventricular dysfunction: Evidence for the "hibernating myocardium." J Am Coll Cardiol 1986; 8:1467–70.

54. de Feyter PJ, Serruys PW, Beatt K, van den Brand M, Hugenholtz P. Effects of successful percutaneous transluminal coronary angioplasty on global and regional left ventricular function in unstable angina pectoris. Am J Cardiol 1987; 60:993–7.

55. Sabbah HN, Brymer JF, Gheorghiade M, Stein PD, Khaja F. Left ventricular function after successful percutaneous transluminal coronary angioplasty for post-infarction angina pectoris. Am J Cardiol 1988; 62:358–62.

56. Wohlgelernter D, Cleman M, Highman HA, Zaret BL. Percutaneous transluminal coronary angioplasty of the "culprit lesion" for management of unstable angina pectoris in patients with multivessel coronary artery disease. Am J Cardiol 1986; 58:460–4.

57. de Feyter PJ, Serruys PW, Arnold A, et al. Coronary angioplasty of the unstable angina related vessel in patients with multivessel disease. Eur Heart J 1986; 7:460–7.

58. Ahmed M, Thompson R, Seabra-Gomes R, Rickards A, Yacoub M. Unstable angina. A clinicoarteriographic correlation and longterm results of early myocardial revascularization. J Thorac Cardiovasc Surg 1980; 79:609.

59. Brawley RK, Merrill W, Gott VL, Donahoo JS, Watkins L, Gardner TJ. Unstable angina pectoris. Factors influencing operative risk. Ann Surg 1980; 19:745.

60. Rankin JS, Newton JR, Califf RM, Jones RH, Wechsler AS, Oldham HN, Wolfe WG, Lowe JE. Clinical characteristics and current management of medically refractory unstable angina. Ann Surg 1984; 200:457–64.

61. Rahimtoola SH, Nunley D, Grunkemeier G, Tepley J, Lambert L, Starr A. Ten year survival after coronary bypass surgery for unstable angina. N Engl J Med 1983; 308:676–81.

62. Cohn LH, O'Neill A, Collins JJ. Surgical treatment of unstable angina up to 1984. In: Hugenholtz PG, Goldman BS, eds. Unstable angina—Current concepts and management. New York: Schattauer-Suttgart, 1985:279–86.

63. Goldman HE, Weisel RD, Christakis G, Katz A, Scully HE, Mickleborough LM, Baird RJ. Predictors of outcome after coronary artery bypass graft surgery for stable and unstable angina pectoris. In: Hugenholtz PG, Goldman BS, eds. Unstable angina—Current concepts and management. New York: Schattauer-Stuttgart, 1985:319–29.

64. McCormick JR, Schick EC, McGabe CH, Kronmal RA, Ryan TJ. Determinants of operative mortality and longterm survival in patients with unstable angina. J Thorac Cardiovasc Surg 1985; 89:683–8.

65. Luchi RJ, Scott SM, Deupree RH, et al. Comparison of medical and surgical treatment for unstable angina. N Engl J Med 1987; 316:977–84.

14

Coronary Angioplasty in Patients with Unstable Angina and Depressed Left Ventricular Function

Germano Di Sciascio and George Vetrovec

Medical College of Virginia Hospitals
Virginia Commonwealth University
Richmond, Virginia

INTRODUCTION

Coronary angioplasty (PTCA) is a revascularization technique that is applied to a wide spectrum of patients with coronary disease, including those with anatomical and clinical situations originally considered contraindications for the procedure. Among the latter are patients with depressed left ventricular function, who, although at higher risk for both the surgical and nonsurgical approach, may nevertheless be in need of revascularization because of unstable symptoms. In fact, the majority of patients with left ventricular dysfunction in whom revascularization is indicated have unstable angina refractory to medical treatment (1), most often with left ventricular dysfunction in the myocardial territory supplied by the affected artery (2), with potential for improvement with successful revascularization (3,4). These patients are increasingly referred for coronary angioplasty because they are deemed unfavorable candidates for bypass surgery (5). Patients with unstable angina represent a large share of the population undergoing PTCA in experienced laboratories: in the most recent National Heart Lung and Blood Institute Registry report, unstable angina was the indication for angioplasty in 50% of the patients (6). Therefore, the results and natural history of angioplasty in unstable angina remain an important subject of clinical research in interventional cardiology (7–10).

The goal of this chapter is to discuss the application of coronary angioplasty to the subset of patients with refractory angina and left ventricular dysfunction, including strategic considerations, new support devices, identification of viable myocardium, and, consequently, the potential normalization of depressed function.

CORONARY ANGIOPLASTY IN PATIENTS WITH SEVERELY DEPRESSED LEFT VENTRICULAR EJECTION FRACTION

At the Medical College of Virginia, in a retrospective analysis (1) of 1260 PTCA procedures performed between February 1985 and December 1987, 61 patients (5%) had left ventricular ejection fraction (EF) < 35%. Unstable angina was present in 70%, and 74% had multivessel coronary artery disease; 39% had recent myocardial infarction (occurring < 15 days from the procedure) with subsequent postinfarction angina; the mean left ventricular EF was 29 ± 6%, with 20% of patients having EF < 20%. All patients had severe ischemic symptoms prompting consideration for revascularization despite expected increased risk, and coronary angioplasty was performed because they were deemed unfavorable candidates for bypass surgery: in many cases, this decision was reached with mutual agreement between the ''angioplaster'' and the cardiac surgeon after joint review of the films (Figs. 1–3). Angioplasty was successful in 55/61 patients (90%), 109/121 lesions (90%), and 81/88 vessels (92%), with a 6.4% incidence of myocardial infarction and a 3.2% mortality; no patient required emergency bypass surgery.

These results are in agreement with a preliminary report by Dorros (11) (Table 1), who obtained 86% success in a series of 101 patients with EF < 35%, with a

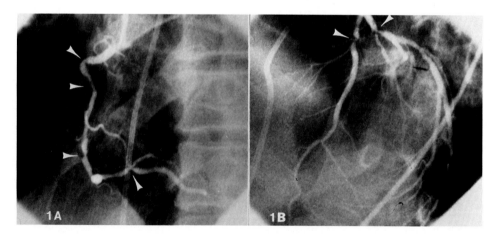

Figure 1   (A, B) Three-vessel CAD in a patient with severe angina and poor left ventricular function, considered an unfavorable candidate for bypass surgery. Pre-PTCA: there is diffuse RCA disease, and severe proximal discrete LAD and LCX lesions.

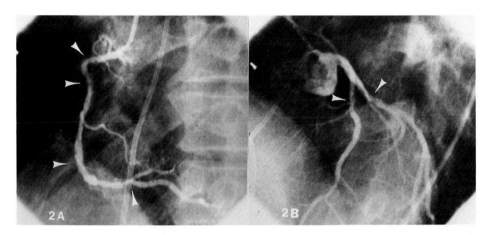

Figure 2 (A, B) Post-PTCA: excellent improvement in lumen diameter at all dilated sites.

4.0% incidence of acute myocardial infarction (MI), 3.0% emergency coronary artery bypass graft (CABG) surgery, and 4.0% mortality. Similarly, a recent study from St. Louis University (12) of PTCA in patients with LVEF < 40% (mean 34%) reports a success rate of 82%, with 4% MI rate, 1.3% emergency bypass surgery, and 4% acute mortality. The largest series, published by the Mid-America Heart Institute Group (13), describes results in 664 patients with ejection fraction < 40%; success was achieved in 93%, with 0.7% acute MI rate, 2% emergency bypass surgery, and a mortality rate of 2.7%.

Data are also available on the natural history of patients with severe left ventricular dysfunction after successful angioplasty (Table 2). In our series (1), follow-up > 1 year (mean 21 months) was available in all 55 successful patients; clinical recurrence (defined as return of symptoms and angiographic evidence of restenosis at dilated sites) was observed in 11 patients (20%), and in keeping with our experience with the general angioplasty population, the majority of them (82%) underwent a successful repeat PTCA, with one patient having a cardiac transplant after 6 months because of worsening heart failure. However, late mortality was high: 13 patients (23%) died during the follow-up period, 10 (18%) of cardiac causes (sudden death); death occurred from 1.9 to 31 months after angioplasty. Actuarial survival was 77% and 70% at 24 and 36 months, respectively. In Dorros' series (11), at a mean follow-up time of 3.3 years, there were 22 late deaths (25%) and a 21% clinical reccurrence rate; the survival rate was 71% at 6 years. In the St. Louis study (12), the 4-year estimated survival was 57 ± 8% and was most adversely affected by the presence of congestive heart failure and LVEF < 30%.

Therefore, from available experience with angioplasty in patients with severe

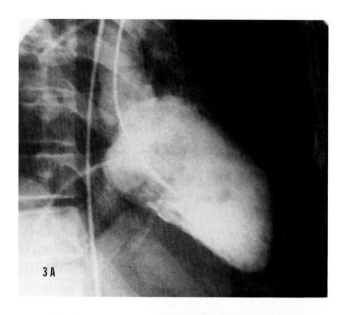

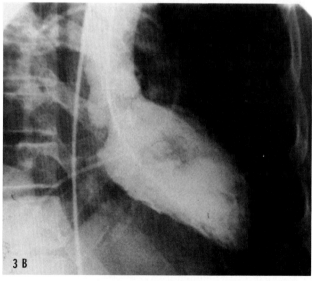

Figure 3   (A, B) Same patient 30° RAO left ventriculography. (A) Diastole; (B) systole. The LV contractility is severely depressed, EF calculated = 18%. Despite successful PTCA, the patient underwent cardiac transplant 6 months later for progressive heart failure.

Table 1 PTCA in Depressed LV Function: Immediate Results

	Ref.	No. pts	EF	Success	Complications		
					MI	CABG	Death
MCV	1	61	<35%	90%	3.3%	0	3.2%
Dorros	11	101	<35%	86%	4.0%	3.0%	4.0%
St. Louis	12	73	<40%	82%	4.0%	1.3%	4.0%
Hartzler	13	664	<40%	93%	0.7%	2.0%	2.7%

Table 2 PTCA in Depressed LV Function: Follow-up

	Ref.	Duration (years)	Clin. recurr.	Nonfatal			Survival rate
				Death	MI	CABG	
MCV	1	2.2	20%	18%	0%	4%	81% (4 yr)
Dorros	11	3.3	21%	25%	0%	3%	71% (6 yr)
St. Louis	12	2.2	13% (?)	14%	4%	7%	57% (4 yr)

left ventricular dysfunction, we can conclude that the immediate angiographic and clinical results are comparable to those obtained with routine angioplasty; however, the complication rate is higher, with an expected acute mortality of approximately 3%, compared to a <1% mortality in routine PTCA in experienced centers. Furthermore, mortality remains high during follow-up and most often presents as sudden cardiac death. Although comparisons with bypass surgery may be difficult, because of differences in patient selection and baseline characteristics, the CASS study (14) reports a 63% actuarial 5-year survival rate for patients with LVEF $\leq$ 26% treated with bypass surgery, versus 43% in medically managed patients.

STRATEGIC APPROACH TO ANGIOPLASTY IN PATIENTS WITH DEPRESSED LEFT VENTRICULAR EJECTION FRACTION

Patients with depressed left ventricular function represent a high-risk population in whom a careful strategic approach to angioplasty is in order. Left ventricular function should be optimized prior to PTCA, with appropriate use of vasodilators, diuretics, pharmacological inotropic support; in addition, hemodynamic monitoring with Swan-Ganz catheterization during the procedure is indicated. Although we have used intra-aortic balloon pumping in our original series in two patients only (one prophylactically because of extremely low ejection fraction, one for hypotension during the procedure), some authors recommend prophylac-

tic counterpulsation if the EF is < 30% or if the hemodynamics are unstable pre-
or during PTCA (15,16). We believe that, although intra-aortic balloon does not
provide direct myocardial protection, it is valuable as systemic support when
hemodynamic instability is present pre-PTCA or when it ensues during the
procedure, especially when newer assist devices are not available.

In patients with left ventricular dysfunction and complex multivessel coronary
disease, choice of vessels to treat and dilatation sequence is of paramount
importance.

In the Medical College of Virginia's experience, more than two-thirds of
patients had multivessel disease, but only 33% had PTCA of multiple vessels.
The remainder underwent dilatation of the "culprit" lesion only (17). In general,
a complete revascularization of all proximal lesions in major vessels is the
preferred approach in our institution (18); however, left ventricular dysfunction
is often the clinical setting in which even an incomplete revascularization, aimed
at the interruption of refractory ischemia by treating the acute vessel only, can be
considered adequate, because of the higher risk of multivessel angioplasty in the
context of decreased left ventricular reserve (Table 3). When critical lesions are
present in multiple vessels requiring revascularization, a "staged" approach may
be preferable (19). The procedure is best performed in two separate sessions,
especially in patients with recent myocardial infarction (20); in those cases, the
infarct-producing vessel is dilated first and the other vessels are treated later in
the hospital course (Figs. 4 and 5). This enables the operator to ascertain the
persistent patency of the previously dilated segment and allows the myocardium
to potentially improve from its "stunned" state; furthermore, vessels "protected" by collateral supply are usually dilated first, and severe lesions in vessel-
supplying collaterals are dilated subsequently (21). The same strategy is applied
in patients with collateralized total occlusions and multivessel coronary disease
(22); the safer approach consists in dilating the occluded coronary first; once
patency is reestablished, this vessel in turn may function as collateral source to
other vessels.

ASSIST DEVICES IN HIGH-RISK PTCA

An important decision in PTCA of patients with poor LV function relates to the
utilization, prophylactic or standby, of a number of assist devices that are
currently investigational or already available in clinical practice as support to
high-risk angioplasty (23) (see also Chapters 20 and 21).

Percutaneous cardiopulmonary bypass [femorofemoral, with its variations:
left atrial-aortic (24), or left atrial-femoral (25)] provides excellent systemic
support even during cardiac arrest or ventricular fibrillation. A multicenter study
recently published (26) confirms its usefulness in patients who would otherwise
be at prohibitive risk for surgical revascularization or routine angioplasty. How-

Table 3 PCA in Severe LV Dysfunction: Strategic Approach

Optimize and monitor LV function pre-PTCA.
Prophylactic IABP if EF < 30% or if hemodynamics unstable during PTCA.
PTCA of ''culprit'' lesion only (incomplete revascularization = adequate
  revascularization).
Stage PTCA when necessary.
Standby assist devices.

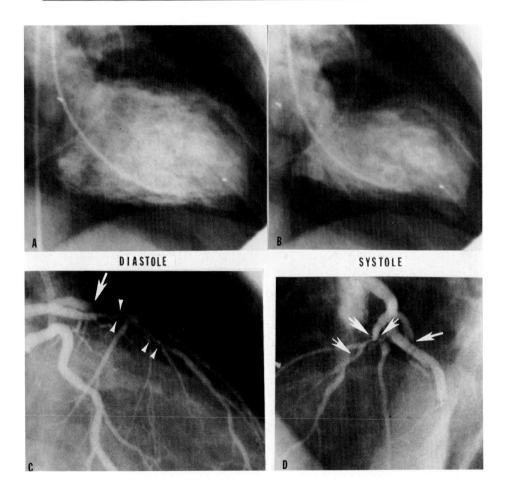

Figure 4 Early post-MI patient. (A, B) Left ventriculography showing severe anterolateral hypokinesis (''stunned'' myocardium). (C, D) Left coronary angiography: there is
a totally occluded large diagonal branch (arrow), with severe bifurcational disease
involving LAD and a large second diagonal. (From Ref. 19. Courtesy of Futura Publishing Company, Mt. Kisco, N.Y.)

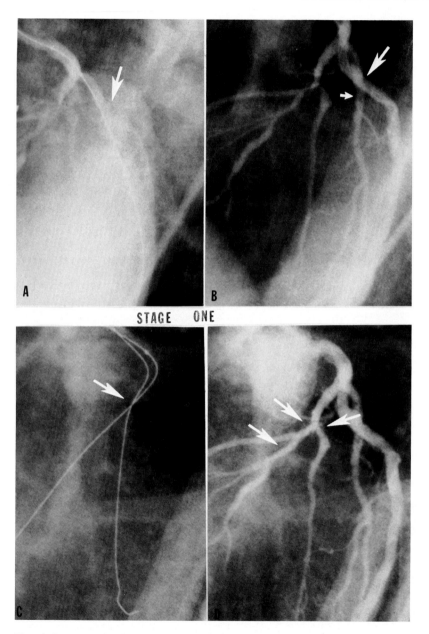

STAGE ONE

Figure 5 (A, B) PTCA, stage 1: the MI-producing vessel was dilated first (diagonal). (C, D) Five days later the LAD diagonal lesion was dilated with the double-wire technique (stage 2). (From Ref. 19. Courtesy of Futura Publishing Company, Mt. Kisco, N.Y.)

ever, major limitations include cost, significant vascular morbidity, and potential complications related to extracorporeal circulation. For these reasons, it appears that a usage in standby mode would be more appropriate than prophylactic application in all patients with expected high risk. The Nimbus hemopump is also an effective device for systemic circulatory support but is not yet available for percutaneous use (27).

Coronary sinus retroperfusion has been applied to limit ischemia during angioplasty, but is also fraught with potential problems that may limit its use, such as difficult cannulation and inadequate protection for vessels other than left anterior descending (28). Antegrade perfusion of the distal coronary bed provides direct myocardial protection during balloon inflation and appears to be very effective in reducing or eliminating clinically detectable ischemia or wall motion abnormalities during angioplasty. It can be performed with passive autoperfusion catheters (29) or with flow-adjusted active perfusion pumps, utilizing the patient's autologus blood (30,31) or oxygen carriers such as Fluosol (32).

PTCA IN SEVERE LEFT VENTRICULAR DYSFUNCTION: UNRESOLVED ISSUES

Coronary angioplasty is feasible in selected patients with depressed ventricular function and vessels amenable to dilation with reasonable probability of success, and a number of support devices may facilitate the procedure and even extend the option of revascularization to patients with refractory symptoms that are deemed inoperable. However, some unresolved issues remain.

After successful completion of the procedure, acute reclosure may still occur when the patient has left the catheterization laboratory; in such situations, hemodynamic decompensation may be difficult to control, especially when the only remaining vessel was dilated, and the support devices that allowed the procedure to be safely performed initially may not be readily reinstituted. Furthermore, the high mortality (sudden death) during follow-up remains of concern; this may be due to residual ischemia from nondilated arteries, but a more intriguing hypothesis is that death may be a fatal manifestation of restenosis in these patients with minimal cardiac reserve. This could be the explanation of the relatively ''low'' (20%) clinical restenosis rate observed in our patients with severely depressed left ventricular function and may indicate the need for routine angiographic follow-up in this high-risk group to detect and treat even silent angiographic restenosis.

Thus, appropriate patient selection is mandatory; the clinical indication for angioplasty should be interruption of ischemia refractory to medical therapy, in the presence of lesions with high probability of successful dilatation; lesions with expected lower success, higher complications, and higher recurrence, such as type C lesions of the ACC/AHA classification (33), should probably be avoided in the setting of a severely dysfunctional myocardium, unless there is absolute contraindication to bypass surgery.

A possible extended application of PTCA in patients with depressed left ventricular function may be, as a temporizing revascularization measure, an alternative to bypass surgery until cardiac transplant; the procedure, however, should be limited to patients with severe ischemic manifestations; in fact, the persistence of elevated mortality during follow-up appears to indicate that the ventricular function improvement may be elusive.

To date, there are no direct randomized comparative studies between bypass surgery and coronary angioplasty in patients with symptomatic coronary disease and poor left ventricular function, and such study should probably be considered.

REVERSAL OF LEFT VENTRICULAR DYSFUNCTION BY PTCA

Reversal of preexisting left ventricular dysfunction has already been documented with coronary bypass surgery (34). Only recently, the attention of many investigators has been directed to the effects of coronary angioplasty on cardiac contractility and PTCA's potential to improve left ventricular dysfunction (Fig. 6). Such recovery has been described with direct mechanical recanalization of acute myocardial infarction (35) and after successful coronary angioplasty early after non-Q-wave myocardial infarction (4). Improvement of resting left ventricular function after bypass surgery has been observed in patients with unstable angina but not in those with stable angina (36).

Few studies have investigated the immediate effects of successful PTCA on left ventricular function in patients with unstable angina (3,37). At the Medical College of Virginia, left ventriculography (30° RAO) was performed in 39 patients before and immediately after 42 successful single-vessel PTCA procedures; 24 patients had unstable angina and 18 had stable angina; clinical characteristics and pre-PTCA medications were not different in the two groups. Global and regional ejection fractions were calculated, and segments were classified as "jeopardized," i.e., supplied by the dilated coronary, and "nonjeopardized," i.e., supplied by nonsignificantly stenosed coronary arteries. Global left ventricular ejection fraction improved significantly after PTCA in patients with unstable angina, from a mean of 54% to a mean of 66%, whereas patients with stable angina demonstrated no change in left ventricular ejection fraction from the baseline level of 61%. More important, segmental analysis revealed significant improvement in regional ejection fraction in jeopardized segments from 37% to 52% in patients with unstable angina, but did not change (46% before and after PTCA) in those with stable angina. Improvement also occurred, to a lesser extent, in the nonjeopardized segments in the unstable angina patients.

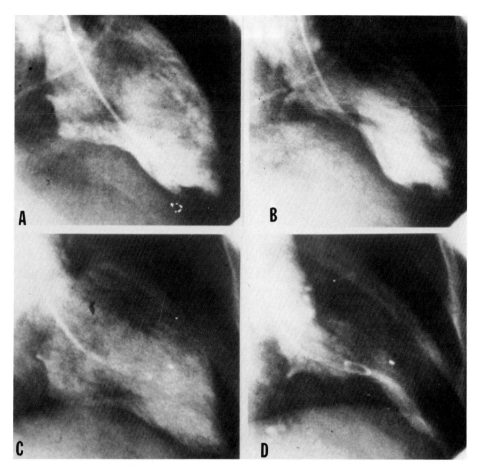

Figure 6 (A, B) Severe anterolateral hypokinesis in a patient with occluded LAD (not shown). (C, D) Six months after successful PTCA of LAD, there is normalization of wall motion.

Depression of regional LV function in the setting of unstable angina can be attributed to "stunned" myocardium, i.e., transient decrease in contractility due to acute ischemia that regains function with improved flow after PTCA (38). The improvement seen in nonjeopardized segments may be artifactual, due to overlapping of the five segments into which the ventricular silhouette was divided for the analysis, but may also be real and correspond to improvement in contractility due to reduction of workload and wall stress on the normal segments, brought about by the resolution of ischemia in the jeopardized segments.

HIBERNATING MYOCARDIUM

A joint study conducted by the Medical College of Virginia and the University of Texas in Dallas provided further evidence of the effectiveness of PTCA in improving contractility, even when applied in the setting of chronically dysfunctional myocardium (39). The study employed 2D echo performed immediately before and 3 days after elective PTCA to evaluate resting left ventricular function in 40 patients. Segmental dysfunction was present in 20 patients pre-PTCA, and 13 of them (65%) had a myocardial infarction in the distribution of the target vessel within the month prior to PTCA. The echo score was significantly improved 3 days post-PTCA in all patients with left ventricular dysfunction, even in those who had wall motion abnormalities with prior MI (83% of the segments in those patients were akinetic prior to revascularization). This study and others (40) provide evidence of myocardial hibernation: chronically ischemic but viable myocardium that improves functionally with increased perfusion (41).

IDENTIFYING VIABLE MYOCARDIUM

The studies described above demonstrate that dysfunctional myocardium, either "stunned" or "hibernating," may improve after angioplasty; in fact, PTCA offers the unique opportunity to evaluate effects of revascularization in the absence of the confounding factors associated with bypass surgery (i.e., cardioplegia, general anesthesia, etc.) . However, detection of reversibility of dysfunction remains largely a post hoc issue; precise methods of identifying a priori the extent of presumed viable myocardium that will benefit from revascularization are not widely available. Reversible perfusion defects at thallium-201 imaging, evidence of improved wall motion after nitroglycerin administration or postextrasystolic potentiation, and absence of Q waves at electrocardiography all have been considered indicative of viability. However, the sensitivity and specificity of those methods are not excellent. At present, positron emission tomography (PET) is the only technique that can identify viable myocardium by monitoring the metabolic activity of fluorine-18 deoxyglucose (42), but its widespread applicability is limited largely by cost.

Ideally, a prospective assessment of reversible dysfunction would be invaluable for guiding revascularization decisions. Clinical situations in which it could be applied are patients with severe global depression of left ventricular function to evaluate their potential for recovery and consequently their long-term prognosis, but also patients early after acute MI. In the latter case, in the presence of an infarct-related vessel that is persistently occluded, the decision to perform a late recanalization with PTCA depends heavily on tissue viability considerations. Current existing evidence suggests that even late reperfusion may be associated with better prognosis (43); this would support an extension of the indications for PTCA to any phase of an ischemic syndrome and may justify recanalization attempts even late after an acute MI (44). Reliable methods for identifying viable myocardium are being investigated and should prove determinant for guiding revascularization decisions in patients with reversibly depressed left ventricular function.

REFERENCES

1. Kohli RS, DiSciascio G, Cowley MJ, Nath A, Goudreau E, Vetrovec GW. Coronary angioplasty in patients with severe left ventricular dysfunction. J Am Coll Cardiol 1990; 16:807–11.
2. Warner M, Kazziha S, Goudreau E, Nath A, Sabri MN, Kohli RS, DiSciascio G, Cowley MJ, Vetrovec GW. Incidence of left ventricular stunning in the distribution of unstable coronary stenoses. J Am Coll Cardiol 1991; 17:256A (Abstract).
3. Carlson EB, Cowley MJ, Wolfgang TC, Vetrovec GW. Acute changes in global and regional rest left ventricular function after successful coronary angioplasty: Comparative results in stable and unstable angina. J Am Coll Cardiol 1989; 13:1262–9.
4. Suryapranata H, Serruys PW, Beatt K, De Feyter PJ, Van Den Brand M, Roelandt J. Recovery of regional myocardial dysfunction after successful coronary angioplasty early after a non-Q wave myocardial infarction. Am Heart J 1990; 120:261–9.
5. Taylor GJ, Robinovich E, Mikell FL, Moses WH, Dove JT, Batchelder JE, Wellons HA, Schneider JA. Percutaneous transluminal coronary angioplasty as palliation for patients considered poor surgical candidates. Am Heart J 1986; 111:840–4.
6. Detre K, Holubkov R, Kelsey J, et al. Percutaneous transluminal coronary angioplasty in 1985–86 and 1977–81: The NHLBI registry. N Engl J Med 1988; 318:265–70.
7. Williams DO, Riley RS, Singh AK, Gewirtz H, Most AS. Evaluation of the role of coronary angioplasty in patients with unstable angina pectoris. Am Heart J 1981; 102:1–9.
8. De Feyter PJ, Serruys PW, Van Den Brand M, Balakumaran K, Mochtar B, Soward AL, Arnold AER, Hugenholtz PG. Emergency coronary angioplasty in refractory unstable angina. N Engl J Med 1985; 313:342–7.
9. De Feyter PJ, Suryapranata H. Serruys PW, Beatt K, Van Domburg R, Van Den Brand M, Tijssen JJ, Azar AJ, Hugenholtz PG. Coronary angioplasty for unstable angina: Immediate and late results in 200 consecutive patients with identification of risk factors for unfavorable early and late outcome. J Am Coll Cardiol 1988; 12:324–33.
10. Morrison DA. Coronary angioplasty for medically refractory unstable angina within 30 days of acute myocardial infarction. Am Heart J 1990; 120:256–60.
11. Dorros G, Lewin R, Mathiak L. Percutaneous transluminal coronary angioplasty in patients with severe left ventricular dysfunction (LV<35%). Cathet Cardiovasc Diagn 1989; 17:62 (Abstract).
12. Serota H, Deligonul U, Lee WH, Aguirre F, Kern MJ, Taussig SA, Vandormael MG. Predictors of cardiac survival after percutaneous transluminal coronary an-

gioplasty in patients with severe left ventricular dysfunction. Am J Cardiol 1991; 67:367–72.

13. Hartzler GO, Rutherford BD, McConahay DR, Johnson WL, Giorgi LV. High risk percutaneous transluminal coronary angioplasty. Am J Cardiol 1988; 61:33G–37G.

14. Alderman EL, Fischer LD, Litwin P, et al. Results of coronary artery surgery in patients with poor left ventricular function (CASS). Circulation 1983; 68:785–95.

15. Kahn JK, Rutherford BD, McConahay DR, Johnson WL, Giorgi LV, Hartzler GD. Supported ''high risk'' coronary angioplasty using intraaortic balloon pump counterpulsation. J Am Coll Cardiol 1990; 15:1151–5.

16. Voudris V, Marco J, Morice MC, Fajadet J, Royer T. ''High risk'' percutaneous transluminal coronary angioplasty with preventive intra-aortic balloon counterpulsation. Cathet Cardiovasc Diagn 1990; 19: 160–4.

17. Wohlgelernter D, Clemon M, Highman HA, Zaret BL. Percutaneous transluminal coronary angioplasty of the ''culprit lesion'' for management of unstable angina pectoris in patients with multi-vessel coronary disease. Am J Cardiol 1986; 58: 460–4.

18. DiSciascio G, Cowley MJ: Multivessel coronary disease. In: Brest A, ed. Coronary Angioplasty—Cardiovascular clinics. Philadelphia: F. A. Davis, 1987:101–14.

19. DiSciascio G, Cowley MJ, Goudreau E, Vetrovec GW, Kelly KM. Staged approach to multivessel coronary angioplasty: Strategic considerations and results. J Interven Cardiol 1988; 1:175–80.

20. Nath A, DiSciascio G, Kelly K, Vetrovec GW, Testerman C, Goudreau E, Cowley MJ. Multivessel coronary angioplasty early after acute myocardial infarction. J Am Coll Cardiol 1990; 16:545–50.

21. DiSciascio G, Cowley MJ, Vetrovec GW, Kelly K, Lewis SA. Triple vessel coronary angioplasty: Acute outcome and longterm results. J Am Coll Cardiol 1988; 12:42–8.

22. DiSciascio G, Vetrovec GW, Cowley MJ, Wolfgang T. Early and late outcome of percutaneous transluminal coronary angioplasty for subacute and chronic total coronary occlusion. Am Heart J 1986; 111:833–9.

23. Linkoff AM, Popma JJ, Ellis SG, Vogel RA, Topol EJ. Percutaneous support devices for high risk or complicated coronary angioplasty. J Am Coll Cardiol 1991; 17:770–80.

24. Babic UU, Grujic S, Djurisic Z, Vucinic M. Percutaneous left atrial-aortic bypass with a roller pump. Circulation 1989; 80(Suppl II):II–271 (Abstract).

25. Glassman E, Chinitz L, Levine H, Slater J, Winer H. Partial left heart bypass support during high risk angioplasty. Circulation 1989; 85(Suppl II):II–272 (Abstract).

26. Vogel RA, Showl F, Tommaso C, et al. Initial report of the National registry of elective cardiopulmonary bypass supported coronary angioplasty. J Am Coll Cardiol 1990; 15:23–9.

27. Frazier OH, Nalcatan T, Duncan JM, Parnis SM, Fuqua JM. Clinical experience with hemopump. ASAIO Transact 1989; 35:604–6.

28. Corday E, Kar S, Drury JK, et al. Coronary versus retroperfusion for support of ischemic myocardium. Cardiovasc Rev Rep 1988; 9:50–3.

29. Quigley PJ, Hinoara T, Phillips HR, Peter RH, Behar VS, Kong Y, Simonton CA,

Perez JA, Stack RS. Myocardial protection during coronary angioplasty with an autoperfusion balloon catheter in humans. Circulation 1988; 78:1128–34.

30. Heibig J, Angelini P, Leachman R, Beall MM, Beall AC. Use of mechanical devices for distal hemoperfusion during balloon catheter coronary angioplasty. Cathet Cardiovasc Diag 1988; 15:143–9.

31. DiSciascio G, Angelini P, Vandormael M, Brinker J, Cowley M, Dean L, Lembo N, Douglas J. Reduction of ischemia with a new flow-adjustable hemoperfusion pump during coronary angioplasty. J Am Coll Cardiol (in press).

32. Cowley MJ, Snow FR, DiSciascio G, Kelly K, Guard C, Nixon JF. Perfluorochemical perfusion during coronary angioplasty in unstable and high-risk patients. Circulation 1990; 81 (Suppl IV):IV-27–IV-34.

33. Ryan TJ, Faxon DP, Gunnar RM, Ward Kennedy J, King SB, Coop FD, Peterson KL, Reeves TJ, Williams DO, Winters WL. Guidelines for percutaneous transluminal coronary angioplasty. A report of the ACC/AHA Task Force on assessment of diagnostic and therapeutic cardiovascular procedures (subcommittee on percutaneous transluminal coronary angioplasty). J Am Coll Cardiol 1988;12:529–45.

34. Brundage RH, Massie BM, Botvinick EH. Improved regional ventricular function after successful surgical revascularization. J Am Coll Cardiol 1984; 3:902–8.

35. O'Neil W, et al. A prospective randomized clinical trial of intracoronary streptokinase versus coronary angioplasty for acute myocardial infarction. N Engl J Med 1986; 314:812.

36. Kolibash AJ, Goodenow JS, Bush CA, Tatalman MR, Lewis RP. Improvement of myocardial perfusion and left ventricular function after coronary bypass grafting in patients with unstable angina. Circulation 1979; 57:66.

37. De Feyter PJ, Suryapranata H, Serruys PW, Beatt K, Van Den Brand M, Hugenholtz PG. Effects of successful percutaneous transluminal coronary angioplasty on global and regional left ventricular function in unstable angina pectoris. Am J Cardiol 1987; 60:993–7.

38. Braunwald E, Kloner RA. The stunned myocardium: Prolonged, postischemic ventricular dysfunction. Circulation 1982; 66:1146–9.

39. Vandenberg EK, Popma JJ, Dehmer GJ, Snow FR, Lewis SA, Vetrovec GW, Nixon JV. Reversible segmental left ventricular dysfunction after coronary angioplasty. Circulation 1990; 81:1210–6.

40. Cohen M, Charney R, Hershman R, Fuster V, Gorlin R, Francis X. Reversal of chronic ischemic myocardial dysfunction after transluminal coronary angioplasty. J Am Coll Cardiol 1988; 12:1193–8.

41. Braunwald E, Rutherford JD. Reversible ischemic left ventricular dysfunction: Evidence for the "hibernating myocardium." J Am Coll Cardiol 1986; 8:1467–70.

42. Tillish J, Brunken R, Marshall R, Schwaiger M, Mandelkorn M, Phelps M, Schelbert H. Reversibility of cardiac wall motion abnormality predicted by position tomography. N Engl J Med 1986; 314:884–8.

43. Braunwald E. Coronary artery patency in patients with myocardial infarction. J Am Coll Cardiol 1990; 16:1550–2.

44. Sabri NM, DiSciascio G, Cowley MJ, et al. Non acute recanalization of occluded infarct-related arteries. Immediate and long term results with coronary angioplasty. Am J Cardiol (in press).

15

Coronary Angioplasty for Early Postinfarction Angina

Harry Suryapranata and Pim J. de Feyter

University Hospital Rotterdam-Dijkzigt and
Erasmus University
Rotterdam, The Netherlands

Patrick W. Serruys

Interuniversity Cardiological Institute
of The Netherlands and
Erasmus University
Rotterdam, The Netherlands

INTRODUCTION

The clinical course of patients with postinfarction angina has been reported to carry a poor short- and long-term prognosis (1–6) and seems to be related to unstable angina or subsequent recurrent myocardial infarction (MI) in the same area, particularly in patients with non-Q-wave MI. Persistent or recurrent angina early after MI implies that the cardiac event is not yet complete and has understandably led some to recommend more aggressive evaluation and treatment strategies for this subset of patients in order to improve clinical status and salvage myocardium (7,8). However, despite marked improvement in pharmacological therapy and substantial improvement in revascularization techniques (coronary bypass surgery and coronary angioplasty), management of these patients remains a challenge. So far, there is still no consensus as to the relative merits of revascularization in the early post-MI phase and many centers continue to manage these patients pharmacologically.

This chapter reviews the natural history, potential predictors of early mortality, pathogenesis, and angiographic findings, as well as the short- and long-term results of coronary angioplasty in patients with early postinfarction angina, with particular emphasis on patients with non-Q-wave MI.

NATURAL HISTORY

The incidence of recurrent angina after sustained MI during the hospitalization period is reported between 18 and 57% and is considered to have a poor short- and long-term prognosis (1–6,9–13). Postinfarction ischemia may be localized either to the border zone of the infarct (ischemia in the infarct zone) or to a distant vascular bed (ischemia at a distance) (10). The latter patients have been shown to have a much worse prognosis. Despite marked improvement in pharmacological therapy, the incidence of recurrent MI remains high, ranging between 19 and 34% (1,3,4,6,12–14) and is associated with an in-hospital mortality of 20–36% versus 9–13% for patients without recurrent MI (1,5,6,9,15–17). The 1-year survival rate was 76% for those with versus 91% for those without recurrent MI (5). In particular, non-Q-wave MIs have been shown to be associated with a higher incidence of recurrent MI (1,9,12–14,18).

The reported incidence of non-Q-wave MI varies between 20 and 36% of all acute MI's (1,3,13–20) and seems to be increasing (21) probably as a result of pharmacological interventions before or during the acute symptomatic phase of acute MI that may minimize the extent of acute myocardial damage. Although non-Q-wave and Q-wave MI as classified by electrocardiographic results cannot always be anatomically differentiated (12,22), it seems likely that they differ clinically, physiologically, and prognostically (23). In particular, non-Q-wave MI is generally associated with smaller amounts of myocardial necrosis, better left ventricular function, and a lower incidence of in-hospital mortality, compared to Q-wave MI. But despite this initially favorable prognosis, evidence has accumulated that long-term mortality in these patients is similar to or even greater than that in patients with Q-wave MI (Table 1) (7,20,21,24–27). The relatively high mortality rate of patients with non-Q-wave MI seems to be related to subsequent unstable angina or recurrent MI in the same area (1,3,12,13,15,16,27,28). In a prospective study designed to determine the prognosis of 50 consecutive patients with non-Q-wave MI, Madigan et al. (9) found that unstable angina occurred in 46% of patients before discharge and that recurrent MI occurred in 21% of the patients, which was associated with a poor prognosis. Maisel et al. (15) reported a high mortality, both early and late, for patients with subsequent extension following a non-Q-wave MI. The in-hospital mortality rate in this subset of patients was 43%, and in those with Q-wave MI it was 15% while the 1-year cumulative survival rates for patients with Q- and non-Q-wave MI without extension were similar: 82 and 84%, respectively. For those with extension, however, 1-year survival rates were 66 and 35%, respectively. These findings were supported by others (1,5,14,16,17,27) and recently confirmed by Schechtman et al. (6), who reported that patients with in-hospital recurrent MI were more than 4 times as likely to die during the early period as were patients without in-hospital recurrent MI. However, none of these patients reported were treated with thrombolysis, and because its frequent use may

Table 1 Incidence and Mortality in Non-Q- and Q-Wave Myocardial Infarction

	Incidence		Short-term mortality		Long-term mortality		Follow-up (months)
	Non-Q MI (n)	Q MI (n)	Non-Q MI (%)	Q MI (%)	Non-Q MI (%)	Q MI (%)	
Norris (24)	205	437	12	31	46	48	72
Szklo (25)	283	953	18	30	28	27	36
Boxall (26)	70	259	1	11	16	22	32
Hutter (7)	67	129	9	20	52	42	29
Marmor (27)	125	215	10	23	27	30	9
Goldberg (21)	882	1577	12	25	15	12	12
Nicod (20)	444	1425	8	12	14	9	12

change the course of non-Q-wave MI, further studies will be needed in this subset of patients.

Finally, in the current thrombolytic era, early administration of intravenous thrombolytic agents to patients with acute MI has markedly reduced the in-hospital mortality of selected patient groups (29–32). However, because none of these agents removes the underlying stimulus for thrombus formation, a propensity for recurrent thrombosis and ischemia remains. Recurrent ischemia occurs in up to 20% of patients in this setting (29,33,34) and has been shown to be associated with an increase in in-hospital mortality (35,36). Ellis et al. (37) have recently shown that the in-hospital mortality in patients with successful initial reperfusion and no clinically evident recurrent ischemia was extremely low (2%) and in those with initially successful reperfusion but subsequent recurrent ischemia was 15%, while patients without successful reperfusion had a very high mortality (32%). In addition, among those patients with subsequent recurrent ischemia, successful early (≤90 min) treatment of recurrent ischemia was associated with a significantly lower in-hospital mortality (0%) than in patients with late successful (21%) or unsuccessful reperfusion (24%) (37).

POTENTIAL PREDICTORS OF EARLY RECURRENT MI AND MORTALITY (Table 2)

On the other hand, several studies have also reported that non-Q-wave MI is not necessarily associated with adverse long-term prognosis. Predischarge exercise test characteristics, coronary anatomy, and the late incidence of subsequent major cardiac events (recurrent MI, coronary bypass surgery, and mortality) at

Table 2 Predictors of Early Recurrent MI and Mortality

Clinical risk factors
  Recurrent angina
  Age > 70 years
  Congestive heart failure
  Previous MI
Electrocardiographic/radionuclide
  Persistent ST-segment depression
  Left ventricular hypertrophy
  Inadequate systolic blood pressure response to exercise testing
  Residual viable myocardial mass
Angiographic
  Infarct-related artery supplying a large area of viable myocardium at risk
  Multivessel disease
  Left main coronary artery disease
  Left ventricular ejection fraction < 40%

1-year follow-up have recently been reported to be similar in patients with Q- or non-Q-wave MI (19,20,28). Differences between studies may be due to a number of factors. Despite the high incidence of previous MI usually seen in patients with non-Q-wave MI (14,20), which is associated with a high prevalence of multivessel disease and recurrent angina (3,14,19,20), many studies did not separate patients with or without previous MI. Similarly, differences in age between groups of patients were often not accounted for. Also, many studies included small numbers of patients or reported only in-hospital or postdischarge clinical outcome. Subgroup analysis, as reported in several studies (3,19,20,28), has shown favorable short- and long-term clinical outcome in patients <70 years of age with a first non-Q-wave MI.

Schechtman et al. (6), from the Diltiazem Reinfarction Study Group, have shown that persistent in-hospital ST-segment depression is a major independent predictor of in-hospital recurrent MI and early mortality, which is reported to be 27.2 times as high as that among patients with no ST-segment depression. These findings are consistent with the hypothesis that ST-segment depression is, in part, an indication of prolonged ischemia (11,13,38–41) and strongly suggest that these patients warrant aggressive early management. Paradoxically, as also observed in other studies (38,42), one-third of all non-Q-wave MI patients in the same study group (43) exhibited ST-segment elevation on admission to the hospital. Subgroup analysis further showed that of patients presenting with ST-segment elevation, 80% did not evolve new Q waves, while in the subgroup presenting with ST-segment depression or T-wave inversion or both, 85% of the patients did not evolve new Q waves (43). The essential finding of these studies is that it is apparent that the specificity of early ST-segment elevation in the diagnosis of evolving Q-wave MI is much less than previously suspected, that ST-segment elevation, while clearly a marker of transmural ischemia, may not invariably culminate in transmural infarction and subsequent Q-wave evolution, and that ST-segment depression should not be considered inherently more ''benign'' than ST-segment elevation. These observations may have important clinical implications, particularly in deciding which MI patients should be selected for acute thrombolytic therapy, since ST-segment depression is generally regarded as an exclusion criterion. However, the role of thrombolytic therapy in patients with evolving MI characterized chiefly by ST-segment depression remains to be evaluated.

The value of angiography as determinant of prognosis after MI has also been investigated (44–47). Sanz et al. (47) found that ejection fraction and the extent of coronary artery disease were the only independent invasive predictors of survival during a follow-up study of 60 months. Patients with a normal ejection fraction, regardless of the number of diseased vessels, lived longest. The probability of survival of patients with an ejection fraction of 21–49% ranged from 78%, for patients with three-vessel disease, to 95%, for those with single-vessel disease. The poorest prognosis corresponded to an ejection fraction less than 20%: 30–75% depending on the number of diseased vessels. According to the 30-month follow-up study of Taylor et al. (44), univariate analysis showed that low ejection fraction, proximal left anterior descending coronary artery disease, and three-vessel disease were associated with a high risk of sudden cardiac death. However, multivariate analysis of 30 clinical and laboratory variables identified previous MI and an ejection fraction less than 40% as predictors of death. Additional information was not provided by the other variables once these two variables were considered. According to de Feyter et al. (45), patients with an ejection fraction less than 30% and three-vessel disease formed a high-risk group for cardiac death. During a mean follow-up of 28 months, 10 of the 11 cardiac deaths occurred in this high-risk group. Roubin et al. (46) showed that three-vessel disease had a lower survival rate at 1 year than two- and one-vessel disease. Also, although not at a significant level, an ejection fraction lower than 50% was associated with a lower 1-year survival rate. Thus, it appears that cardiac death in survivors of acute MI is related to the extent of coronary artery disease and the severity of left ventricular dysfunction.

Furthermore, univariate and multivariate analysis, in patients treated with and without thrombolytic therapy for acute MI, has recently shown the following determinants of mortality after hospital discharge: age exceeding 60 years, congestive heart failure, a history of previous MI, large enzymatic infarct size, left ventricular ejection fraction <40%, contraindications for or inadequate systolic blood pressure response to exercise testing, and multivessel disease (48). It has been further concluded from this study (48) that coronary angiography did not improve the predictors of mortality after hospital discharge.

PATHOGENESIS

The long-term prognosis of patients with postinfarction angina may be related to the degree of potentially jeopardized myocardium. Patients with non-Q-wave MI appear to have more residual myocardial mass at risk, as determined by exercise scintigraphy (13,42), for subsequent ischemia or necrosis. The prevalence and extent of quantitatively determined thallium-201 redistribution within the infarct zone on exercise scintigraphy was greater in patients with non-Q-wave MI than in those with Q-wave MI (60% versus 36%) (13). Furthermore, a recent study (49) of regional myocardial metabolism and blood flow assessed by positron emission tomography demonstrated metabolic integrity (residual viable tissue) in 91% of infarcted regions without Q waves, whereas only 36% of the infarcted regions with Q waves showed metabolic activity. This jeopardized myocardium may be tenuously preserved by the collateral circulation, thereby favoring the development of angina, recurrent MI, and malignant ventricular arrhythmias. The pathophysiological basis of the apparent greater clinical instability after non-

Q-wave MI and the reason for loss of the initial prognostic advantage have been supported by several studies that found greater rates of angina, recurrent MI, and sudden death among hospital survivors of non-Q-wave MI than among those with Q-wave MI (1,3,12–18,27).

The pathogenesis of non-Q-wave MI may involve spontaneous coronary reperfusion characterized by a lower and shorter time to peak creatine kinase (CK) level and smaller enzymatic infarct size as well as a higher prevalence of patient infarct-related vessel, which may result in better left ventricular function and regional perfusion, compared to the Q-wave MI (42). Figures approach the findings in our thrombolytic trials (29,50). In this controlled randomized trial of intracoronary streptokinase, it was found that recanalization of an initially occluded infarct-related artery was associated with a significant improvement in resting regional myocardial function of the infarct zone, implying reperfusion-related limitation in infarct size. However, the incidence of recurrent MI in the same area as the initial injury was found higher after successful thrombolytic therapy compared with the control group. In most other trials, a higher incidence of recurrent MI was also reported after thrombolytic therapy than among controls (51–54). Again, a smaller infarct size after thrombolytic therapy and thus more viable myocardium in the territory of the infarct-related vessel after thrombolysis is the most likely explanation. Of note, data from another intracoronary strep-tokinase study (55) also indicated more extensive exercise-induced peri-infarction ischemia in patients with open versus closed infarct-related vessel at 5–6 weeks after onset of MI. These findings suggest similarities between thrombolysis-treated infarcts and the naturally evolving non-Q-wave MI. As such, it seems likely that as fibrinolytic therapy becomes more widely used, the pool of patients with incomplete infarctions who are at increased risk of recurrent MI will increase. Furthermore, this finding supports the concept that acute ST-segment elevation without progression to Q waves is indicative of coronary obstruction with subsequent early recanalization and attendant myocardial salvage.

There is also evidence that postinfarction angina and unstable angina may share a common pathogenesis. Several clinical, angiographic, and pathological studies have emphasized the important pathophysiological link between unstable angina and postinfarction angina (56–62). In unstable angina, the pathophysiological process is limited to endothelial ulceration, platelet aggregation, and thrombus formation, which may be intermittent or more permanent in the presence of an adequate collateral supply. Acute MI is related to the same process but with the formation of a totally occlusive thrombus. When the balance between intracoronary thrombus and antithrombotic natural and pharmacological factors leans toward continued thrombus formation, persistent total coronary occlusion leading to acute MI may occur. If the coronary artery remains occluded for a long period (more than 15 min), then myocardial necrosis will occur. If very early clot lysis occurs with or without embolization to the distal coronary bed, or if an adequate collateral supply is present, infarction will be limited (non-Q-wave MI), whereas it will be extended (Q-wave MI) when no or late clot lysis occurs.

ANGIOGRAPHIC FINDINGS AND LEFT VENTRICULAR FUNCTION IN SURVIVORS OF ACUTE MI

Only a few prospective angiographic studies after acute MI have been performed, which give insight into the overall spectrum of coronary anatomy in post-MI patients. Most studies tend to be biased toward high-risk patients, as coronary angiography has not been routinely performed in asymptomatic patients after MI. In Table 3, the prevalence of multivessel disease in survivors of acute MI is summarized from those prospective studies (44–46,63). The prevalence of multivessel disease seems to be similar between survivors of Q- and non-Q-wave MI, while the prevalence of multivessel disease is significantly higher in survivors of a Q-wave inferior wall MI than in a Q-wave anterior wall MI and is significantly higher in patients with early postinfarction angina (79–92%) than in those without angina (45–70%). Furthermore, in patients with a previous MI the presence of multivessel disease is higher (73–100%) than in those with a first MI (31–64%).

In contrast to Q-wave MI, total coronary occlusion of the infarct-related vessel is infrequently observed in the early hours of a non-Q-wave MI, but it increases moderately in frequency over the next several days (56). Several angiographic studies (9,13,19,42,56,64) have demonstrated that patients with non-Q-wave MI had a lower incidence of a totally occluded infarct-related vessel, ranging from 32 to 48%, compared to those with Q-wave MI. In Q-wave MI, the frequency of a total occlusion within 6 hr after onset of symptoms is reported between 80 and 91%, at 6–24 hours 67%, at 2 weeks 53%, and at 4 weeks 45% (65–72), while the incidence of collateral circulation to the area supplied by occluded vessel in patients with non-Q-wave MI was higher, ranging from 85 to 93%, compared to those with Q-wave MI. The essential finding of these studies is that some degree of perfusion, either antegrade or by means of collateral vessels, is present soon after non-Q-wave MI, although it is insufficient to prevent the initial necrosis. Thus, it appears that the anatomical distribution of coronary artery disease in those with non-Q-wave MI resembles that of patients with Q-wave MI, but that viable amounts of myocardium may be protected from further necrosis by the presence of a subtotal occlusion or collateral circulation. These findings have been supported by postmortem studies (73,74).

Furthermore, a specific angiographic morphology frequently present in patients with unstable angina, as described by Ambrose et al. (61), is also found in

Table 3 Prevalence of Multivessel Disease (MVD) in Survivors of Acute MI

	Taylor et al. (44)		Turner et al. (63)		de Feyter et al. (45)		Roubin et al. (46)	
	n	MVD (%)	n	MVD (%)	n	MVD (%)	n	MVD (%)
Q-wave MI	64	72	94	76	143	54	148	37
Non-Q-wave MI	42	76	23	74	21	48	78	32
Anterior MI	29	59			62	41	114	31
Inferior MI	35	83			81	73	108	39
With early post-MI angina			26	92	52	79		
Without early post-MI angina			91	70	127	45		
With previous MI	28	100	15	73	24	75		
Without previous MI	78	64	164	53	202	31		

patients with non-Q-wave MI. This eccentric convex intraluminal obstruction with a narrow neck resulting from one or more irregular overhanging edges was found in 65% of ischemia-related coronary arteries in patients with non-Q-wave MI (61). This similarity in coronary morphology suggests once again a similar pathogenesis, as previously suggested. Therefore, the management of patients with non-Q-wave MI should be similar to that of patients with unstable angina.

It has been shown in several prospective studies (44–46,72) that ejection fractions of <30%, 30–49%, and >50% are observed in, respectively, 7–17%, 44–55%, and 31–48% of the patients after acute MI. Similar data were also found with radionuclide-determined ejection fractions (75). The global ejection fraction is significantly lower in patients with multivessel disease than in those with single-vessel disease (45,72). In patients with a totally occluded infarct-related vessel, the ejection fraction is lower and the impairment of regional left ventricular function is higher than in those with a lesser degree of obstruction of the infarct vessel (50,72,76,77). Left ventricular dysfunction is more severe with anterior MI than with inferior MI (44,45,50,72,76,77), particularly in patients with a history of previous MI. Apparently, a well-developed collateral circulation improves the ejection fraction and decreases the size of dyskinetic regional segments (72,78). Wackers et al. (79) demonstrated spontaneous improvement in left ventricular ejection fraction within the first 24 hr of Q-wave MI in 52 patients not treated with thrombolytic agents. This improvement may be associated with spontaneous recanalization, as evidenced by rapid release of CK-MB, as suggested by Ong et al. (80). de Feyter et al. (76) showed a better left ventricular function in patients with spontaneous recanalization than with persisting occlusion of the infarct-related vessel in patients with a first Q-wave acute MI who were catheterized 6–8 weeks after the acute event. These findings are consistent with the results achieved in several thrombolytic trials (29,50,77,81).

THERAPEUTIC IMPLICATIONS

Randomized trials in postinfarction patients using long-term beta-adrenergic blockade have yielded conflicting results when data are analyzed according to the presence or absence of electrocardiographic Q waves. The Beta-blocker Heart Attack Trial (82) demonstrated reduced mortality with propranolol compared with placebo in 2858 patients with Q-wave MI, but showed no effect in 873 patients with non-Q-wave MI. By comparison, the Norwegian Timolol Trial (83) found prolonged survival in timolol-treated patients regardless of infarct type; however, the incidence of reinfarction was reduced only in patients with Q-wave MI. Although several animal studies have shown that calcium-channel blockers can protect ischemic myocardium at risk for MI (84–86), only a few clinical trials of patients with non-Q-wave MI have been reported. The results of a recently published study indicated that treatment with diltiazem has a protective effect against reinfarction and recurrent angina (87).

The problem of definitive therapy and the timing of therapy are more difficult. Persistent or recurrent angina early after MI implies that the cardiac event is not yet complete and suggests that more aggressive management might improve patients' clinical status and salvage myocardium. The occurrence of severe or refractory postinfarction angina has been a primary indication for urgent revascularization. In the acute situation, however, when a patient presents with chest pain and electrocardiographic signs of ischemia early after acute MI, the distinction between ischemia and recurrent MI is often difficult, since the electrocardiographic and enzymatic patterns of the evolving initial MI are blurring the diagnosis of recurrent MI. Treatment of patients in this situation is facilitated by the fact that the initial goal of therapy is the same: to resolve myocardial ischemia and to prevent further necrosis. In practice this means the preservation or early restoration of antegrade flow in the ischemia-related artery. To this end, coronary bypass surgery and coronary angioplasty have been shown to be effective in the management of patients with postinfarction angina (88–92).

The first reports (93–100) of patients undergoing surgical revascularization early after MI noted an increased operative mortality compared with that in other patients undergoing revascularization months or years after MI. Patients treated surgically within the first 7 days after MI experienced twice the mortality of those treated surgically after 8–30 days and more than threefold the mortality of those treated surgically more than 30 days after MI (98). These patients are more likely to require inotropic support and intra-aortic balloon counterpulsation and have a higher incidence of significant arrhythmia's and perioperative MI rates than those operated on later (92). However, continuing improvement in surgical techniques, development of effective methods of intraoperative myocardial protection, and improvement in postoperative care, associated with the consequent lower mortality and better long-term results, have restored enthusiasm among some surgeons for revascularization in patients with angina early after MI. Several investigators (Table 4) (92,101–110) have demonstrated that surgical intervention within the first 30 days after MI can be accomplished with an acceptable operative mortality in selected patients, although overall mortality (up to 16%) and morbidity (up to 15% MI) rates remain higher than those reported for elective surgery. The risks of surgery performed at least 1 month after MI appear to be comparable to those of elective surgery (92). Accordingly, current strategy for the management of patients with early postinfarction angina is aimed at delaying surgery to such a time when it can be performed with the least inherent risks. Obviously, such a waiting period incurs its own risks, particularly in unstable patients, with recurrent MI and morbidity despite the intensive treatment itself playing prominent roles.

Coronary angioplasty in this situation has been shown to be an attractive alternative to surgical revascularization (Table 5) (8,88,89,111–113). Particularly in these patients with their brittle condition and large area at risk and persistently insufficient coronary perfusion, the avoidance of additional risks of

Table 4 Surgical Mortality and Perioperative MI in Early (< 30 days) Postinfarction Angina

	n	Perioperative	
		Mortality (%)	MI (%)
Nunley et al. (101)	21	0	—
Williams et al. (92)	92	2	0
Molina et al. (102)	38	10.5	—
Rankin et al. (103)	52	4	4
Baumgartner et al. (104)	34	9	15
Gertler et al. (105)	44	16	—
Singh et al. (106)	108	1.8	4.6
Brower et al. (107)	34	3	12
Breyer et al. (108)	75	8	—
Jones et al. (109)	107	8.5	8.5
Stuart et al. (110)	225	5.3	—

major anesthesia is attractive. However, careful analysis of the published reports and our own experience indicates that coronary angioplasty in patients with early postinfarction angina is associated with increased risks of major complications (Table 5) compared with elective coronary angioplasty in stable angina. A procedure-related mortality is reported up to 2% and incidence of acute MI occurs in up to 8%, while acute surgery is required in up to 12% of the patients. The reasons for this relatively high major complication rate are apparently related to the preexisting underlying pathophysiology, with ongoing platelets, fibrin, thrombus, or thromboxane A_2 activities leading to clinical instability and an increased risk of abrupt closure due to the formation of an occlusive thrombus, as discussed previously. After initially successful angioplasty, however, the prognosis is excellent, with a low incidence of late mortality and a low occurrence of late nonfatal MI, while recurrent angina appears to be comparable to that of patients with stable angina (Table 5). Thus, the available data suggest that coronary angioplasty performed early after acute MI is an effective procedure in a subset of patients who have preserved but jeopardized left ventricular function, predominant single-vessel disease, and an anatomy suitable for angioplasty. However, it remains to be determined whether the same benefits can be achieved in those who have multivessel disease and reduced left ventricular function. Furthermore, it may be preferable, as an initial approach, to produce a stable state in selected patients with multivessel disease by dilating the ischemia-related vessel only (114). However, this strategy is associated, not unexpectedly, with a higher incidence of residual angina, which may necessitate subsequent bypass surgery or coronary angioplasty of other vessels on a more elective basis with less risks.

Table 5 Coronary Angioplasty for Early (< 30 days) Postinfarction Angina

	n	Success rate (%)	Major complication rate			Major events after successful angioplasty			
			Death (%)	MI (%)	Acute surgery (%)	Death (%)	MI (%)	Angina (%)	F/U (months)
de Feyter et al. (8)	53	89	0	8	8	0	4	26	9
Holt et al. (111)	70	76	2	5	12	2	4	21	27
Gottlieb et al. (112)	47	91	2	4	2	3	3	18	16
Safian et al.[a] (88)	68	87	0	1.5	1.5	0	2	41	17
Hopkins et al. (113)	54	81	0	0	4	0	2	25	11
Suryapranata et al.[a] (89)	60	85	0	5	7	0	5	23	20

[a]Patients with non-Q-wave MI.

In addition, the results of our previous study (7) have shown that the initially depressed regional myocardium in patients with early postinfarction angina is capable of recovering function and has the potential to achieve normal contraction after adequate reperfusion with coronary angioplasty, resulting in a significant improvement in global ejection fraction. These findings support once again the concept of myocardial salvage through recanalization to prevent further loss of myocardium, for one might postulate that these patients are left with an "incomplete" MI with an area of the myocardium "at risk" and might therefore benefit from revascularization of the relevant artery, resulting in reduced disability and improved survival (89). The salutary results of revascularization in patients with myocardial dysfunction emphasize the importance of detecting the reversibility of the regional myocardial dysfunction. Determining whether revascularization will improve abnormal resting wall motion has depended on the demonstration of reversible flow abnormalities on exercise thallium-201 scintigraphy (115) or on evidence of improved wall motion after nitroglycerin infusion (116), with exercise (117) or inotropic stimulus, such as postextrasystolic potentiation during contrast or radionuclide angiography (118), or the infusion of a sympathomimetic amine (119). Positron emission tomography and echocardiography during dobutamine infusion have also been reported to be reliable for identification of viable myocardium (49,120–122).

RECOMMENDATIONS AND CONCLUSIONS

The relative safety of cardiac catheterization performed early after a sustained MI has been established with low procedure-related deaths and major complication rates (44,45,63,71). However, the crucial question remains whether coronary angiography should be performed before discharge in all survivors of MI in an attempt to guide therapy to assess prognosis. Although patients recovering from acute MI who are symptomatic should be appropriately evaluated, which may include coronary and left ventricular angiography, the need for angiography in asymptomatic post-MI patients remains conflicting. Multivariate analysis study (48) has recently shown that coronary angiography does not improve the prediction of mortality after hospital discharge. Low-risk patients (47% of the total patient population), characterized in this study by the absence of recurrent ischemia or signs of congestive heart failure, without a history of previous MI, and with an adequate systolic blood pressure response to exercise, have an excellent prognosis in the first year after hospital discharge and are unlikely to benefit from predischarge angiography. Furthermore, previous studies (123–126) have shown that surgery or coronary angioplasty in this subset of patients is not superior to medical treatment for improving survival rates. On the other hand, to assess prognosis and to identify high-risk patients, clinical variables or noninvasive tests such as exercise electrocardiographic and radionuclide studies appear to be appropriate, and therefore only those with early postinfarction angina and those with evidence of inducible ischemia, despite optimal pharmacological therapy, which constitutes a high-risk subgroup of patients and may demand early intervention, are recommended for early angiography and subsequent revascularization.

However, as within the same patients different pathophysiological mechanisms may occur at different times and in succession, it will be difficult to decide what optimal therapy for that particular stage of the disease at that particular moment in time for that patient consists of. The uncertainty of outcome in a specific patient forces one to provide "maximal" treatment. Despite the substantial improvement in surgical techniques and postoperative care associated with the consequent lower mortality and better long-term results (Table 4), there is still no consensus as to the relative merits of surgery in the early post-MI phase, and many centers continue to manage these patients pharmacologically. It has been demonstrated that coronary angioplasty can be performed safely and effectively in patients with early postinfarction angina (Table 5). The capability of recovering regional myocardial function after adequate reperfusion with coronary angioplasty in patients with postinfarction angina (7) further indicates that more aggressive management might salvage myocardium and improve prognosis. However, the results of coronary angioplasty cannot be compared with those obtained with surgery, since patients who undergo angioplasty are a selection from the whole spectrum of patients with early postinfarction angina. Selected for coronary angioplasty are those with predominantly single-vessel disease and well-preserved left ventricular function. Furthermore, given the facts that up to 20% of patients treated with intravenous thrombolytic therapy will have recurrent ischemia (29,33,34) associated with increased in-hospital mortality (35,36) and that early treatment of recurrent ischemia appears to improve survival (37), it has been recommended that patients treated with intravenous thrombolytic therapy should have rapid access to facilities where secondary reperfusion can be readily obtained (37), particularly since there is no single reliable marker of reperfusion available and there are no angiographic parameters that allow accurate prediction of reocclusion. Although preliminary reports suggest high initial patency, but also frequent recurrent ischemia, when tissue-type plasminogen activator is readministered (127), it is still unknown whether a second administration of a thrombolytic regimen can match the results achieved with coronary angioplasty in this setting.

Therefore, randomized studies are perhaps the only way to provide clear insight into the relative merits of current pharmacological treatment, bypass surgery, and coronary angioplasty in the management of patients with early postinfarction angina. More important, future studies should be directed toward defining a subgroup of patients who will most likely benefit from revascularization procedure after MI—more specifically, to identify the high-risk group of patients likely to have recurrent ischemia with its major consequences. Until further information becomes available, we propose the following practical approach. This approach is based on the history of angina, the time interval between ischemic attack, the instituted therapy, and the initial acute MI, the presence of persistent electrocardiographic ST-segment depression, the response to pharmacological treatment, and the coronary anatomy and left ventricular function. Patients with early postinfarction angina should initially receive prompt management with pharmacological therapy in an attempt to achieve stability. If this approach fails and ischemic episodes continue, despite maximal medical management, prolongation of what must be regarded as ineffective treatment should be avoided, and early angiography and a more definitive attempt at myocardial revascularization should be instituted without delay to prevent progression to recurrent MI and thus improve prognosis. Coronary angioplasty is indicated when a stenosis, technically suitable for angioplasty, is found to be responsible for the unstable state. The decision in favor of coronary angioplasty in patients with single-vessel disease is easy to make, but in the presence of multivessel disease some uncertainty remains. Patients with left main stem disease or severe multivessel disease should be scheduled for coronary artery bypass surgery. However, in selected patients with multivessel disease, dilatation of the ischemia-related vessel only is acceptable as an initial approach to achieve stability, and if necessary, subsequent complete revascularization procedure (bypass surgery or angioplasty of other vessels) can be performed on a more elective basis.

REFERENCES

1. Marmor A, Sobel BE, Roberts R. Factors presaging early recurrent myocardial infarction ("extension"). Am J Cardiol 1981; 48:603–10.
2. Floretti P, Brower RW, Balakumaran K. Early post-infarction angina. Incidence and prognostic relevance. Eur Heart J 1986; 7:73–7.
3. Krone RJ, Friedman E, Thanavaro S, Miller JP, Kleiger RE, Oliver GC. Long-term prognosis after first Q-wave (transmural) or non-Q-wave (nontransmural) myocardial infarction: analysis of 593 patients. Am J Cardiol 1983; 52:234–9.
4. Stenson RE, Flamm MD, Zaret BL, McGowan RG. Transient ST-segment elevation with postmyocardial infarction angina: prognostic significance. Am Heart J 1975; 89:449–54.
5. Fraker TD, Wagner GS, Rosati RA. Extension of myocardial infarction: incidence and prognosis. Circulation 1979; 60:1126–9.
6. Schechtman KB, Capone RJ, Kleiger RE, Gibson RS, Schwartz DJ, Roberts R, Boden WE and the Diltiazem Reinfarction Study Group. Differential risk patterns associated with 3 month as compared with 3 to 12 month mortality and reinfarction after non-Q-wave myocard infarction. J Am Coll Cardiol 1990; 15:940–7.
7. Suryapranata H, Serruys PW, Beatt K, de Feyter PJ, van den Brand M, Roelandt J.

Recovery of regional myocardial dysfunction after successful coronary angioplasty early after a non-Q wave myocardial infarction. Am Heart J 1990; 120:261–9.

8. de Feyter PJ, Serruys PW, Soward A, van den Brand M, Bos E, Hugenholtz PG. Coronary angioplasty for early postinfarction unstable angina. Circulation 1986; 6:1365–70.

9. Madigan NP, Rutherford BD, Frye RL. The clinical course, early prognosis and coronary anatomy of subendocardial infarction. Am J Med 1976; 60:634–41.

10. Schuster EH, Bulkley BH. Early postinfarction angina: ischemia at a distance and ischemia in the infarct zone. N Engl J Med 1981; 305:110–5.

11. Bosch X, Théroux P, Waters D, Pelletier GB, Roy D. Early postinfarction ischemia: Clinical, angiographic, and prognostic significance. Circulation 1987; 75:988–95.

12. Hutter AM, De Sanctis RW, Flynn T, Yeatman LA. Nontransmural myocardial infarction: A comparison of hospital and late clinical course of patients with that of matched patients with transmural anterior and transmural inferior myocardial infarction. Am J Cardiol 1981; 48:595–602.

13. Gibson RS, Beller GA, Gheorghiade M, et al. The prevalence and clinical significance of residual myocardial ischemia 2 weeks after uncomplicated non-Q-wave infarction: a prospective natural history study. Circulation 1986; 73:1186–98.

14. Ogawa H, Hiramori K, Haze K, et al. Comparison of clinical features of non-Q wave and Q wave myocardial infarction. Am Heart J 1986; 111:513–8.

15. Maisel AS, Ahnve S, Gilpin E, et al. Prognosis after extension of myocardial infarct: the role of Q-wave or non-Q wave infarction. Circulation 1985; 71:211–7.

16. Hollander G, Ozick H, Greengart A, Shani J, Lichstein E. High mortality early reinfarction with first nontransmural myocardial infarction. Am Heart J 1984; 108:1412–6.

17. Buda AJ, MacDonald IL, Dubbin JD, Orr SA, Strauss HD. Myocardial infarct extension: Prevalence, clinical significance, and problems in diagnosis. Am Heart J 1983; 105:744–9.

18. Cannom DS, Levy W, Cohen LS. The short- and long-term prognosis of patients with transmural and nontransmural myocardial infarction. Am J Med 1976; 61:452–8.

19. Fox JP, Beattie JM, Salih MS, Davies MK, Littler WA, Murray RG. Non-Q wave infarction: Exercise test characteristics, coronary anatomy, and prognosis. Br Heart J 1990; 63:151–3.

20. Nicod P, Gilpin E, Dittrich H, et al. Short- and long-term clinical outcome after Q wave and non-Q wave myocardial infarction in a large patient population. Circulation 1989; 79:528–36.

21. Goldberg RJ, Gore JM, Alpert JS, Dalen JE. Non-Q wave myocardial infarction: Recent changes in occurrence and prognosis—A community-wide perspective. Am Heart J 1987; 113:273–9.

22. Savage RM, Wagner GS, Ideker RE, Podolsky SA, Hackel DB. Correlation of postmortem anatomic findings with electrocardiographic changes in patients with myocardial infarction: Retrospective study of patients with typical anterior and posterior infarcts. Circulation 1977; 55:279–85.

23. Spodick DH. Q-wave infarction versus ST infarction: Non-specificity of electro-cardiographic criteria for differentiating transmural and nontransmural lesions. Am J Cardiol 1983; 51:913–5.

24. Norris RM, Caughey DE, Deeming LW, Mercer CJ, Scott PJ. Coronary prognostic index for predicting survival after recovery from acute myocardial infarction. Lancet 1970; 2:485–7.

25. Szklo M, Goldberg R, Kennedy HL, Tonascia JA. Survival of patients with nontransmural myocardial infarction: a population-based study. Am J Cardiol 1978; 42:648–52.

26. Boxall J, Saltups A. A comparison of nontransmural and transmural myocardial infarction. Aust NZ J Med 1980; 10:176–9.

27. Marmor A, Geltman EM, Schechtman K, Sobel BE, Roberts R. Recurrent myocardial infarction: Clinical predictors and prognostic implications. Circulation 1982; 66:415–21.

28. Stone PH, Raabe DS, Jaffe AS, et al. Prognostic significance of location and type of myocardial infarction: Independent adverse outcome associated with anterior location. J Am Coll Cardiol 1988; 11:453–63.

29. Simoons ML, Serruys PW, van den Brand M, et al. Early thrombolysis in acute myocardial infarction: Limitation of infarct size and improved survival. J Am Coll Cardiol 1986; 7:717–28.

30. Gruppo Italiano per lo Studio della Streptoochinasi nell'Infarto Miocardio (GISSI). Effectiveness of intravenous thrombolytic treatment in acute myocardial infarction. Lancet 1986; 1:397–402.

31. Second International Study of Infarct Survival (ISIS-2) Collaborative Group. Randomized trial of intravenous streptokinase, oral aspirin, both or neither among 17,187 cases of suspected acute myocardial infarction: ISIS-2. Lancet 1988; 2:349–60.

32. AIMS Trial Study Group. Effect of intravenous APSAC on mortality after acute myocardial infarction: preliminary report of a placebo-controlled clinical trial. Lancet 1988; 1:545–9.

33. Chesebro JH, Knatterud G, Roberts R, et al. Thrombolysis in Myocardial Infarction (TIMI) Trial, Phase I. A comparison between intravenous tissue plasminogen activator and intravenous streptokinase clinical findings through hospital discharge. Circulation 1987; 76:142–54.

34. Topol EJ, Califf RM, George BS, et al. Coronary arterial thrombolysis with combined infusion of recombinant tissue type plasminogen activator and urokinase in patients with acute myocardial infarction. Circulation 1988; 77:1100–7.

35. Ohman EM, Califf RM, Topol EJ, et al. Characteristics and importance of reocclusion following successful reperfusion therapy in acute myocardial infarction. Circulation 1990; 82:781–91.

36. Ellis SG, O'Neill WW, Bates ER, et al. Implications for patient triage from survival and left ventricular function recovery analyses in 500 patients treated with coronary angioplasty for acute myocardial infarction. J Am Coll Cardiol 1989; 13:1251–9.

37. Ellis SG, Debowey D, Bates, ER, Topol EJ. Treatment of recurrent ischemia after thrombolysis and successful reperfusion for acute myocardial infarction: Effect on

in-hospital mortality and left ventricular function. J Am Coll Cardiol 1991; 17:752–7.

38. Willich S, Stone PH, Muller JE, et al. High-risk subgroups of patients with non-Q wave myocardial infarction based on direction and severity of ST segment deviation. Am Heart J 1987; 114:1110–9.
39. Ogawa H, Hiramori K, Haze K, et al. Classification of non-Q wave MI according to electrocardiographic changes. Br Heart J 1985; 54:73–8.
40. MacDonald RG, Hill JA, Feldman RL. ST segment response to acute coronary occlusion: coronary hemodynamic and angiographic determinants of direction of ST segment shift. Circulation 1986; 74:973–9.
41. Fuchs RM, Achuff SC, Grunwald L, Yin FCP, Griffith LSC. Electrocardiographic localization of coronary artery narrowings: Studies during myocardial ischemia and infarction in patients with one-vessel disease. Circulation 1982; 66:1168–76.
42. Huey BL, Gheorghiade M, Crampton RS, et al. Acute non-Q wave myocardial infarction associated with early ST segment elevation: Evidence for spontaneous coronary reperfusion and implications for thrombolytic trials. J Am Coll Cardiol 1987; 9:18–25.
43. Boden WE, Gibson RS, Schechtman KB, Kleiger RE, Schwartz DJ, Capone RJ, Roberts R and The Diltiazem Reinfarction Study Research Group. ST segment shifts are poor predictors of subsequent Q wave evolution in acute myocardial infarction: A natural history study of early non-Q wave infarction. Circulation 1989; 79:537–48.
44. Taylor GJ, Humphries JO, Mellits ED, et al. Predictors of clinical course, coronary anatomy and left ventricular function after recovery from acute myocardial infarction. Circulation 1980; 62:960–70.
45. de Feyter PJ, van Eenige MJ, Dighton DH, Visser FC, de Jong J, Roos JP. Prognostic value of exercise testing, coronary angiography and left ventriculography 6–8 weeks after myocardial infarction. Circulation 1982; 66:527–36.
46. Roubin GS, Harris PJ, Bernstein L, Kelly DT. Coronary anatomy and prognosis after myocardial infarction in patients 60 years of age and younger. Circulation 1983; 67:743–9.
47. Sanz G, Castaner A, Betriu A, et al. Determinants of prognosis in survivors of myocardial infarction: A prospective clinical angiographic study. N Engl J. Med 1982; 306:1065–70.
48. Arnold AER, Simoons ML, Detry JMR, et al., for the European Cooperative Study Group. Prediction of mortality after hospital discharge in patients with and without recombinant tissue plasminogen activator for myocardial infarction: Is there a need for coronary angiography? Thesis: Benefits and risks of thrombolysis for acute myocardial infarction. Erasmus Universiteit, Rotterdam, 1990:135–53.
49. Hashimoto T, Kambara H, Fudo T, et al. Non-Q wave versus Q wave myocardial infarction: Regional myocardial metabolism and blood flow assessed by positron emission tomography. J Am Coll Cardiol 1988; 12:88–93.
50. Serruys PW, Simoons ML, Suryapranata H, et al. Preservation of global and regional left ventricular function after early thrombolysis in acute myocardial infarction. J Am Coll Cardiol 1986; 7:729–42.
51. Schröder R, Neuhaus KL, Leizorovicz A, et al. A prospective placebo-controlled

double-blind multicenter trial of intravenous streptokinase in acute myocardial infarction (ISAM): Long-term mortality and morbidity. J Am Coll Cardiol 1987; 9:197–203.

52. Simoons ML, Vos J, Tijssen JGP, et al. Long-term benefit of early thrombolytic therapy in patients with acute myocardial infarction. J Am Coll Cardiol 1989; 14:1609–15.

53. Kennedy JW, Ritchie JL, Davis KB, et al. The Western Washington randomized trial of intracoronary streptokinase in acute myocardial infarction: A 12 month follow-up report. N Engl J Med 1985; 321:1073–8.

54. Dalen JE, Gore JM, Braunwald E, et al. Six and twelve months follow-up of the phase I thrombolysis in myocardial infarction (TIMI) trial. Am J. Cardiol 1988; 62:179–85.

55. Melin JA, DeCoster PM, Renkin J, Detry J-MR, Beckers C, Col J. Effects of intracoronary thrombolytic therapy on exercise-induced ischemia after acute myocardial infarction. Am J Cardiol 1985; 56:705–11.

56. De Wood MA, Stifter WF, Simpson CS, et al. Coronary arteriographic findings soon after non-Q wave myocardial infarction. N Engl J Med 1986; 315:417–23.

57. Davies MJ, Thomas DC: Plaque fissuring—The cause of acute myocardial infarction, sudden ischemic death and crescendo angina. Br Heart J 1985; 53:363–71.

58. Falk E. Unstable angina with fatal outcome: Dynamic coronary thrombosis leading to infarction or sudden death. Circulation 1985; 71:699–708.

59. Ambrose JA, Winters SL, Arora RR, et al. Coronary angiographic morphology in myocardial infarction: A link between the pathogenesis of unstable angina and myocardial infarction. J Am Coll Cardiol 1985; 6:1233–8.

60. Gorlin R, Fuster V, Ambrose JA. Anatomic-physiologic link between acute coronary syndromes. Circulation 1986; 74:6–9.

61. Ambrose JA, Hjemdahl-Monsen CE, Borrico S, Gorlin R, Fuster V. Angiographic demonstration of a common link between unstable angina pectoris and non-Q wave acute myocardial infarction. Am J Cardiol 1988; 61:244–7.

62. Mandelkorn JB, Wolff NM, Singh S, et al. Intracoronary thrombus in non-transmural myocardial infarction and in unstable angina pectoris. Am J Cardiol 1983; 52:1–6.

63. Turner JD, Rogers WJ, Mantle JA, Rackley CE, Russell RO. Coronary angiography soon after myocardial infarction. Chest 1980; 77:58–64.

64. Nicholson MR, Roubin GS, Bernstein L, Harris PJ, Kelly DT. Prognosis after initial non-Q wave myocardial infarction related to coronary arterial anatomy. Am J Cardiol 1983; 52:462–5.

65. De Wood MA, Spores J, Notske R, et al. Prevalence of total coronary occlusion during the early hours of transmural myocardial infarction. N Engl J Med 1980; 303:897–902.

66. Ganz W, Buchbinder N, Marcus H, et al. Intracoronary thrombolysis in evolving myocardial infarction. Am Heart J 1981; 101:4–13.

67. Rutsch W, Scharti M, Mathey D, et al. Percutaneous transluminal coronary recanalization: Procedure, results and acute complications. Am Heart J 1981; 102:1178–81.

68. de Feyter PJ, Eenige van MJ, de Jong JP, van der Wall EE, Dighton DH, Roos JP.

Experience with intracoronary streptokinase in 36 patients with acute evolving myocardial infarction. Eur Heart J 1982; 3:441–8.

69. Timmis GC, Gangadharan V, Hauser AM, Ramos RC, Westveer DC, Gordon S. Intracoronary streptokinase in clinical practice. Am Heart J 1982; 104:925–38.

70. Cowley MJ, Hastillo A, Vetrovec GW, Hess ML. Effects of intracoronary streptokinase in acute myocardial infarction. Am Heart J 1981; 102:1149–58.

71. Bertrand ME, Lefebvre JM, Laisne CL, Rousseau MF, Carre AG, Lekieffre JP. Coronary arteriography in acute transmural myocardial infarction. Am Heart J 1979; 97:61–9.

72. Betriu A, Castaner A, Sanz GA, et al. Angiographic findings 1 month after myocardial infarction: A prospective study of 259 survivors. Circulation 1982; 65:1099–1105.

73. Davies MJ, Woolf N, Robertson WB. Pathology of acute myocardial infarction with particular reference to occlusive coronary thrombi. Br Heart J 1976; 38:659–64.

74. Freifeld AG, Schuster EH, Bulkley BH. Nontransmural versus transmural myocardial infarction: A morphologic study. Am J Med 1983; 75:423–32.

75. Gibson RS, Watson DD, Craddock JB, et al. Prediction of cardiac events after uncomplicated myocardial infarction: A prospective study comparing predischarge exercise thallium-201 scintigraphy and coronary angiography. Circulation 1983; 68:321–36.

76. de Feyter PJ, van Eenige MJ, van der Wall EE, et al. Effects of spontaneous and streptokinase-induced recanalization on left ventricular function after myocardial infarction. Circulation 1983; 67:1039–44.

77. Suryapranata H, Serruys PW, Vermeer F, et al. Value of immediate coronary angioplasty following intracoronary thrombolysis in acute myocardial infarction. Cathet Cardiovasc Diagn 1987; 13:223–32.

78. Rentrop P, Smith H, Painter L, Holt J. Changes in left ventricular ejection fraction after intracoronary thrombolytic therapy. Circulation 1983; 68(suppl I):55–60.

79. Wackers FJ, Berger HJ, Weinberg MA, Zarett BL. Spontaneous changes in left ventricular function over the first 24 hours of acute myocardial infarction: Implications for evaluating early therapeutic interventions. Circulation 1982; 66:748–54.

80. Ong L, Reiser P, Coromillas J, Scherr L, Morrison J. Left ventricular function and rapid release of creatine kinase MB in acute myocardial infarction. Evidence for spontaneous reperfusion. N Engl J Med 1983; 309:1–6.

81. Van de Werf F, Arnold AER, and the European Cooperative Study Group. Intravenous tissue plasminogen activator and size of infarct, left ventricular function, and survival in acute myocardial infarction. Br Heart J 1988; 297:1374–9.

82. Beta-Blocker Heart Attack Research Group. A randomized trial of propranolol in patients with acute myocardial infarction: mortality results. JAMA 1982; 247:1707–14.

83. Norwegian Multicenter Study Group. Timolol-induced reduction in mortality and reinfarction in patients surviving acute myocardial infarction. N Engl J Med 1981; 304:801–7.

84. Yellon DM, Hearse DJ, Maxwell MP, Chambers DE, Downey JM. Sustained limitations of myocardial necrosis 24 hours after coronary artery occlusion: Ve-

rapamil infusion in dogs with small myocardial infarcts. Am J Cardiol 1981; 51:1409.

85. Klein HH, Schubothe M, Nebendahl K, Kreuzer H. The effects of two different diltiazem treatments on infarct size in ischemic, reperfused porcine hearts. Circulation 1984; 69:1000–5.

86. Melin JA, Becker LC, Hutchins GM. Protective effects of early and late treatments with nifedipine during myocardial infarction in the conscious dog. Circulation 1984; 69:131–41.

87. Gibson RS, Borden WE, Théroux P, et al. and the Diltiazem Reinfarction Study Group. Diltiazem and reinfarction in patients with non-Q-wave myocardial infarction: Results of a double-blind, randomized multicenter trial. N Engl J Med 1986; 315:423–9.

88. Safian RD, Synder, LD, Synder BA, et al. Usefulness of percutaneous transluminal coronary angioplasty for unstable angina pectoris after non-Q wave acute myocardial infarction. Am J Cardiol 1987; 59:263–6.

89. Suryapranata H, Beatt K, de Feyter PJ, et al. Percutaneous transluminal coronary angioplasty for angina pectoris after a non-Q wave acute myocardial infarction. Am J Cardiol 1988; 61:240–3.

90. Madigan NP, Rutherford BD, Barnhorst DA, Danielson GK. Early saphenous vein grafting after subendocardial infarction: Immediate surgical results and late prognosis. Circulation 1977; 56(Suppl II):1–3.

91. Aintablian A, Hamby RI, Weiss D, Hoffman I, Voleti CO, Wisoff BG. Results of aortocoronary bypass surgery grafting in patients with subendocardial infarction: Late follow-up. Am J Cardiol 1978; 42:183–6.

92. Williams DB, Ivey TD, Bailey WW, Irey SJ, Rideout JT, Stewart D. Postinfarction angina: Results of early revascularization. J Am Coll Cardiol 1983; 2:859–64.

93. Johnson WD, Flemma RJ, Lepley D Jr. Direct coronary surgery utilizing multiple-vein bypass grafts. Ann Thorac Surg 1970; 9:436–44.

94. Cohn LH, Fogarty TJ, Daily PO. Emergency coronary artery bypass. Surgery 1972; 10:821–9.

95. Favaloro RG, Effler DB, Cheanvechai C. Acute coronary insufficiency (impending myocardial infarction and myocardial infarction): Surgical treatment by the saphenous vein graft technique. Am J Cardiol 1971; 28:598–613.

96. Piffarre R, Spinazzola A, Nemickas R, Scanlon PJ, Tobin JR. Emergency aortocoronary bypass for acute myocardial infarction. Arch Surg 1971; 103:525–8.

97. Sustaita H, Chatterjee K, Matloff JM. Emergency bypass surgery in impending and complicated acute myocardial infarction. Arch Surg 1972; 105:30–5.

98. Dawson JT, Hall RJ, Hallman GL, Cooley DA. Mortality in patients undergoing coronary artery bypass surgery after myocardial infarction. Am J Cardiol 1974; 33:483–6.

99. Hill JD, Kerth WJ, Kelly JJ, et al. Emergency aortocoronary bypass for impending or extending myocardial infarction. Circulation 1971; 43/44 (Suppl I):105–10.

100. Reul GJ, Morris GC, Howell, JF, Crawford ES, Sterlter WJ. Emergency coronary artery bypass grafts in the treatment of myocardial infarction. Circulation 1973; 47/48 (Suppl III):127–31.

101. Nunley DL, Grunkemeier GL, Teply JF, et al. Coronary bypass operation following acute complicated myocardial infarction. J Thorac Cardiovasc Surg 1983; 85:485–91.

102. Molina JE, Dorsey JS, Emanuel DA, Reyes J. Coronary bypass operation for early postinfarction angina. Surg Gynaecol Obstret 1983; 157:455–60.

103. Rankin JS, Newton JR, Califf RM, et al. Clinical characteristics and current management of medically refractory unstable angina. Ann Surg 1984; 200:457–64.

104. Baumgartner WA, Borkon AM, Zibulewsky J, et al. Operative intervention for postinfarction angina. Ann Thorac Surg 1984; 38:265–7.

105. Gertler JP, Elefteriades JA, Kopf GS, Hashim SW, Hammond GL, Geha AS. Predictors of outcome in early revascularization after acute myocardial infarction. Am J Surg 1985; 149:441–4.

106. Singh AK, Rivera R, Cooper GN, Karlson KE. Early myocardial revascularization for post infarction angina: results and longterm follow-up. J Am Coll Cardiol 1985; 6:1121–5.

107. Brower RA, Fioretti P, Simoons ML, Haalebos M, Rulf ENR, Hugenholtz PG. Surgical versus non surgical management of patients soon after acute myocardial infarction. Br Heart J 1985; 54:460–5.

108. Bryer RH, Engelman RM, Rousou JA, Lemeshow S. Postinfarction angina: an expanding subset of patients undergoing bypass surgery. J Thorac Cardiovasc Surg 1985; 90:532–40.

109. Jones RN, Pifarre R, Sullivan HJ, et al. Early myocardial revascularization for postinfarction angina. Ann Thorac Surg 1987; 44:159–62.

110. Stuart RS, Baumgartner WA, Soule L, et al. Predictors of perioperative mortality in patients with unstable postinfarction angina. Circulation 1988; 78(Suppl I): 163–5.

111. Holt GW, Gersh BJ, Holmes DR, et al. The results of percutaneous transluminal coronary angioplasty (PTCA) in post infarction angina pectoris (abstract). J Am Coll Cardiol 1986; 7:62A.

112. Gottlieb SO, Brim KP, Walford GD, McGaughey M, Riegel MB, Brinker JA. Initial and late results of coronary angioplasty for early postinfarction unstable angina. Cathet Cardiovasc Diagn 1987; 13:93–9.

113. Hopkins J, Savage M, Zaluwski A, Dervan JP, Goldberg S. Recurrent ischemia in the zone of prior myocardial infarction: Results of coronary angioplasty of the infarct related artery. Am Heart J 1988; 115:14–9.

114. de Feyter PJ. Coronary angioplasty for unstable angina. Am Heart J 1989; 118:860–8.

115. Brundage BH, Massie BM, Botvinick EH. Improved regional ventricular function after successful surgical revascularization. J Am Coll Cardiol 1984; 3:902–8.

116. Bodenheimer MM, Banka VS, Hermann GA, Trout RG, Pasdar H, Helfant RH. Reversible asynergy: histopathology and electrographic correlations in patients with coronary heart disease. Circulation 1976; 53:792–6.

117. Rozanski A, Berman D, Gray R, et al. Preoperative prediction of reversible myocardial asynergy by postexercise radionuclide ventriculography. N Engl J Med 1982; 307:212–6.

118. Popio KA, Gorlin R, Bechtel D, Levine JA. Postextrasystolic potentiation as a predictor of potential myocardial viability: Preoperative analyses compared with studies after coronary bypass surgery. Am J Cardiol 1977; 39:944–53.

119. Nesto RW, Cohn LH, Collins JJ Jr, Wynne J, Holman L, Cohn PF. Inotropic contractile reserve: A useful predictor of increased 5 year survival and improved postoperative left ventricular function in patients with coronary artery disease and reduced ejection fraction. Am J Cardiol 1982; 50:39–44.

120. Marshall RC, Tillisch JH, Phelps ME, et al. Identification and differentiation of resting myocardial ischemia and infarction in man with positron computed tomography: ^{18}F-labeled flurodeoxyglucose and N-13 ammonia. Circulation 1983; 67:766–78.

121. Tillisch J, Brunken R, Marshall R, et al. Reversibility of cardiac wall motion abnormalities predicted by positron tomography. N Engl J Med 1986; 314:884–8.

122. Piérard LA, de Landsheere CM, Berthe C, Rigo P, Kulbertus HE. Identification of viable myocardium by echocardiography during dobutamine infusion in patients with myocardial infarction after thrombolytic therapy: Comparison with positron emission tomography. J Am Coll Cardiol 1990; 15:1021–31.

123. Norris RM, Agnew TM, Brandt PWT, et al. Coronary surgery after recurrent myocardial infarction: Progress of a trial comparing surgical with non-surgical management for asymptomatic patients with advanced disease. Circulation 1981; 63:785–92.

124. CASS principal investigators and their associates. Coronary Artery Surgery Study (CASS): A randomized trial of coronary artery bypass surgery. Survival data. Circulation 1983; 68:939–50.

125. Simoons ML, Arnold AER, Betriu A, et al. Thrombolysis with tissue plasminogen activator in acute myocardial infarction: No additional benefit from immediate percutaneous coronary angioplasty. Lancet 1988; 1:197–204.

126. TIMI Research Group. Immediate vs delayed catheterization and angioplasty following thrombolytic therapy for acute myocardial infarction. JAMA 1988; 260:2849–58.

127. Barbash GI, Hod H, Roth A, et al. Repeat infusions of recombinant tissue-type plasminogen activator in patients with acute myocardial infarction and early recurrent myocardial ischemia. J Am Coll Cardiol 1990; 16:779–83.

16

Percutaneous Balloon Angioplasty of Saphenous Vein Bypass Grafts
A Clinical and Morphological Review

Cass A. Pinkerton

*St. Vincent Hospital and Health Care Center
Indianapolis, Indiana*

Bruce F. Waller

*Indiana University School of Medicine,
St. Vincent Hospital, and The Indiana Heart Institute
Indianapolis, Indiana*

INTRODUCTION

Percutaneous balloon angioplasty (PBA) has demonstrated its usefulness in nonoperative treatment of obstructed coronary arteries. Further usefulness of PBA has been demonstrated in dilating obstructed aortocoronary saphenous vein bypass grafts and narrowed internal mammary arteries used as bypass conduits. This chapter will focus on clinical results of PBA on saphenous vein bypass grafts and provide a review of the anatomical basis for and pathological changes resulting from saphenous vein balloon angioplasty.

CLINICAL RESULTS OF BALLOON ANGIOPLASTY OF SAPHENOUS VEIN BYPASS GRAFTS: THE NASSER, SMITH AND PINKERTON CARDIOLOGY EXPERIENCE

Patient Population

An extensive clinical angioplasty data base has been developed over the last decade recording various angioplasty procedures performed at Nasser, Smith and Pinkerton Cardiology. A review of the angioplasty database disclosed 205 patients who had undergone balloon angioplasty procedures of aortocoronary saphenous vein bypass grafts. Of these 205 patients, 159 (78%) were men and 46

(22%) were women. Patient age ranged from 35 to 82 years (average 60 years). Of the 205 patients dilated, 23 (11%) were aged 70 years or older.

Clinical Observations

Of the 205 patients, 251 saphenous vein bypass graft lesions underwent attempted balloon angioplasty and 239 (95%) were successfully dilated (Tables 1–3). Of the 205 patients, 42 (20%) had significant left ventricular dysfunction and two had left main coronary arteries dilated.

Procedural Data

Procedural data involving saphenous vein bypass dilation are summarized in Table 1. Inflation atmospheres ranged from 5 to 13 and inflation duration ranged from 1 to 16 min. Of the saphenous vein graft lesions dilated with four or more inflations, the success rate was slightly higher than for lesions receiving less than four inflations. Successful dilation was more successful when inflation atmospheres were 8 or higher (99%) compared to less than 8 atmospheres (90%). Successful dilation was also greater when inflation time was 3 min or longer (99%) compared to inflation under 3 min (93%) (Table 1). Successful angioplasty was twice as common in grafts dilated *without* the associated use of thrombolytic agents.

Table 1   Procedural Data of Bypass Graft Angioplasty

		Attempted	Success	%
1.	Inflation frequency	1–13 (mean 4)		
2.	Inflation atmospheres	5–13 (mean 11)		
3.	Inflation duration (min)	1–16 (mean 2)		
4.	Number of inflations	Attempted	Success	%
	<4	113	106	94
	≥4	138	135	98
5.	Atmospheres of inflation			
	<8	88	79	90
	≥8	163	162	99
6.	Duration of inflation (min)			
	<3	125	116	93
	≥3	127	125	99
7.	Thromboltyic agent			
	Yes	9	4	49
	No	242	235	97
8.	Angio evidence of distal emboli			
	Yes	8	5	62
	No	242	234	96

Table 2 Location of Lesion and Results of Balloon Angioplasty

Site of bypass graft	# attempted lesions	# successful	% successful
Proximal anastomosis	57	52	91
Mid (body)	48	45	94
Distal anastomosis	130	127	98
Ostial	16	15	94
Total	251	239	95

RESULTS OF ANGIOPLASTY EARLY AFTER THE PROCEDURE (PRIMARY RESULTS)

Saphenous balloon angioplasty was most successful in grafts to the left anterior descending (LAD) (90%), followed by bypass grafts to the obtuse margin branch (Ob Marg) and main left circumflex (LCx) arteries (94%, 93% respectively) (Table 2). Results of balloon angioplasty according to site of vein dilation are summarized in Table 3. The site of most successful angioplasty was at the distal anastomosis (coronary–saphenous vein anastomosis) (98%), followed by the midportion (body of graft) (94%), and least successful was the proximal anastomotic site (aorta–saphenous vein anastomosis) (91%).

Complications

Complications of saphenous vein bypass graft dilation were limited. No distal *emboli* were recognized angiographically. However, myocardial infarction occurred in seven cases (3.4%). Urgent bypass surgery was performed in six patients (2.8%) and four patients (2%) died. Of the four deaths, two patients had dilation of saphenous vein grafts during an evolving acute myocardial infarction and two patients were dilated under "shock" conditions (salvage angioplasty).

Table 3 Site Results of Balloon Angioplasty

Bypassed vessel	# attempted lesions	# successful	% successful
LAD	72	69	96
LCx	30	28	93
Ob Marg	50	47	94
Diag	14	13	93
LM	2	2	100
Total	251	239	95

Diag = diagonal; LAD = left anterior descending, LCx = left circumflex; LM = left main; Ob Marg = obtuse marginal.

Table 4 Saphenous Vein Graft Dissections Following Balloon Angioplasty
[$n = 14/127$ (11%)]

1.	Inflation duration (min)			
	Minutes	Attempted	Dissected	%
	≤4	60	6	10
	>4	67	7	10
2.	Atmospheres of inflation			
	Atmosphere	Attempted	Dissected	%
	≤8	51	5	10
	>8	76	9	12
3.	Age of graft (years)			
	≤4	55	5	9
	>4	69	10	15
4.	Over 4 balloon inflations			
	≤4 years old	52	28	52
	>4 years old	62	35	57
5.	Over 8 atmospheres			
	≤4 years old	52	34	65
	>4 years old	63	35	56
6.	Over 3 min inflation			
	≤4 years old	47	20	43
	>4 years old	62	30	48

Saphenous vein *dissection* during angioplasty occurred in 13 of 127 attempts (20%) (Table 4). Analysis of dissections by inflation duration and atmospheres of inflation disclosed dissections were similar whether inflation lasted more or less than 4 min (10% each group) and whether atmospheres of inflation were more or less than 8 (12%, 10% respectively) (Table 4). Older grafts were nearly twice as frequently associated with angioplasty dissection (15%) compared to grafts aged under 4 years (9%) (Table 4). Older grafts also required longer duration of inflation. Younger grafts (under 4 years) generally required higher atmospheres to dilate (Table 5).

RESULTS OF ANGIOPLASTY LATE AFTER THE PROCEDURE (RESTENOSIS)

Follow-up clinical and angiographic information is available on 123 patients. Of the 123 patients, 68 (55%) had angiographic (>20% decrease diameter reduction) and/or clinical (positive thallium treadmill, recurrence of angina) evidence of restenosis. Age of saphenous vein grafts ranged from 1 to 7.3 years.

Clinical Factors Associated with Restenosis

Several factors were studied to determine "risk factors" for restenosis of saphenous vein bypass grafts previously undergoing PBA. Age of graft (≤6, >6

Table 5 Clinical Variables of Graft Restenosis After Balloon Angioplasty

1.	Age of graft		
	<6 years	42 (53%)	NS
	≥6 years	20 (60%)	
2.	Family history of CAD		
	Yes	52 (60%)	NS
	No	15 (42%)	
3.	Systemic hypertension (>140/>90)		
	Yes	44 (68%)	$p = 0.006$
	No	24 (4%)	
4.	Cigarette smoking		
	Yes	38 (51%)	NS
	No	30 (61%)	
5.	Hyperlipidemia		
	Yes	27 (52%)	NS
	No	41 (58%)	
6.	Diabetes mellitus		
	Yes	15 (48%)	NS
	No	53 (58%)	

years), family history of coronary disease, systemic hypertension, cigarette smoking, hyperlipidemia, and diabetes mellitus were analyzed (Table 5). Only the presence of systemic hypertension (defined as systolic > 140 mmHg and/or diastolic > 90 mmHg) was significantly related to angioplasty restenosis of saphenous vein grafts.

Procedural Variable in Restenosis

Several procedural variables were studied to assess the risk for restenosis of saphenous vein angioplasty sites, including number of inflations (≤4, >4), atmospheres of inflation (≤8, >8), duration of balloon inflation (≤3 min, >3 min), and the severity of saphenous vein preangioplasty lesion (≤95%, >95%) (Table 6). None of these variables was significantly related to the occurrence of restenosis at the saphenous vein angioplasty site.

Site of Graft Angioplasty Restenosis

In view of the differences in primary success rate of saphenous vein angioplasty at the proximal anastomosis, mid (body), or distal anastomoses, a similar analysis was undertaken for restenosis. No significant differences of restenosis were noted between the sites but the *mid* lesions had the highest frequency (68%), followed by the distal (52%) and proximal (46%) anastomotic sites (Table 7). No specific difference in restenosis was found between the various coronary arteries and/or coronary artery branches bypassed.

Table 6 Procedural Variables and Bypass Graft Restenosis After Angioplasty

1.	Number of inflations		
	>4	28 (55%)	NS
	≤4	35 (56%)	
2.	Inflation atmospheres		
	≤8	18 (50%)	NS
	>8	47 (59%)	
3.	Duration of inflation		
	>3 min	31 (52%)	NS
	≤3 min	28 (57%)	
4.	Severity of SV pretreatment lesion		
	≤95% DR	33 (51%)	NS
	>95% DR	34 (60%)	

MORPHOLOGICAL RESULTS OF BALLOON ANGIOPLASTY OF SAPHENOUS VEIN BYPASS GRAFTS

This section describes morphological changes following angioplasty in morphological observations in young and old saphenous vein grafts (1–28). Operatively excised segments of saphenous vein bypass grafts from two patients undergoing PBA of the bypass graft early (≤1 year) and late (>1 year) after aortocoronary bypass surgery served as the basis of this study. Clinical and morphological data from the two patients are summarized in Table 8 and Figures 1–9.

ANGIOPLASTY OF SAPHENOUS VEIN GRAFT EARLY AFTER BYPASS SURGERY (22)

Clinical Features

A 63-year-old man (see Table 8) with angina pectoris underwent PBA of the LAD coronary artery. Approximately 30 min after successful dilation, the LAD

Table 7 Site of Graft Angioplasty and Frequency of Restenosis

1.	Artery bypassed	
	LAD	20 (54%)
	LCx	6 (67%)
	R	24 (55%)
	OBM	12 (50%)
	DIAG	5 (63%)
2.	Location of lesion	
	Proximal anastomosis	10/22 (46%)
	Mid	17/25 (68%)
	Distal anastomosis	35/67 (52%)

Abbreviations as in Table 3.

Table 8 Clinical and Morphological Data in Two Patients Who Underwent Percutaneous Transluminal Balloon Angioplasty of Stenotic Saphenous Vein Bypass Conduits *Early* (≤1 Year) and *Late* (>1 Year) After Aortocoronary Bypass Operation

Observation	Early conduit (63-year-old man)	Late conduit (41-year-old man)	
		Dilation procedure	
		#1	#2
1. Age (months) of SV conduit	3	56	
2. Interval (months) from bypass operation to PTA	2	52	54
3. Interval (months) from PTA to SV conduit excision	1	4	2
4. Angiography-angioplasty data:			
a. Maximal SV conduit narrowing (% DR) (location) before PTA	95 (proximal)	95 (mid)	95 (mid)
b. Maximal SV conduit narrowing (% DR) after PTA (total ↓)	10 (85%)	25 (70%)	10 (85%)
c. Mean intraconduit pressure (mmHg) before → after PTA (total ↓)	37 4 (33)	60 15 (45)	60 10 (50)
d. Number of balloon inflations	Multiple	4	8
e. Maximal balloon inflation pressure (atmospheres)	12	9	10
f. Duration (sec) balloon inflation	60	90	90
g. Dilating catheter(s)	S25–30	G20–30	G20–20 G20–30 S37–25
h. Angiographic "dissection" or "splint"	0	0	+
i. Maximal SV conduit narrowing (% DR) prior to SV excision	85		95

Table 8 (*Continued*)

Observation	Early conduit (63-year-old man)	Late conduit (41-year-old man)
5. Morphological data		
a. Maximal SV conduit narrowing (% XSA)	76–100	76–100
b. Conduit narrowing (% XSA) at site of PTA	76–100	76–100
c. Cause of conduit narrowing	IFT	IFT + AP
d. Calcific deposits	0	+
e. Evidence of PTA	+[a]	+[b]

[a] Loss of endothelial lining in area of balloon dilation but no tears, breaks, or cracks.
[b] Healing intimal separation (intimal flap).
AP = atherosclerotic plaque; DR = diameter reduction; IFT = intimal fibrous thickening; PTA = percutaneous transluminal angioplasty; SV = saphenous vein; XSA = cross-sectional area.
Source: Ref. 22.

coronary artery suddenly closed, and the patient became hypotensive and developed ventricular tachycardia and fibrillation. An angioplasty balloon was inserted, the vessel was successfully reopened, and the patient was stabilized. Despite multiple balloon inflations, the LAD coronary artery continued to reclose, and the patient underwent aortocoronary saphenous vein bypass grafting to the LAD coronary artery. Seven weeks after bypass surgery, the patient had recurrent angina pectoris. Cardiac catheterization disclosed 95% symmetrical diameter reduction of the saphenous vein bypass graft at the proximal (aortic) anastomotic site (Fig. 1). The vein graft was dilated with a steerable 25–30 balloon, with multiple inflations of up to 60-sec duration resulting in a marked increase in graft luminal diameter (Fig. 1). Four weeks after successful bypass graft angioplasty (3 months after graft insertion), the patient had recurrent angina. Repeat angiography disclosed severe graft narrowing (restenosis) at the previous dilation site. This time, however, the stenotic segment was not smooth and symmetrical, but irregular and asymmetrical. Because of the angiographic appearance of the stenotic segment and the rapid recurrence of stenosis, the patient underwent repeat bypass grafting. The proximal portion of the graft was excised at operation.

Morphological Features

The operatively excised portion of saphenous vein graft (Fig. 2) measured 40 mm in length and was free of calcific deposits. The excised segment included the site of maximal balloon inflation and a short distal portion in which the catheter

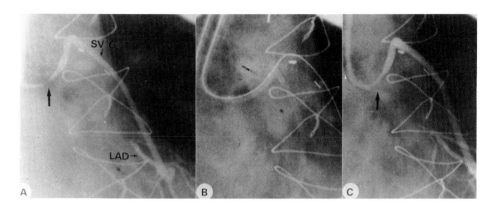

Figure 1   Angiographic frames of a saphenous vein bypass graft (SV G) before and after transluminal balloon angioplasty 1 month before graft excision and 2 months after graft insertion. (A) Severe luminal narrowing of the bypass graft near the aortic anastomotic site (arrow). (B) Inflated angioplasty balloon located within the proximal saphenous vein graft. (C) Marked increase in luminal diameter of saphenous vein graft following angioplasty (arrow). LAD = left anterior descending coronary artery. [From Waller et al. (22), with permission.]

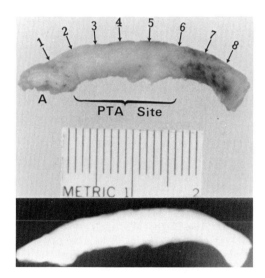

Figure 2   Operatively excised portion of a 3-month-old saphenous vein graft (Table 6). (Top) The diameter of the proximal portion (aortic anastomotic end) (A) subjected to transluminal balloon angioplasty is slightly wider than the diameter of the distal, nondilated segment. The numbers represent sites of transverse sections appearing in Figure 5. (Bottom) Radiograph of specimen discloses *no* calcific deposits. [From Waller et al. (22), with permission.]

and guidewire had passed but in which balloon inflation did not occur. The external diameter (about 7 mm) of the proximal 30 mm of graft (the portion subjected to angioplasty) was slightly wider compared with the external diameter (about 5 mm of the distal nondilated segment) (Fig. 2). The entire specimen was cut transversely into eight 5-mm segments numbered 1–8. Segments 1–6 were from areas of previous PBA, and segments 7 and 8 were from nondilated areas.

Angioplasty of Saphenous Vein Graft Late After Bypass Surgery

A 42-year-old man (Table 8) was hospitalized with acute myocardial infarction. Continued chest pain prompted coronary angiography and subsequent double aortocoronary saphenous vein bypass grafting to the left circumflex coronary artery (margin branch and distal left circumflex). About 1 year later, he had recurrent chest pain, which worsened over the next 2 years. Repeat angiography 3 years later disclosed total occlusion of the graft to the distal left circumflex coronary artery and 50% diameter reduction in the midportion of the graft to the distal left circumflex marginal branch. Two years later, a third coronary angiogram disclosed progressive narrowing of all three major coronary artery systems and 50% diameter reduction of the bypass graft to the marginal branch of the left circumflex coronary artery. The patient underwent repeat aortocoronary bypass operation with insertion of new grafts to the LAD and right coronary systems. Two months later, angina pectoris recurred. Repeat angiography showed that the graft to the right coronary artery was open, the graft to the left anterior descending system was closed, and the graft to the left circumflex marginal branch now was narrowed 95% in diameter (Fig. 3).

The patient underwent PBA of the left circumflex graft (52 months after graft insertion) (Table 8) resulting in decreased graft luminal narrowing (95% to 20%) and decreased transstenotic mean pressure gradient (60 mmHg to 15 mmHg). Two months later, he had recurrent angina. Repeat angiography disclosed lumi-

---

Figure 3 Serial angiographic frames of a saphenous vein (SV) bypass graft (G) before and after two transluminal balloon angioplasty (TBA) procedures. (A) Severe luminal narrowing in the midportion of the SV G (arrow) 52 months after insertion. TBA (not shown) resulted in decreased luminal narrowing (from 95% to 20%). LC = left circumflex coronary artery. (B) Restenosis at graft 2 months later at previous TBA site (arrow). (C–I) Second TBA (54 months after insertion) showing serial dilations (D#1 to D#3) using progressively larger balloons and variable inflation pressures and inflation durations. F and I show a localized "break," "fracture," or "dissection" line at the site of TBA (small arrows). The second TBA resulted in decreased luminal narrowing (from 95% to 10%). (J) Restenosis of the graft 2 months later (56 months after insertion) at the previous TBA sites. The boxed area indicates the operatively excised segment (Ex Sg) of the saphenous vein graft. Numbers in each frame indicate month and year. [From Waller et al. (22), with permission.]

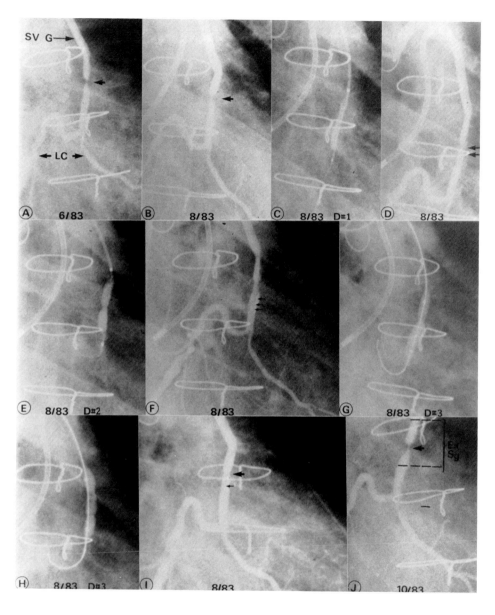

nal irregularities of the right graft and 95% diameter narrowing of the left circumflex graft at the site of previous PBA (Fig. 3). The patient underwent a second angioplasty of the left circumflex graft (Fig. 3). Serial dilations using progressively larger balloons, variable inflation pressure (6–9 atmospheres), and balloon inflation durations (10–90 sec) (Table 8) resulted in decreased graft luminal narrowing (95% to 10%) and decreased mean transstenotic pressure gradient (60 mmHg to 10 mmHg). Furthermore, graft angiograms disclosed a localized dissection ("break," "crack," "fracture") at the angioplasty site (Fig. 3). The patient had recurrent angina 2 months later, when the sixth coronary angiogram disclosed restenosis (95% diameter reduction) of the graft to the left circumflex marginal branch (Fig. 3) and total occlusion of the right graft. The patient underwent a third aortocoronary bypass operation. The midportion of the left circumflex conduit was excised at operation, and despite successful regrafting, the patient died at operation.

Morphological Features

The operatively excised portion of saphenous graft (Fig. 4) measured 42 mm in length and had foci of calcific deposits in the area of dilation. The entire specimen was cut transversely into eight 5-mm segments numbered 1–8. Segments 4–6 were from the site of maximal balloon inflation. The area of the angioplasty dissection notes angiographically (Fig. 3) was specifically localized on the excised saphenous vein specimen (Fig. 12, segments 4–6).

Morphological Observations in the Early Saphenous Vein Graft

The lumen of each of the eight 5-mm saphenous vein segments was narrowed more than 75% in cross-sectional area by intimal thickening (Fig. 5). Histologically, the diffuse intimal thickening of both dilated and nondilated segments consisted of cellular fibrocollagenous tissue without foam cells or cholesterol clefts (intimal "fibrous hyperplasia," "fibrous proliferation"). Segments 1–6 were serially sectioned at $10\text{-}\mu$ intervals to search for sites of "splits," "tears," or "cracks" or other morphological evidence of previous PBA. Control segments 7 and 8 were also sectioned in a similar fashion. Histological assessment by light microscopy did not disclose any distinctive morphological lesion(s) in the intimal, medial, or adventitial layers of dilated or nondilated segments of the saphenous vein graft.

Ultrastructural evaluation of segments 2 (dilated) and 6 (nondilated) (Fig. 6) disclosed the absence of endothelial luminal cells in the dilated segment compared with their presence in the nondilated segment. Cells lining the graft lumen in the *dilated* segment had features of myofibroblasts (cytoplasmic filaments with focal condensations and abundant rough endoplasmic reticulum). Fibrin-like extracellular material (possible representing residual basement membrane) condensed along the luminal border of these myofibroblasts. The endothelial

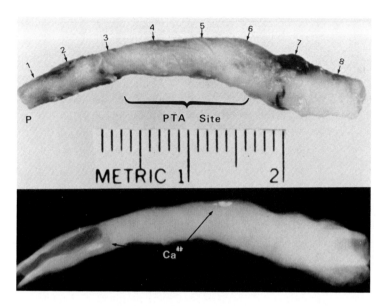

Figure 4 Operatively excised portion of a 56-month-old saphenous vein graft (Table 6). (Top) Brackets indicate the site of two TBA procedures located in the midportion of the graft. P = proximal end. The numbers represent sites of transverse sections appearing in Figure 7. (Bottom) Radiograph of transverse section discloses foci of calcific (Ca^{2+}) deposits. [From Waller et al. (22), with permission.]

cells lining the lumen of the distal *nondilated* segment had luminal and abluminal micropinocytotic vesicles and well-formed intercellular junctions (Fig. 6). No distinctive differences in myofibroblasts or collagen fibrils were noted between segments 2 and 8.

Morphological Observations in the Late Saphenous Vein Graft

The lumen of each of the eight 5-mm saphenous vein segments had diffuse but variable degrees of intimal thickening (Fig. 7). The maximal cross-sectional area luminal reduction by intimal thickening occurred in segments 3, 5, and 6. Histologically, the intimal thickening in segments 4–6 consisted of foam cells, cholesterol clefts, fibrocollagenous tissue, foci of myofibroblasts, and calcific deposits characteristic of atherosclerotic plaque (Fig. 8). Intimal thickening of segments 1–3 and 7 was predominantly fibrocollagenous except for occasional foci of foam cells, cholesterol clefts, and calcium. The site of angioplasty dissection (segments 4–6) (Fig. 8) had partial separation of the intima from the media. This ''intimal flap'' had begun to reattach to the wall of the graft, representing healing of a localized plaque ''tear'' or ''fracture.''

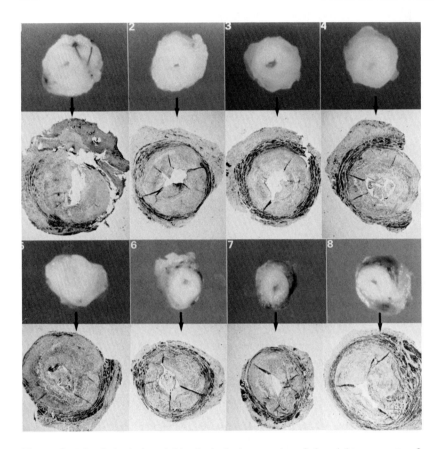

Figure 5 Morphological and histological photographs of the eight segments of saphenous vein graft corresponding to the sites labeled in Figure 2. Segments 1–6 are from
the area of balloon inflation and dilation and segments 7 and 8 are from nondilated
portions of the graft (i.e., "controls"). Each of the eight segments had diffuse and severe
cross-sectional area luminal narrowing by intimal thickening consisting of fibrocollagenous tissue. No segments contained atherosclerotic plaque or calcium deposits. No
distinctive histological changes were observed in the segments subjected to transluminal
balloon angioplasty compared with control segments (elastic stains, ×6). [From Waller et
al. (22), with permission.]

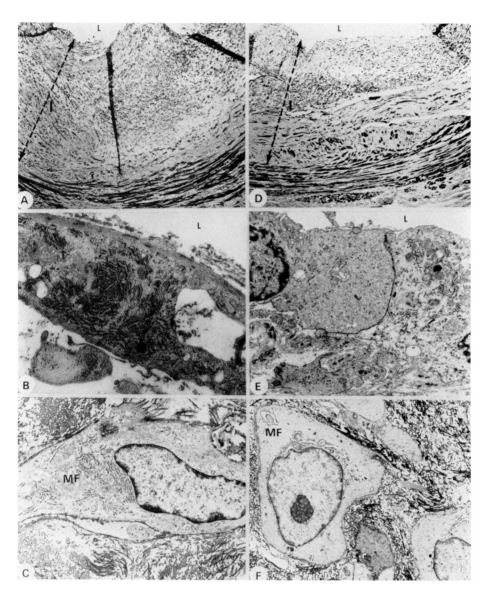

Figure 6 Light and electron micrographs of dilated (A–C) (segment 2 from Fig. 5) and nondilated (D–F) (segment 8 from Fig. 5). Portions of the saphenous vein graft. (A and D) Light micrographs of dilated (A) and nondilated (D) segments show that both segments have marked intimal thickening composed of smooth muscle cells and fibrocollagenous tissue (elastic stains, ×40). (B and E) Electron micrographs at the luminal border of dilated (B) and nondilated (E) segments show a loss of endothelial cells, with micropinocytotic vesicles bordering the lumen in E. A short segment of basement membrane is visible at the lower right (×8300). (C and F) Electron micrographs from deeper portions of the intimal thickening of the dilated (C) and nondilated (F) segments show similar types of myofibroblastic cells (MF) and dense bundles of collagen fibrils (×8300). [From Waller et al. (22), with permission.]

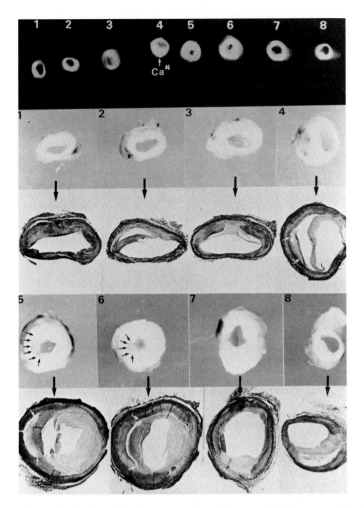

Figure 7 Radiographs (upper panel) and photographs (lower panel) of morphological and histological segments of saphenous vein graft corresponding to the sites labeled in Figure 4. Each of the segments shows diffuse but variable degrees of intimal thickening composed of atherosclerotic plaque. The segment with the most severe luminal narrowing (5) corresponds to the area of previous transluminal balloon angioplasty procedures (small arrows). [From Waller et al. (22), with permission.]

Clinical-Morphological Correlations

Each of the patients just described had one or more clinically successful percutaneous transluminal angioplasty dilations of a stenotic saphenous vein bypass graft *early* (2 months) or *late* (52 and 54 months) after graft insertion.

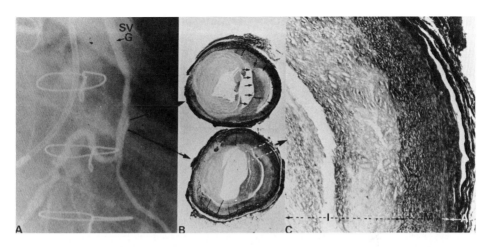

Figure 8 Angiographic-morphological-histological correlation at the site of angioplasty dissection 2 months before graft excision. (A) Angiographic frame of saphenous vein bypass graft (SV G) following transluminal balloon angioplasty showing a line of dissection. (B) Corresponding morphological segments of SV G in area of angiographic dissection showing severe luminal cross-sectional area narrowing with an "intimal flap" (small arrows) and a partially healed intimal "fracture." (C) Higher magnification ($\times 80$) of boxed area in B showing the intimal (I) fracture site. The intimal thickening is composed of fibrocollagenous tissue, foam cells, and cholesterol clefts (M = media; A = adventitia) (elastic stains). [From Waller et al. (22), with permission.]

Angiographic similarities between the early and late saphenous vein grafts included an increase in luminal diameter associated with a decrease in mean transstenotic pressure gradient following angioplasty and restenosis of the graft at the site of previous dilation 1 or 2 months later. *Angiographic differences* between the grafts included the absence of "cracks," "breaks," or "splits" following dilation in the early graft, but the presence of an intimal "split" following the second angioplasty procedure in the late graft. An additional angiographic difference between the grafts was the location of stenosis. The site of stenosis in the early graft was at the proximal end of the graft (aortic anastomosis), whereas the site of stenosis in the late graft was in the graft body (midportion).

Morphological similarities between the grafts included diffuse intimal thickening by fibrocollagenous tissue with fibrotic medial and adventitial layers. *Morphological differences* between the grafts were distinctive: the early graft had thickened intima without atherosclerotic plaque changes or calcific deposits and no morphological evidence of previous dilations, whereas the late graft had thickened intima typical of atherosclerotic plaque with focal calcific deposits and morphological evidence of PBA injury.

Therapeutic Implications for Saphenous Vein Angioplasty Derived from Morphological Observations

The fate of an aortocoronary saphenous vein bypass graft appears to be dependent on several factors relevant to the time interval from bypass grafting to graft obstruction (1–27). Graft occlusion developing *within 1 month* of bypass graft insertion is almost invariably secondary to graft thrombosis related to technical factors such as stenosis at aortic or coronary anastomotic sites, intraoperative vein trauma, or poor distal runoff secondary to severe atherosclerosis or reduced caliber of the distal native vessel (5,24). These technical factors and the nature of the obstruction material (thrombus) appear to limit the role of PBA in successfully relieving saphenous vein graft obstruction occurring within 1 month of bypass operation.

Functionally significant graft stenoses developing *between 1 month and 1 year* following graft insertion nearly always are characterized by intimal thickening histologically composed of cellular or acellular fibrocollagenous tissue. The venous medial and adventitial layers become fibrotic, and the graft resembles a thick, fibrous tube. Focally stenotic lesions produced by this intimal thickening appear amenable to dilation by PBA, as illustrated in the first patient described earlier. However, in view of the histological composition of the intima, the dilating mechanism is probably not "intimal compression" but rather graft "stretching" (Fig. 9). Depending on the degree of graft stretching, the dilating procedure may have limited therapeutic success (weeks to months), with graft "restenosis" representing gradual "restitution of tone" of an overstretched graft segment.

Saphenous vein graft stenoses occurring *beyond 1 year* and generally after 3 years following graft insertion usually consists of atherosclerotic plaque in addition to intimal fibrous thickening (12,20). The atherosclerotic plaque in saphenous vein grafts appears morphologically similar to that observed in native coronary arteries: foam cells, cholesterol clefts, blood product debris, fibrocollagenous tissue, and calcific deposits (12,27). Focal stenoses produced by this type of lesion also appear amenable to dilation by PBA, as illustrated in the second patient described earlier. The mechanism(s) of conduit dilation in this setting appears similar to that proposed for coronary artery angioplasty: plaque "splitting," "cracking," or "breaking" with or without localized intimal-medial dissection (Fig. 9). Therapeutic limitations in dilating saphenous vein grafts narrowed by atherosclerotic plaque should be similar to those observed in atherosclerotic coronary arteries subjected to PBA.

In addition to the *age* of the bypass graft, at least two other anatomical factors appear to influence the therapeutic success of PBA of saphenous vein grafts: (a) the *length* of stenosis and (b) the *location* of stenosis. *Long* stenotic segments of saphenous vein (>15–20 mm) are frequently technically more difficult to dilate and are associated with a lower primary therapeutic success compared with *short*

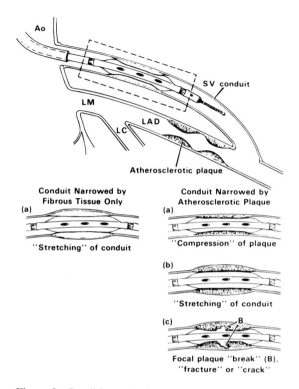

Figure 9   Possible mechanisms of luminal balloon angiography in stenotic aortocoronary saphenous vein (SV) bypass grafts. Two types of lesions characterize the SV stenoses depending on the interval from graft insertion to early obstruction. *Early* (≤1 year) grafts (A, left) contain intimal thickening composed primarily of fibrocollagenous tissue without calcium, and dilation is accomplished by conduit "stretching." *Late* (≥1 year) grafts (A–C, right) contain intimal thickening composed of atherosclerotic plaque and calcium, and dilation is accomplished by "plaque compression" (unlikely), graft "stretching," or plaque "fracture" or "break" (most likely). Ao = aorta; LAD = left anterior descending coronary artery; LC = left circumflex coronary artery; LM = left main coronary artery. [From Waller, et al. (22), with permission.]

stenotic segments (<5 mm). Graft stenoses may be located at the *anastomotic sites* (aorta-graft or coronary artery–graft) or *within the body* of the graft. Angiographic studies have suggested that saphenous vein graft stenoses at the coronary artery–graft anastomotic site have the best therapeutic results, followed by lesions in the graft body and at the aorta-graft anastomotic site, respectively. An anatomical factor supporting the relatively high success rate at dilating stenotic coronary artery–graft anastomotic sites is the presence of atherosclerotic plaque in the coronary portion of the anastomosis (24). Stenoses in the graft body or aortic-graft anastomotic site are less likely to have the potential angioplasty advantage of associated atherosclerotic plaque unless the graft is over 3 years old.

Clinical Results of Percutaneous Transluminal Angioplasty of Saphenous Vein Grafts

The angiographic results of at least 72 saphenous vein bypass grafts subjected to PBA have been previously reported in four studies (22). Ford and colleagues (3,4) dilated nine saphenous vein grafts 4–84 months (mean, 46 months) after insertion. Primary angiographic success occurred in six of the nine grafts, with only late success (>9 months) in two of the six initial successes. Of the two late successes, one graft was 18 months old at initial angioplasty and the other was 5 months old. Famularo and colleagues (1) recently reported morphological observations in an unsuccessful dilation of a saphenous vein conduit with atherosclerotic plaque. Although the age of the graft was not provided, morphology of the angioplasty site showed intimal tears of atherosclerotic plaque. Douglas and associates (28) recently reported their angioplasty results in 62 bypass grafts. Of 62 grafts, 40 (65%) were dilated early after insertion (≤1 year) and 22 (35%) were dilated late after insertion (>1 year). Of the early grafts, primary success occurred in 37 grafts, primary success occurred in 21 grafts (95%), with the same restenosis rate as with the early grafts (24%). Breakdown of the early and late grafts according to stenosis location revealed that the distal graft stenoses (early and late) had a high initial dilation success and lower restenosis rate. Graft stenoses located in the body or proximal end had a slightly lower initial dilation success, but three times the restenosis frequency compared with the distal sites (39% versus 13%). The morphological and histological observations in grafts from the two patients described earlier provide anatomical support for these clinical results.

REFERENCES

1. Famularo M, Vasilomanolakis EC, Schrager B, et al. Percutaneous transluminal angioplasty of aortocoronary saphenous vein graft: Morphologic observations. JAMA 1983; 249:3347–50.
2. Finley JP, Beaulieu RG, Nanton MA, et al. Balloon catheter dilatation of coarctation of the aorta in young infants. Br Heart J 1983; 50:411–5.
3. Ford WB, Wholey MH, Zikria EA, et al. Percutaneous transluminal angioplasty in the management of occlusive disease involving the coronary arteries and saphenous vein bypass grafts. J Thorac Cardiovasc Surg 1980; 79:1–11.
4. Ford WB, Wholey MH, Zikria EA, et al. Percutaneous transluminal dilation of aortocoronary saphenous vein bypass grafts. Chest 1981; 79:529–35.
5. Griffith LSC, Bulkley BH, Hutchins GM. Occlusive changes at the coronary artery-

bypass graft anastomosis. Morphologic study of 95 grafts. J Thorac Cardiovasc Surg 1977; 73:668–79.

6. Gruntzig AR, Senning A, Siegenthaler WE. Nonoperative dilation of coronary artery stenosis. N Engl J Med 1979; 301:61–8.

7. Kan JS, White RI, Mitchell SE, et al. Percutaneous balloon valvuloplasty: A new method for treating congenital pulmonary valve stenosis. N Engl J Med 1982; 370:540–3.

8. Kent KM, Bentivoglio LG, Block PC, et al. Percutaneous transluminal coronary angioplasty: Report from the registry of the National Heart, Lung, and Blood Institute. Am J Cardiol 1982; 49:2011–20.

9. Kimbiris D, Iskandrian AS, Goel I, et al. Transluminal coronary angioplasty complicated by coronary artery perforation. Cathet Cardiovasc Diagn 1982; 8: 481–7.

10. Lababidi Z, Jiunn-Ren W, Walls JT. Percutaneous balloon aortic valvuloplasty: Results in 23 patients. Am J Cardiol 1984; 53:194–7.

11. Lee G, Ikeda RM, Joye JA, et al. Evaluation of transluminal angioplasty of chronic coronary artery stenosis. Value and limitations assessed in fresh human cadaver hearts. Circulation 1980; 61:77–83.

12. Lie JT, Lawrie GM, Morris GC Jr. Aortocoronary bypass saphenous vein graft atherosclerosis. Anatomic study of 99 vein grafts from normal and hyperlipoproteinemic patients up to 75 months postoperatively. Am J Cardiol 1977; 40:906–13.

13. Lock JE, Bass JL, Amplatz K, et al. Balloon dilation angioplasty of aortic coarctations in infants and children. Circulation 1983; 68:109–16.

14. Lock JE, Castaneda-Zuniga WR, Fuhrman BP, et al. Balloon dilation angioplasty of hypoplastic and stenotic pulmonary arteries. Circulation 67:962–7.

15. Lock JE, Castaneda-Zuniga WR, Bass JL, et al. Balloon dilation of excised aortic coarctation. Radiology 1982; 143:689–91.

16. Lock JE, Niemi T, Burke BA, et al. Transcutaneous angioplasty of experimental aortic coarctation. Circulation 1982; 66:1280–6.

17. Pepine CJ, Gessner IH, Feldman RL. Percutaneous balloon valvuloplasty for pulmonic valve stenosis in the adult. Am J Cardiol 1982; 50:1442–5.

18. Saffitz JE, Rose TE, Oaks JB, et al. Coronary arterial rupture during coronary angioplasty. Am J Cardiol 1983; 51:902–4.

19. Singer MI, Rowen M, Dorsey TJ. Transluminal aortic balloon angioplasty for coarctation of the aorta in the newborn. Am Heart J 103:131–2.

20. Smith SH, Greer JC. Morphology of saphenous vein–coronary artery bypass grafts. Seven to 116 months after surgery. Arch Pathol Lab Med 1983; 107:13–8.

21. Waller BF. Early and late morphologic changes in human coronary arteries after percutaneous transluminal coronary angioplasty. Clin Cardiol 1983; 6:363–72.

22. Waller BF, Rothbaum DA, Gorfinkel JH, et al. Morphologic observations following percutaneous transluminal balloon angioplasty of early and late aortocoronary saphenous vein bypass grafts. J Am Coll Cardiol 1984; 4.

23. Waller BF, Girod DA, Dillon JC. Transverse aortic wall tears in infants following balloon angioplasty. Relation of aortic wall damage to diameter of inflated angioplasty balloon and aortic lumen in 7 necropsy infants. J Am Coll Cardiol (in press).

24. Waller BF, Roberts WC. Amount of luminal narrowing in bypassed and non-bypassed native coronary arteries in necropsy patients early and late after aorto-coronary bypass operations. In: Mason DT, Collins JT Jr, (eds.) Myocardial revascularization. Medical and surgical advances in coronary disease. New York: Yorke, 1981: 503–13.

25. Waller BF, Dillon JC, Crowley MH. Plaque hematoma and coronary dissection with percutaneous transluminal coronary angioplasty (PTCA) of severely stenotic lesions: Morphologic coronary observations in 5 men within 30 days of PTCA. Circulation 1983; 68(Suppl III):III–144.

26. Waller BF, McManus BM, Gorfinkel HJ, et al. Status of the major coronary arteries 80 to 150 days after percutaneous transluminal coronary angioplasty. Analysis of 3 necropsy patients. Am J Cardiol 1983; 51:81–4.

27. World Health Organization. Classification of atherosclerotic lesions—Report of a study group. Technical Report Series. Publication 143. Geneva: World Health Organization, 1958: 3–20.

28. Douglas JS, Gruntzig AR, King SB, et al. Percutaneous transluminal angioplasty in patients with prior coronary surgery. J Am Coll Cardiol 1983; 2:745–54.

VI
BRIDGE TECHNIQUES FOR REVASCULARIZATION

17

Assisted Angioplasty
Adjuvant Techniques in Coronary Angioplasty

Carl L. Tommaso

Northwestern University Medical School and
Veterans Administration Lakeside Medical Center
Chicago, Illinois

Robert A. Vogel

University of Maryland Hospital
Baltimore, Maryland

INTRODUCTION

The application of coronary angioplasty has been significantly broadened. The technique was originally used as treatment for discrete single-vessel lesions in patients with good ventricular function (1), but new advances in balloon technology and new techniques such as lasers and arthrectomy have made it possible to treat many more coronary lesions and patients. Additionally, there has been broadening of angioplasty indications, with multivessel angioplasty being the rule. Many patients with severe left ventricular dysfunction, some felt not to be candidates for surgery, are being treated with angioplasty.

The purpose of this chapter is to discuss the clinical application of some newer technologies to the management of patients with medically refractory unstable angina. Specifically, this chapter will be devoted to a description of the tools available to the interventionalist to support the systemic and/or coronary circulation during angioplasty when the anatomy is so threatening that any compromise such as acute closure or even myocardial ischemia during balloon inflation may threaten the survival of the patient.

DEFINITION OF HIGH-RISK ANGIOPLASTY

A significant amount of data has been accumulated on factors that contribute to risk in patients undergoing coronary artery bypass surgery. In regard to angioplasty, while much experience has accumulated concerning the morphological parameters that determine lesion success, relatively little work has been done on factors that determine the risk to a patient undergoing angioplasty. Reasons for this include the continual evolution of technique and apparatus and the lack of controlled or randomized studies comparing angioplasty to medical or surgical treatment.

The factors determining the risk of coronary angioplasty can be classified two ways: (a) technical/anatomical risks and (b) clinical parameters (2). Technical/anatomical risk is a function of the morphology of the target lesion. These factors determine the likelihood of procedural success and include lesion severity, length, calcification, vessel tortuosity, and branching. Although these factors were crucial for the early angioplasty success utilizing primitive equipment, more recent data from the National Heart, Lung and Blood Institute Percutaneous Transluminal Coronary Angioplasty (PTCA) Registry suggest that these factors are of decreasing importance for operators with high skill levels (3).

It appears that patient procedural mortality is determined by more general clinical features. Hartzler et al. (4) described the clinical parameters defining low- and high-risk patients (Table 1). The two most important factors determining procedural mortality are amount of left ventricular myocardium perfused by the target lesion and overall left ventricular function. Factors such as multivessel angioplasty, recent myocardial infarction, and patient age greater than 70 also appear to increase risk. In addition to procedural mortality, dilatation of vessels perfusing large amounts of myocardium exposes patients to higher subsequent mortality due to vessel restenosis or occlusion.

Table 1 Coronary Angioplasty Procedural Mortality

	Procedural risk (%)
All patients	0.7
Low risk[a]	0.25
High risk	.
PTCA 3 vessels	1.3
Age > 70 years	1.4
Left main equivalent	2.6
Ejection fraction < 40%	2.9
Left main stenosis	3.4

[a] Low-risk group has none of the "high-risk" characteristics.
Source: Adapted from Hartzler et al. (4).

However, there appears to be an important role for myocardial and/or systemic circulatory support for many high-risk patients. In addition to decreasing overall procedural mortality and morbidity, the goals of myocardial and systemic circulatory protection include a decrement in chest pain, electrocardiographic changes, and rhythm disturbances caused by myocardial ischemia, which limit the duration and repetition of balloon dilatations.

Parameters to define high-risk procedures have not been studied prospectively, but rather have been drawn from retrospective review of large patient populations.

There remains controversy surrounding the definition of high-risk patients. Data from Bergelson et al. (5) suggested that angiographic criteria, including ostial stenosis of the left anterior descending, angled, sequential, bifurcation, thrombus, and jeopardized collaterals, and clinical parameters, including age, concomitant illness, and left ventricular ejection fraction, could not discriminate between high and low risk, although complications, including abrupt closure, hemodynamic compromise, and need for coronary bypass surgery, were higher in the presence of a risk factor.

Few data exist on the risk of coronary angioplasty in patients undergoing dilatation of vessels perfusing substantial amounts of myocardium. Dilatation of a proximal stenosis in a vessel providing collaterals to another major distribution that was totally occluded would be an example of two distributions supplied by a target lesion; however, factors such as myocardial viability, vessel size, and objectively quantifying myocardium at risk make it difficult to determine amount of jeopardized myocardium. Tierstein et al. (6) reported that dilatation of the left coronary artery in the presence of a totally occluded right coronary artery carried no increase in procedural risk in a small group of patients.

Therefore, it appears that the major factors that determine procedural risk include the amount of viable myocardium tended by the "culprit vessel" and the preexisting left ventricular function. Other factors, such as age and proximity to acute myocardial infarction, are also important, although not as critical as the amount of viable myocardium and left ventricular function.

With this in mind, a number of adjunctive tools, both pharmacological and mechanical, have been used in an effort to reduce the procedural risk of an angioplasty.

ADJUNCTS TO ANGIOPLASTY

Pharmacological Agents

Myocardial ischemia during balloon inflation may be limited by reduction in regional oxygen consumption and augmentation of collateral flow. Several pharmacological agents have been studied. Dorrey et al. (7) found nitroglycerin prolonged the time to the onset of angina slightly following balloon occlusion and reduced the increase in left-ventricular end-diastolic pressure.

Kern et al. (8) studied the effects of sublingual nifedipine administration and concluded that the beneficial effects most likely occur through a reduction in vessel spasm or reduction of myocardial oxygen demand, rather than directly by augmenting coronary blood flow through the collateral circulation.

It was found by Serruys et al. (9) that regional nifedipine administration was associated with a negative inotropic effect and decreased anaerobic metabolism. Piessens et al. (10) found that intravenously administered diltiazem delayed the onset of ischemic pain and ST-segment elevation. The onset of myocardial ischemia was prevented or delayed after administration of intravenous nicardipine in 7 of 10 patients studied by Feldman et al. (11). In contrast to previous studies, residual great cardiac vein blood flow increased during left anterior descending occlusion in 9 of 10 patients following nicardipine administration, suggesting an increase in collateral perfusion.

Beta-adrenergic blockers have also been used both systematically and regionally to prevent ischemia during balloon occlusion. Feldman et al. (12) found that intravenous propranalol prevented or delayed myocardial ischemia in 10 of 16 patients undergoing left anterior descending angioplasty. Zalewski et al. (13) evaluated the regional effect of propranalol and found that the timing and magnitude of ST-segment elevation were favorably affected.

In summary, nitroglycerin, calcium channel blockers, and beta-adrenergic blockers appear to reduce myocardial ischemia during coronary angioplasty through local reduction in myocardial oxygen consumption. Although these methods are effective, they may not cause a significant increase in safety to be universally adopted.

Myocardial Perfusion

An obvious method of reducing myocardial ischemia during balloon inflation would be to maintain blood or nutrient flow to the distal coronary. Several approaches to distal coronary perfusion during angioplasty have been developed. These include the use of (a) autoperfusion catheter, (b) pump perfusion of blood, and (c) perfusion of Fluosol-DA, 20%. Characteristics of these three approaches are summarized in Table 2 (14).

Preservation of ventricular function and metabolism has been demonstrated using autologous blood pumped through a balloon catheter in both experimental and clinical studies. Autologous blood perfusion at 60 ml/min has been shown to reduce anginal pain and ST-segment depression during clinical coronary angioplasty (15–19). Meier et al. (15) infused blood through the lumen of an angioplasty catheter during prolonged balloon occlusion in dogs and noted preservation of ventricular function; however, also noted was the development of

Table 2 Antegrade Perfusion During Angioplasty

	Autoperfusion catheter	Blood perfusion	Fluosol perfusion
O$_2$ capacity	Normal	Normal	Decreased
Viscosity	High	High	Moderate
Additional vascular access	No	Yes	Yes
Pump necessary	No	Yes	Yes
Disadvantages	———————— Need control of lesion ————————		
	High profile requires sufficient perfusion pressure	Hemolysis, thrombosis	Reduced O$_2$ delivery

Source: Adapted from Rossen (14).

thrombosis and hemolysis. Farcot et al. (17) demonstrated the utility of a system that provided phasic pulsatile flow through low-profile balloon catheters.

Although not widely employed, antegrade perfusion has been used in unstable patients and in those undergoing dilatation of vessels supplying substantial amounts of myocardium. Guidewire removal and use of at least moderately large profile catheters to preclude hemolysis and thrombosis are necessary. Hence, antegrade blood or pharmacological agent perfusion requires larger profile balloon catheters and "control" of the artery and lesion with guidewire and balloon prior to the infusion.

In an attempt to eliminate hemolysis and thrombosis, antegrade oxygen-carrying fluorocarbon perfusion has been used. The most commonly used oxygen carrier is Fluosol-DA, 20%, which is a moderate-viscosity emulsion of perfluorodecaline and perfluorotripropylamine. It has a lower oxygen affinity than blood and requires hyperoxygenation at a pO$_2$ of 600 mmHg to carry approximately one-third of oxygen-saturated blood concentration. In experimental studies, Fluosol infusion has improved regional left ventricular dysfunction during balloon occlusion but was less effective than autologous blood perfusion (20–24).

In an attempt to eliminate the need for additional arterial access and pump technology, autoperfusion balloon catheter systems have been evaluated in experimental and clinical studies (25–30). Autoperfusion balloon catheters have multiple shaft side holes proximal and distal to the balloon and a central lumen, which allows blood to flow passively across the lesion. Distal coronary perfusion is directly related to perfusion pressure, and flows of 40–60 ml/min are provided only with near-normal systemic blood pressure. Under these conditions, autoperfusion appears adequate during prolonged balloon inflations to maintain near-normal ventricular function. Under hypotensive conditions inadequate perfusion may result.

The use of autoperfusion balloons has been effective following acute vessel closure (29). The utility of the perfusion balloon catheter as an adjunct to high-risk angioplasty has yet to be established.

MECHANICAL SUPPORT

Coronary Sinus Interventions

In addition to working in the coronary artery, it has been demonstrated that coronary support can be achieved via the cardiac venous system as well (31–34). The investigators for the MultiCenter Coronary Venous Retroperfusion Clinical Trial Group (31) reported good results in using synchronized retrograde perfusion (SRP) to reduce the onset of ischemia and manage patients when prolonged balloon inflation was necessary. Angina occurred in 44% of SRP-treated inflations at average time of 47 sec versus 58% at 38 sec in a control group.

These methods have the disadvantage of requiring cannulation of the coronary sinus, which in some patients may be difficult.

Intra-aortic Balloon Pump

Almost all centers have used intra-aortic balloon pump (IABP) support during coronary angioplasty (4,35–37). Most angiographers are familiar with IABP and have performed PTCA in patients who have been placed on IABP for hemodynamic or ischemia control and have required PTCA. Many centers have also used the IABP prophylactically in patients undergoing PTCA. Hartzler et al. (4) recommend IABP in the following cases:

1. In patients with moderate to severe LV dysfunction
2. During PTCA of any remaining patent artery

Table 3 Comparison of Intra-aortic Balloon Pump with Percutaneously Inserted Cardiopulmonary Bypass

	Intra-aortic balloon pump	Cardiopulmonary bypass
Arterial access	10–12 F	16–20 F
Venous access	None	18–20 F
Augmentation of cardiac output	20–30%	4–6 L/min
Rhythm dependent	Yes	No
Duration of support	Days	Hours
Ventricular unloading	Yes	Yes

3. During PTCA of unprotected left main stenosis or protected left main stenosis with moderately depressed LV function
4. During PTCA in patients with anterior infarctions, elevated LVEDP, or extensive wall motion abnormalities
5. In patients with uncontrollable hypotension during PTCA

Alcan et al. (36) reported the circumstances of adjunctive IABP to PTCA in 14 patients. These included:

1. Clinically unstable situations such as left main disease, multivessel disease, unstable syndromes, and cardiogenic shock
2. Preoperative insertion following unsuccessful PTCA
3. Hemodynamic instability following abrupt vessel closure
4. Late vessel closure following initially successful PTCA

The mechanism for ischemic relief by IABP appears to be the reduction of myocardial oxygen consumption, rather than the enhancement of coronary blood flow. Data from Williams et al. (38) demonstrate reduction in rate-pressure product with variable change in regional coronary blood flow in patients having symptomatic relief of unstable angina. There appears to be a 20–30% increase in cardiac output in patients with low-output syndromes and a significant amount of afterload reduction, as demonstrated in reduction of mitral regurgitation.

The use of down-sized catheters (8.5–12 F) and sheaths and percutaneous insertion has reduced the vascular complications of IABP. There remains a 5–10% complication rate (39), most commonly ischemia of the lower extremity. As many as 30% of patients may have symptomatic lower extremity ischemia which will improve with catheter removal, and 10% may require an additional vascular procedure. Other complications include acute aortic dissection, which is rare, and hemolysis and platelet destruction, particularly after prolonged use.

Significant advantages of IABP are the ease of use, such that a trained CCU nurse can manage the device, and the fact that it can be used for several days to weeks if necessary.

Percutaneous Cardiopulmonary Bypass

For a number of years, development of a device for cardiopulmonary bypass that could be rapidly initiated without thoracotomy has been underway. Not until 1986 was a device available for use clinically (40–44). The initial indication was as a replacement or adjunct for cardiopulmonary resuscitation in patients with failing hemodynamics due to a variety of reasons, including trauma, drug overdose, and so forth. With further experience, the device has been used extensively in cardiology for a variety of reasons (45–56).

The percutaneous cardiopulmonary bypass (PCBP) system utilizes several components, including cannulae, connecting tubing, pump, heat exchanger, and oxygenator, which will be described (Fig. 1).

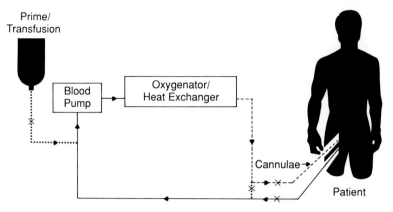

Figure 1 Diagram of cardiopulmonary bypass system used for percutaneous femoro-femoral support.

There are two cannulae, a venous and an arterial, which are inserted either percutaneously or by cutdown (Fig. 2). The sheaths are available in #16–#20 French sizes and are inserted over a tapered dilator. The venous sheath is about 75 cm in length and has multiple (>30) sideholes in addition to the large endhole. It is inserted via a femoral vein and placed such that the distal end lies in the right atrium. The arterial sheath is about 32 cm in length. The lines are then connected to a BioMedicus (Eden Prairie, MN) pumphead and pump. A membrane oxygenator and heat exchanger are in series between the arterial and venous cannulae (Fig. 3). This pump differs from the usual roller pumps used in cardiopulmonary bypass because it is a conical rotating centrifugal pump. It provides negative pressure for venous outflow as well as positive pressure for arterial flow.

Although the pump is quite simple, it does require a trained perfusionist to operate. The addition of a perfusionist on-site limits the procedure to facilities with open-heart capability.

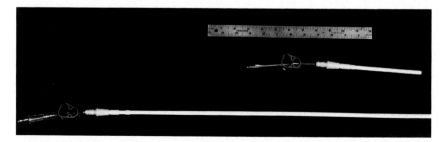

Figure 2 Cannulae used for femorofemoral bypass.

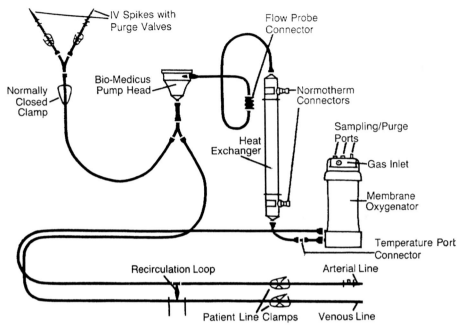

Figure 3 Schematic of circuit used for the percutaneously inserted cardiopulmonary bypass.

The coupling of percutaneously inserted cardiopulmonary bypass and angioplasty (supported angioplasty) was begun in 1987 and has gone through some modifications and refinements, particularly in regard to insertion and removal of cannulae and indications for the procedure.

In the initial experience, the cannulae were inserted via surgical cutdown, but the trend has recently been toward percutaneous insertion. In several centers a cutdown is still used. The percutaneous technique most commonly used is based on that as described by Shawl et al. (57) and is similar to that described by Vignola et al. (58) for insertion and removal of intra-aortic balloon pumps.

When the system is inserted electively, iliac/femoral angiography is performed using 20 ml of contrast (at the rate of 10 ml/sec) of the femoral artery into which percutaneous bypass will be inserted. This is done to ascertain patency of the vessel, to identify the femoral rather than the profunda artery, and to check for tortuosity, which may limit insertion of the sheath and the flow rate. The venous cannula is positioned so the distal end lies in the upper portion of the right atrium.

The arterial sheath is inserted similarly after entering the vessel. Once inserted, the arterial and venous cannulae and connector are mated. Heparin, 300 U/kg, is then administered for full anticoagulation.

A number of methods are available for removal of the cannulae. The cardio-pulmonary bypass system can then be removed once it is ascertained that the patient is stable or after a several-hour delay to allow some resolution of the heparin. Some centers have placed the cannulae percutaneously and removed them via a cutdown and direct vessel repair. If cutdown was performed for insertion, the vessels are secured, and once the lines are removed, hemostasis is maintained and the vessels are sutured as appropriate.

In the fully percutaneous method of Shawl et al. (57), the patient is then transferred to a stretcher with a full metal base and positioned near the edge of the stretcher. The sheaths then can be withdrawn and a C-clamp Compressor System (Instromedix, Hillsboro, OR) applied to the point where no bleeding is noted but where pulses are still present by either Doppler or palpation (57).

Reversal of heparin has not been routinely used for fear of thrombosis at the recent PTCA site, although we have reversed heparin for other procedures such as valvuloplasty. Titration of heparin by measurement of activated clotting times is reasonable, but not reported.

Other users have kept the sheaths in for 4–6 hr to allow metabolism of heparin and then pulled them and maintained hemostasis manually (1–1.5 hr).

Because of thrombophlebitis and late acute closure (24–72 hr) that has been noted, heparin is usually continued and the patient is often placed on oral anticoagulants for 4–6 weeks.

Although interventional cardiologists are well versed in cardiopulmonary physiology, the use of cardiopulmonary bypass in the catheterization laboratory presents a new technology and physiological state that must be managed.

PCBP can usually provide 5 liters/min or more of retrograde aortic blood flow as cardiopulmonary bypass depending on cannulae size. It appears that the venous cannulae may be more limiting, and therefore a larger venous cannula may be mated to a smaller arterial cannula.

During bypass because of nonpulsatile flow, vasodilation occurs. Patients often experience a marked warmth and perspiration. Due to the unloading nature of the pump and the vasodilation, pulmonary artery, pulmonary capillary wedge, and systemic pressures often drop markedly. It is our practice to maintain mean systemic pressures in the range of 60–70 mmHg to maintain coronary perfusion and perfusion of other organ systems. Use of pure short-acting vasoconstrictors such as neosynephrine and volume replacement may be necessary.

Since the PCPB system as currently does not vent the left ventricle, the use of cooling and cardioplegic solutions cannot be recommended at this time.

It is suggested by the low incidence of electrocardiographic changes or chest pain during PTCA balloon inflation that PCPB reduces ischemia. Cardiopulmonary bypass in the conscious patient may reduce ischemia by significantly reducing afterload and wall tension. It may have an additional beneficial action on increasing coronary flow by raising aortic diastolic pressures and reducing left ventricular diastolic pressures, hence increasing coronary artery perfusion gradient. However, data suggest that although PCPB favorably affects hemodynamic determinants of myocardial oxygen demand, it causes anaerobic metabolism and does not prevent myocardial ischemia (59). This may be largely due to the acute anemia and reduced oxygen-carrying capacity due to the hemodilution from the priming "dead space." Some centers have circumvented this by priming with blood.

Since the effect of PCPB on myocardial ischemia may be variable, in the event of acute closure efforts to maintain coronary flow through use of "bailout" or autoperfusion catheter should be used. However, these devices depend on the presence of systemic pressure to provide perfusion. In the hypotensive patient, PCPB inserted prophylactically or urgently may be helpful in maintaining systemic pressure to further facilitate use of these devices.

In the cardiac catheterization laboratory this system may be quickly employed in patients who have unexpected complications of either diagnostic cardiac catheterization or interventional procedures when hemodynamic collapse appears or in lieu of CRP (60–63). In our experience, this system can be inserted in several minutes (4–6) by the experienced operator with the assistance of a perfusionist familiar with the equipment.

A number of complications are possible, as listed in Table 5. Because of the large bore of these catheters, vascular occlusion and bleeding are certainly possible complications that must be treated expectantly. A number of patients have had subsequent thrombophlebitis, and hence, it is recommended that short-term (4–6 weeks) anticoagulation with Coumadin be used.

Disadvantages of percutaneously inserted cardiopulmonary bypass supported angioplasty are:

1. Left ventricular unloading is incomplete.
2. Segmental ischemia is reduced but not prevented.
3. Circulatory support is limited to about 6 hr (because of use of the membrane oxygenator).

Table 4 Uses of PCPB

Transient, reversible, cardiac, or pulmonary dysfunction
CPR failure
Supported angioplasty
Supported valvuloplasty (aortic)
Postoperative cardiac dysfunction
Unexpected hemodynamic crisis during catheterization
Failed PTCA (hemodynamically unstable)
Mechanical complications of myocardial infarction
Cardiogenic shock
Hemodynamic support during other interventional procedure(s)
Catheter mapping and ablation, etc.

Table 5 Potential Complications of PCBP

Vascular injury
  Perforation
  Thrombosis
  Bleeding
  Thrombophlebitis
  Arteriovenous fistula
  Pseudo aneurysm
Air embolism
Hypotension
Gastrointestinal bleeding
Gastrointestinal ischemia
Acute renal failure
Transient cerebral ischemia
Transfusion
Infection
Skin necrosis
Femoral nerve palsy

4. Removal of the large-diameter cannulae is problematic, especially following high-dose heparin administration.

National Registry for Supported Angioplasty

Following reports of the first supported angioplasty procedures, a number of centers across the nation began performing the procedure. In order to record the results and evaluate the benefits and complications of the procedure, a voluntary national registry was formed. In the first year of the registry, 14 centers entered 105 patients (45). In the second year, 20 centers entered an additional 350 patients (64). Therefore, data on more than 450 patients have been accumulated.

Table 6 National Supported Angioplasty Registry: 1988 Results

	Age > 75 yr	LMCA	EF < 20%	CABG inop	Only patent vessel	Age < 75, no LMCA
Number	17	17	23	20	30	76
LVEF (%)	35	45	16	28	27	28
Mortality (%)	29	29	4	0	7	2.6

LMCA = ≥75% lumen diameter of left main coronary artery; EF = left ventricular ejection fraction; CABG inop = deemed inoperable for coronary artery bypass surgery.
Source: Vogel et al. (45).

The Registry experience suggests that in these patients, who may constitute the largest collection to date of "high risk" patients undergoing angioplasty, results were very encouraging. In each year of the registry, there was a greater than 95% success rate (50% or less final lumen diameter after PTCA of targeted vessel. When the registry considered subgroups, it was noted that patients with very poor ventricular function (less than 20%), those undergoing dilatation of their only patent coronary vessel, and surgically inoperable patients underwent supported angioplasty with a hospital mortality rate of 2–3% (45,64). These data were consistent in the second year as well as the first year of the registry.

However, patients with left main coronary stenosis undergoing dilatation of that or other vessels have experienced high hospital mortality rates (29%). These data were again consistent in the first and second years of the registry and suggested that there was an intrinsic high risk to patients with left main coronary disease not overcome by supported angioplasty.

Vascular complications and general morbidity were initially frequent, but have decreased with additional experience to less than 20%. In the first year of the registry, there was a 39% morbidity rate predominantly due to vascular complications. However, in the second year, the vascular complications fell to less than 18% despite the fact that more than three-quarters of the patients had percutaneous insertion and removal. This aspect of supported angioplasty has shown the steepest improvement, presumably owing to increased familiarity with the procedure (64).

Late follow-up suggests that many of these high-risk patients have had excellent postinterventional courses. Ninety percent of individuals improve their New York Heart Association (NYHA) anginal classification by at least two classes (45), and mean left ventricular ejection fraction increased 7.3%. Shawl et al. reported an 82% 18-month survival, with 87% either asymptomatic or class I (65).

A major limitation of angioplasty in high-risk patients appears to be a 4% incidence of late vessel closure, occurring from 10 hr to 4 days following the

Table 7 Advantages and Disadvantages of Assisted Angioplasty

Advantages
  Broadens indication for PTCA
  Stabilizes hemodynamically unstable patients
  Ease of management of failed PTCA
  Makes interventional procedures safer
Disadvantages
  Arterial venous injury
  Blood loss
  Complex technology needing skilled operator

Table 8 Comparison of 1988 and 1989 Registry Results

	1989	1989
Participating institutions	14	20
Total patients	105	350
Standby use	3.0%	26%
Percutaneous insertion	55%	77%
Total morbidity	39%	18%
Hospital mortality	7.6%	5.8%
Subacute closure mortality	3.8%	3.1%

procedure. Acute myocardial infarction almost invariably results, and death occurs in about half the patients experiencing this complication. The etiology of this late phenomenon is uncertain, but it was present in similar degree in both years of the registry (64).

More recently, standby use of femorofemoral cardiopulmonary bypass, as described above, has been employed for many patients previously utilizing prophylactic support. Emergency initiation of support in the standby situation has been required in the minority of cases and has been performed successfully even during cardiac arrest. Late vessel closure with significant morbidity and mortality has also been observed in patients undergoing standby supported angioplasty (66,67).

The success of supported angioplasty must be tempered by a number of factors. First, the National Registry suffers from all the potential bias that a voluntary registry faces. Second, there is no randomization or comparison to other potential treatment modalities to compare the effectiveness of this procedure.

Nonetheless, it is our feeling that the availability of PCBP used prophylactically or as standby is useful in patients undergoing high-risk PTCA, when it is felt that acute closure or even balloon passage and inflation may lead to sudden profound hemodynamic collapse and make it impossible to complete a procedure. The precise hemodynamic and angiographic features that indicate such use are continuing to be investigated. We recommend prophylactic insertion in patients undergoing dilation of an "only patent vessel" or in patients who have demonstrated hemodynamic instability. In patients who have either left ventricular ejection fractions less than 25% or more than 50% of the "viable" left ventricular myocardium supplied by the target vessel, we recommend "standby support" where in the contralateral vessel (potential insertion site) is angiographed, and the vein is instrumented with small-diameter catheters (5 or 6 F dilators) and the system and pressures are reduced to go on pump. Our estimation in experienced hands is approximately 4–6 min to go on pump in this situation (64).

Table 9 Circulatory Support During Angioplasty Based on Risk

Risk category	Patient characteristics	Suggested strategy
Standard	Single stenosis	Routine
	Normal LV function	
Complex	Multivessel disease	Routine
	Moderate LV dysfunction	May require "staged" PTCA
	Complex lesions	
High	Target vessel supplying $> 1/2$ myocardium	Perfusion balloon, retroperfusion, IABP
	LVEF < 15–25%	Standby support
Manifest	Dilatation only patent vessel	Cardiopulmonary support
	LVEF $< 15\%$	Hemopump
	Hemodynamic collapse during PTCA	

We have evaluated the indications that were originally used for supported angioplasty (LVEF $< 25\%$ or target lesion supplying $> 50\%$ of myocardium). We compared our results in patients who underwent supported angioplasty to an angiographically and clinically similar group of patients who underwent "standby supported angioplasty" where PCBP was available but not used (66). In none of the standby patients was there need for placement to PCBP because of hemodynamic collapse. In a larger group of patients collected from the Supported Angioplasty National Registry, only 5% of patients with these indications needed to go on PCBP, suggesting that the initial indications were too restrictive (66). Based on our experience with supported angioplasty, our current indications and recommendations for the use of adjunctive supportive techniques in PTCA are described in Table 9.

Because the Registry database was collected retrospectively, it is not possible to ascertain how many patients were indeed "medically refractory," but more than two-thirds were in NYHA class IV prior to the procedure. These patients appeared to be a particularly high-risk subset of medically refractory patients, in that they not only were refractory, but had either poor ventricular function or were at high risk for surgical or interventional procedures because of their anatomy and/or ventricular function.

OTHER MECHANICAL SUPPORT DEVICES

Other types of left ventricular support systems are currently being considered for high-risk angioplasty. One uses transseptal cannulation of the left atrium in conjunction with synchronized pumping into the femoral artery (68,69). This approach does not require an oxygenator, therefore reducing the need for high-dose heparin. Large-diameter transseptal cannulation is, however, more difficult to perform than right atrial access and may be particularly difficult in an acutely ill patient.

Another left ventricular support system is the Hemopump (Johnson and Johnson Interventional Systems), which uses a turbine pump placed transfemorally across the aortic valve. This system, capable of 3.5 liters/min output, has been used for intermediate-term circulatory support (70). At present, the pump's 22-F diameter necessitates cutdown vessel entry, but smaller-diameter systems are planned. Loisance et al. (71) reported their experience with this device in assisting angioplasty. Both these approaches are unaffected by intrinsic cardiac output and have been utilized for supporting angioplasty in a few high-risk patients.

CONCLUSIONS

High-risk angioplasty, though defined well on a lesion-by-lesion basis, is not well defined in terms of risk of mortality for the patient undergoing an interventional procedure. Becoming available are an increasing number of tools to assist the interventionalist in performing procedures with less risk and better results; however, indications remain less than perfectly defined and will undergo further refinement in the future.

The medically refractory "hot" patient, who is also a high risk for an interventional procedure because of anatomy or ventricular function, will require painstaking and heroic care.

REFERENCES

1. Gruentzig AR, Senning A, Seigenthaler WE. Non-operative dilatation of coronary artery site: Percutaneous transluminal coronary angioplasty. N Engl J Med 1979; 301:61–8.
2. Tommaso CL. Management of high-risk coronary angioplasty. Am J Cardiol 1989; 64:33E–37E.
3. Bentivoglio LG, VanRaden MJ, Kelsey SF, Detre KM. Percutaneous transluminal coronary angioplasty (PTCA) in patients with relative counterindications: Results of the National Heart, Lung, and Blood Institute PTCA Registry. Am J Cardiol 1984; 53:82C–88C.
4. Hartzler GO, Rutherford BD, McConahay DR, Johnson WL, Giorgi LV. "High-risk" percutaneous transluminal coronary angioplasty. Am J Cardiol 1988; 61:33G–37G.
5. Bergelson BA, Kyller MG, Jacobs AK, Ruocco NA, Ryan TJ, Faxon DP. Inadequacy of current criteria for predicting high risk angioplasty. J Am Cardiol 1990; 15:206A (Abstract).
6. Tierstein P, Giorgi L, Johnson W, McConahay D, Rutherford B, Hartzler G. PTCA of the left coronary artery when the right coronary is chronically occluded. Am Heart J 1990; 119:479–83.

7. Dorrey AJ, Mehmel HC, Schwartz FX, Kubler W. Amelioration by nitroglycerin of left ventricular ischemia induced by percutaneous transluminal coronary angioplasty: assessment by hemodynamic variables and left ventriculography. J Am Coll Cardiol 1985; 6:267–74.
8. Kern MJ, Deligonul U, Labovitz A, Gabliani G, Vandormael M, Kennedy HL. Effects of nitroglycerin and nifedipine on coronary and systemic hemodynamic during transient coronary artery occlusion. Am Heart J 1988; 115:1164–70.
9. Serruys PW, van den Brand M, Brower RW, Hugenholtz PG. Regional cardioplegia and cardio-protection during transluminal angioplasty: Which role for nifedipine? Eur Cardiol J 1983; 4:115–21.
10. Piessens J, Tomasz B, Stammen F, van Haecke J, Vrolix M, DeGeest H. Effect of intravenous diltiazem on myocardial ischemia occurring during percutaneous transluminal coronary angioplasty. Am J Cardiol 1989; 64:1103–7.
11. Feldman RL, McDonald RG, Hill JA, Pepine C. Effect of nicardipine on determinants of myocardial ischemia occurring during acute coronary occlusion produced by percutaneous transluminal coronary angioplasty. Am J Cardiol 1987; 60:267–70.
12. Feldman RL, McDonald RG, Hill JA, Limacher MC, Conti CR, Pepine CJ. Effect of propanalol on myocardial ischemia during acute coronary occlusion. Circulation 1986; 73:727–33.
13. Zalewski A, Goldberg S, Dervan J, Slysh S, Maroko PR. Myocardial protection during transient artery occlusion in man: Beneficial affects of regional beta adrenergic blockade. Circulation 1986; 73:734–9.
14. Rossen JD. Perfusion during coronary angioplasty. Cardiology 1989; 6:103–6.
15. Meier B, Gruentzig AR, Dekmezian RH, Brown JE. Percutaneous perfusion of occluded coronary arteries with blood from the femoral artery: A dog study. Cathet Cardiovasc Diag 1985; 11:81–7.
16. Lehmann KG, Atwood E, Snyder EL, Ellison RL. Autologous blood perfusion for myocardial protection during coronary angioplasty: A feasibility study. Circulation 1987; 76:312–23.
17. Farcot JC, Berland J, Bourdarias JP, Letac B. Physiologic anteroperfusion system during balloon angioplasty: Experimental validation and clinical evaluation in single coronary disease patients. J Am Coll Cardiol 1990; 15:249A (Abstract).
18. Angelini P, Heibig J, Leachman R. Distal hemoperfusion during percutaneous transluminal coronary angioplasty. Am J Cardiol 1986; 58:252–5.
19. Heibig J, Angelini P, Leachman DR, Beall MM, Beall AC Jr. Use of mechanical devices for distal hemoperfusion during balloon catheter coronary angioplasty. Cathet Cardiovasc Diag 1988; 15:143–9.
20. Tokioka H, Miyazoki A, Fung P, Rajagopalan RE, Kar S, Meesbaum S, Corday E, Drury JK. Effects of intra-coronary perfusion of arterial blood or Fluosol-DA 20% on regional myocardial metabolism and function during brief coronary artery occlusions. Circulation 1987; 75:473–81.
21. Anderson HV, Leimgruber PP, Roubin GS, Nelson DL, Gruentzig AR. Distal coronary artery perfusion during percutaneous transluminal coronary angioplasty. Am Heart J 1985; 110:720–6.
22. Cleman M, Jaffee CC, Wohlgelernter D. Prevention of ischemia during percutaneous transluminal coronary angioplasty by transcatheter infusion of oxygenated Fluosol DA 20%. Circulation 1986; 74:555–62.

23. Cleman MW, LaSala JM. Protected PTCA. In: Topol EJ, ed. Textbook of interventional cardiology. Philadelphia: Saunders, 1990:496–514.

24. Lane TA, Lamkin GE. Paralysis of phagocyte migration due to an artificial blood substitute. Blood 1984; 64:400–5.

25. Quigley PJ, Hinohora T, Phillips HR, Peter RH, Behar VS, Kong Y, Simonton CA, Perez JA, Stack RS. Myocardial protection during coronary angioplasty with an autoperfusion balloon catheter in humans. Circulation 1988; 78:1128–34.

26. Turi ZG, Campbell CA, Gottimukkala MV, Kloner RA. Preservation of distal coronary perfusion during prolonged balloon inflation with an autoperfusion angioplasty catheter. Circulation 1987; 75:1273–80.

27. Turi ZG, Pezkalla S, Campbell CA, Kloner RA. Ameliation of ischemia during angioplasty of the left anterior descending coronary artery with an autoperfusion catheter. Am J Cardiol 1988; 62:513–7.

28. Erbel R, Clas W, Bursch U, von Seelen W, Brennecke R, Meyer J. New balloon catheter for prolonged percutaneous transluminal coronary angioplasty and bypass flow in occluded vessels. Cathet Cardiovasc Diag 1986; 12:116–23.

29. Stack RS, Quigley PJ, Collins G, Phillips HR. Perfusion balloon catheter. Am J Cardiol 1988; 61:77G–80G.

30. Kereiakes DJ, Stack RS. Perfusion angioplasty. In: Topol EJ, ed. Textbook of interventional cardiology. Philadelphia: Saunders, 1990:452–66.

31. Kar S, for the Investigators of the MultiCenter Coronary Venous Retroperfusion Clinical Trial Group. Reduction of PTCA induced ischemia by synchronized coronary venous retroperfusion: Results of a multicenter clinical trial. J Am Coll Cardiol 1990; 15:250A (Abstract).

32. Yamazaki S, Drury K, Meerbaum S, Corday E. Synchronized coronary venous retroperfusion: Prompt improvement of left ventricular function in experimental myocardial ischemia. J Am Coll Cardiol 1985; 5:655–63.

33. Drury JK, Yamazaki S, Fishbein MC, Meerbaum S, Corday E. Synchronized diastolic coronary venous retroperfusion; results of a preclinical safety and efficacy study. J Am Coll Cardiol 1985; 6:328–35.

34. Gore JM, Weiner BH, Benotti JR, Sloan KM, Okike ON, Cuenoud HF, Gaca JM, Albert JS, Dalen JE. Preliminary experience with synchronized coronary sinus retroperfusion in humans. Circulation 1986; 74:381–8.

35. Margolis JR. The role of the percutaneous intra-aortic balloon in emergency situations following percutaneous transluminal coronary angioplasty. In: Kaltenbach M, Gruentzig A, Rentrop P, Bassman W-D, eds. Transluminal coronary angioplasty and intracoronary thrombolysis. Berlin: Springer-Verlag, 1982:145–50.

36. Alcan KE, Stertzer SH, Walsh JE, de Pasquale NP, Bruno MS. The role of intra-aortic balloon counterpulsation in patients undergoing percutaneous transluminal coronary angioplasty. Am Heart J 1983; 105:527–30.

37. Szatmary LJ, Marco J, Fajadet J, Caster L. The combined use of diastolic counterpulsation and coronary dilatation in unstable angina due to multivessel disease under unstable hemodynamic conditions. Int J Cardiol 1988; 19:59–66.

38. Williams DO, Korr KS, Gewirtz H, Most AS. The effect of intraaortic balloon counter pulsation on regional myocardial blood flow can oxygen consumption in the presence of coronary artery stenosis in patients with unstable angina. Circulation 1982; 66:593–7.

39. Bolooki H. Current status of circulatory support with an intra-aortic balloon pump. Cardiol Clin 1985; 3:123–33.
40. Proctor E, Kowalik TA. Circulatory support by pump oxygenator in experimental fibrillation and acute left heart failure induced by coronary artery ligation. Cardiovasc Resus 1967; 1:189–93.
41. Evans D, Baird RJ. The effects of closed chest vaso-arterial bypass with oxygenation on cardiopulmonary hemodynamics. J Thorac Cardiovasc Surg 1971; 62:76–82.
42. Kennedy JH. The role of assisted circulation in cardiac resuscitation. JAMA 1988; 197:615–8.
43. Lande AJ, Subramanian VA, Lillehei CW. Clinical experience with emergency use of prolonged cardiopulmonary bypass with a membrane pump-oxygenator. Ann Thorac Surg 1970; 10:409.
44. Phillips J, Ballentine B, Slonine D, Hall J, Vandekorr, Konstanhorn C, Zeff RH, Skinner JR, Peckmok GD. Percutaneous initiation of cardio-pulmonary bypass. Ann Thorac Surg 1983; 36:223–5.
45. Vogel RA, Shawl F, Tommaso CL, et al. Initial report of the national registry of elective supported angioplasty. J Am Coll Cardiol 1990; 15:23–9.
46. Vogel RA. Maryland experience: Angioplasty and valvuloplasty using percutaneous cardiopulmonary support. Am J Cardiol 1988; 62:11k–14k.
47. Vogel R, Tommaso C, Gundry S. Initial experience with angioplasty and aortic valvuloplasty using elective semipercutaneous cardiopulmonary support. Am J Cardiol 1988; 62:811–3.
48. Vogel RA, Gundry SR, Zoda AR, Stafford JL, Johnson RA, Tommaso CL. Supported angioplasty: Initial experience with high risk patients. Clin Res 1988; 36:791.
49. Tommaso CL, Gundry SR, Zoda AR, Stafford JL, Johnson RA, Vogel RA. Supported angioplasty: Initial experience with high risk patients. Clin Res 1988; 36:867A.
50. Tommaso CL, Vogel RA, Stafford JL, Alikhan M, Gundry SR. Use of prophylactic semi-percutaneous cardiopulmonary bypass during aortic balloon valvuloplasty. Clin Res 1988; 36:867A.
51. Tommaso CL, Gundry SR, Zoda AR, Stafford JL, Johnson RA, Vogel RA. Supported Angioplasty; initial experience with high risk patients. J Am Coll Cardiol 1989; 13:159A (Abstract).
52. Shawl FA, Domanski MJ, Punja S, Hernandez TJ. Percutaneous cardiopulmonary bypass support in high-risk patients undergoing percutaneous transluminal coronary angioplasty. Am Heart J 1989; 64:1258–63.
53. Shawl FA, Domanski MJ, Punja S. Hernandez TJ. Emergency percutaneous cardiopulmonary (bypass) support in cardiogenic shock. J Am Coll Cardiol 1989; 13:160A (Abstract).
54. Vogel JHK, Ruiz CE, Janke EJ, et al. Percutaneous (nonsurgical) supported angioplasty in unprotected left main disease and severe left ventricular dysfunction. Clin Cardiol 1989; 12:297–300.
55. Topol EJ. Emerging strategies for failed percutaneous transluminal coronary angioplasty. Am J Cardiol 1989; 63:249–50.
56. Freedman RJ, Wrenn RC, Godley ML, Knoepp JD, Smith C, LaCroix C. Complex

multiple percutaneous transluminal coronary angioplasties with vortex oxygenator cardiopulmonary support in the community hospital setting. Cathet Cardiovasc Diag 1989; 17:237–42.

57. Shawl FA, Domanski MJ, Punja S, Hernandez TJ. Percutaneous institution of cardiopulmonary (bypass) support: Technique and complications. J Am Coll Cardiol 1989; 13:159A (Abstract).

58. Vignola PA, Swaye PS, Gosselin AJ. Guidelines for effective and safe percutaneous intra-aortic balloon pump insertion and removal. Am J Cardiol 1981; 48:660–4.

59. Stack, RK, Pavlides GS, Justeson G, Schreiber TL, O'Neill WW. Hemodynamic and metabolic effects of cardiopulmonary support during PTCA. J Am Coll Cardiol 1990; 15:250A (Abstract).

60. Ballenotz J, Karch S. Closed chest heart-lung bypass for high risk PTC. Am J Cardiol 1988; 5:72–8.

61. Overlie PA, Reichman RT, Smith SC, Dembitsky W, Adamson RM, Jaski BE, Marsh DG, Daily PO. Emergency use of portable cardiopulmonary bypass in patients with cardiac arrest. J Am Coll Cardiol 1989; 13:160A (Abstract).

62. Hartz R, LoCicero, Sanders J, Frederiksen J, Michaelis L. Portable bypass does not improve survival in cardiac arrest patients. J Am Coll Cardiol 1989; 13:121A (Abstract).

63. O'Neill P, Menendez T, Host R, Howell J, Espoda R, Pacifico A. Prolonged ventricular fibrillation salvage using a new percutaneous cardiopulmonary support system. Am J Cardiol 1989; 64:545.

64. Vogel RA, Shawl FA, for the Registry participants. Report of the National Registry of elective supported angioplasty: Comparison of 1988 and 1989 results. Circulation 1990; 82:III-653 (Abstract).

65. Shawl FA, Domanski MJ, Wish M. Cardiopulmonary bypass supported PTCA: Long term follow-up of 85 consecutive patients. Circulation 1990; 82:III-653 (Abstract).

66. Tommaso CL, Johnson RA, Stafford JL, Zoda AR, Vogel RA. Supported coronary angioplasty and standby supported coronary angioplasty for high-risk coronary artery disease. Am J Cardiol 1990; 66:1255–6.

67. Teirstein PS, Vogel RA, Dorros G, Stertzer SH, Vandormael MG, Smith SC, Overlie PA. Prophylactic vs standby cardiopulmonary support for high risk PTCA. Circulation 1990; 82:III680 (Abstract).

68. Shani J, Hollander G, Nathan I, Greengart A, Toproff B, Jacobowitz I, Glassman E, Cunningham J, Lichstein E. Percutaneous left atrial-femoral artery bypass with a pulsatile pump: Initial experience in cardiogenic shock. J Am Coll Cardiol 1989; 13:53A (Abstract).

69. Glassman E, Chinitz L, Levite H, Slater J, Winer H. Partial left heart support during high-risk angioplasty. Circulation 1989; 80:II-272 (Abstract).

70. Smalling RW, Cassidy DB, Merhige M, Felli PR, Wise GM, Barrett RL, Wampler RD. Improved hemodynamic and left ventricular unloading during acute ischemia using the left ventricular assist device compared to intra-aortic balloon counterpulsation. J Am Coll Cardiol 1989; 13:160A (Abstract).

71. Loisance D, Dubois-Rande JL, Deleuze P, Okude J, Cachera JP, Geschwind H. Prophylactic use of hemopump in high risk coronary angioplasty. J Am Coll Cardiol 1990; 15:249A (Abstract).

18

Pharmacological Support of Angioplasty in Unstable Angina

Paul T. Vaitkus and Warren Laskey

*Hospital of the University of Pennsylvania and
University of Pennsylvania School of Medicine
Philadelphia, Pennsylvania*

INTRODUCTION

The role of intracoronary thrombosis in the pathogenesis of unstable angina has been implicated on the basis of pathological (1), angiographic (2), angioscopic (3), and biochemical (4,5) data. Percutaneous transluminal coronary angioplasty (PTCA) undertaken for the treatment of unstable angina is associated with an increased rate of acute occlusion and a diminished success rate (6–9). Furthermore, PTCA performed in the setting of angiographically demonstrated intracoronary thrombus carries an increased risk of acute closure of the dilated vessel (10–12). It is, therefore, not surprising that antiplatelet agents, heparin, and, more recently, thrombolytic therapy have all been utilized as pharmacological adjuncts in efforts to manage intracoronary thrombosis and acute occlusion occurring during PTCA.

This critical link between thrombus formation (and propagation) characteristic of both unstable angina and a procedure that by its very nature is highly thrombogenic presents a dilemma for the invasive approach to the treatment of patients with unstable angina. The substantial incidence of recurrent morbid events as well as mortality in unstable angina is the result of an inexorable occlusive process within the coronary artery. Therefore, any therapeutic modality purporting to be effective and safe in this setting must address these key features of the underlying disease. The substantial intimal disruption, exposure of coronary arterial media and collagen, and hydraulic conditions favorable for highly nonlaminar flow that are the sequelae of PTCA are ideal risk factors in themselves for acute thrombosis and vessel closure. Therefore, it is to be expected that PTCA in the setting of unstable angina should be characterized by an excessive proportion of adverse outcomes.

Recent studies have focused attention on the role of an intact endothelium in maintaining vasodilatory tone in coronary arteries (13). Disruption of endothelium (as occurs in unstable angina) may facilitate vasoconstriction (13,14). The additional deleterious effects of intimal damage during PTCA coupled with the release of platelet-derived factors amplify this risk of coronary vasoconstriction (15). Finally, thrombin formation as the result of activation of the intrinsic and extrinsic components of the coagulation cascade not only enhances platelet aggregation, but is a potent vasoconstrictor in the setting of dysfunctional endothelium (13). Thus, once again, the effects of PTCA in the setting of unstable angina might tend to increase the risk of periprocedural conduit or resistance-vessel constriction.

This complex relationship between vessel wall vasomotor tone, platelet function, and intravascular coagulation has provided interesting new insights into the varied effects of traditional pharmacological agents. For example, the recent demonstration of the ability of nitroglycerin to inhibit platelet deposition (16) supports this complex interplay of the factors responsible for vessel patency with those elements leading to vessel occlusion.

Coronary artery occlusion during PTCA predictably causes myocardial ischemia and ventricular dysfunction. The extent of ischemic ventricular dysfunction varies directly with the size of the area at risk, the extent of collateral flow formation, the duration of occlusion of coronary inflow, and the extent of abnormally functioning myocardium in regions remote from the ischemic coronary bed. Unstable angina represents a unique situation in which there frequently exists a reversibly injured, or stunned, segment of myocardium that is subjected to additional periods of coronary occlusion and, therefore, additional risk of ischemic (or irreversible) myocardial injury. It is this element of the equation, in addition to the rheological–vessel wall interaction noted above, that completes the identification of risk factors for an adverse outcome of PTCA in unstable angina. Therefore, the ability to achieve an optimal coronary angiographic and hemodynamic result is particularly important in this setting. Unfortunately, the operator's inability to control or limit these inevitable consequences of ischemia may preclude his ability to obtain an optimal angiographic result. Therefore, adjunctive techniques allowing for the application of an appropriate duration of balloon occlusion for successful vessel dilation and remodeling, with attenuation of the adverse hemodynamic and metabolic sequalae of myocardial ischemia, is highly desirable. Attempts at pharmacological "myocardial protection" during PTCA have included the administration of beta-blockers, nitrates, calcium blockers, and oxygenated perfluorochemicals.

The following discussion will focus on published techniques designed to improve the outcome of PTCA in the setting of unstable angina. It should be recalled that implicit in these varied approaches is the fact that the clinical outcome of PTCA in this setting, to date, remains significantly different from that in stable angina, We will initially review the experience with therapies designed to minimize occlusive thrombus formation and conclude with a review of approaches designed to attenuate the ischemic response. Clearly, all aspects must be included in a comprehensive solution to the problem.

ANTITHROMBOTIC THERAPY

Anticoagulant Therapy

A number of investigators have examined the role of systemic anticoagulation with intravenous heparin preceding, during, or following PTCA in patients with unstable angina. Table 1 summarizes the published experience dealing with heparin therapy *preceding* PTCA. A preliminary report (17) suggested that a period of heparinization in patients with unstable angina or non-Q-wave myocardial infarction *and* angiographically demonstrated intracoronary thrombus was associated with significant improvement in the appearance of the clot on follow-up angiography. Douglas and associates further suggested that PTCA undertaken in these patients was very likely to be successful, but a suitable control group was not studied (17). Laskey et al. (11) examined the outcome of PTCA in 53 patients with angiographic coronary thrombus. Eighty-one percent of the patients presented with unstable angina. Thirty-five of these patients received 1–7 days of heparin therapy before the procedure, while 18 did not. The heparinized patients more frequently demonstrated improvement in the appearance of the thrombus. Furthermore, PTCA was more frequently successful in the anticoagulated group (94% versus 61%, $p < 0.05$) and was less frequently complicated by acute vessel closure (6% versus 33%, $p < 0.05$) and the need for emergent bypass surgery (0% versus 22%, $p < 0.01$).

Additional preliminary reports have expanded these tentative conclusions regarding improved outcome of PTCA in patients with unstable angina demonstrated to have intracoronary thrombus. Pow et al. enrolled 110 patients with unstable angina of whom 41 received intravenous heparin for 3.7 days (mean) before PTCA while 69 did not (18). The incidence of intraluminal thrombus did not differ between the two groups (10.1% and 14.4%, respectively). The heparinized patients suffered fewer acute closures (0% versus 10.1%, $p < 0.05$) or major clinical complications (myocardial infarction, bypass surgery, or death in 4.9% of treated versus 14.3% in control patients), although the latter trend did not achieve statistical significance. Hartman and colleagues compared the results of PTCA after 22.6 days (mean) of intravenous heparin therapy in 14 patients with unstable angina or non-Q-wave myocardial infarction and intracoronary thrombus to a similar group of 13 patients who did not receive heparin (19). Seventy-one percent of the heparin group versus 0% of the control group

Table 1 Adjunctive Heparin Therapy

Study	Patient population	Heparin						Control					
		n	MI, CABG, or death	PTCA success	Acute occlusion	Thrombus progression	Thrombus improvement	n	MI, CABG, or death	PTCA success	Acute occlusion	Thrombus progression	Thrombus improvement
Douglas (17)	Unstable angina	19		100%	0%	5%	90%						
Laskey (11)	IC thrombus	35	0%	94%	6%	13%	38%	18	22%	61%	33%	25%	0%
Pow (18)	Unstable angina	41	5%		0%			69	14%		7%		
Hartman (19)	IC thrombus	14				14%	71%	13					0%
Hettleman (20)	Unstable angina	62	0%	95%	1.6%			126	19%	78%	10.3%	69%	
Laskey (21)	Unstable angina	135		91%	1.5%			169		81%	8.3%		

IC = intracoronary.

exhibited improvement in the appearance of the thrombus at follow-up angiography. Conversely, 14% of the treated and 69% of the comparison patients revealed a worsening in the appearance of the thrombus. More recently, Hettleman and colleagues compared the outcome of PTCA in 62 patients with unstable angina who received at least 3 days of pre-PTCA heparin to outcome in 126 patients who did not receive heparin (20). The heparin group had a greater frequency of procedural success (95% versus 78%) and a reduction in complications. Specifically, 19% of the nonheparinized group suffered a myocardial infarction, underwent emergency bypass surgery, or died, compared to none of the heparin-treated patients.

In a review of 304 consecutive patients with unstable angina undergoing PTCA, Laskey et al. compared differences in procedural outcome in 135 patients who had received heparin for 2–9 days (mean 5.7) to outcome in 169 patients not receiving heparin (21). They noted a higher angiographic success rate (91% versus 81%, respectively, $p = 0.02$) and lower immediate (thrombotic) vessel occlusion rate (1.5% versus 8.3%, respectively, $p < 0.01$) in patients receiving preprocedural heparin. Of interest was the similar frequency of angiographic coronary arterial dissection, thus emphasizing the specific contribution of thrombosis to outcome.

Several studies have examined the impact of the degree of anticoagulation achieved *during* PTCA on the occurrence of complications. None of these studies was limited to patients with unstable angina. Dean et al. were unable to correlate the occurrence of acute closure to the degree of prolongation of the activated clotting time (ACT) obtained 5 min after a standard 10,000-unit heparin bolus (22). However, their study was small ($n = 80$) and the acute occlusions were few ($n = 3$). Dougherty et al. in a larger study, analyzed their experience with 503 PTCA procedures (23). Patients who required urgent bypass surgery or died during the procedure had lower ACTs (79% with ACT < 250 sec) than those patients who did not suffer a major complication (100% of patients with ACT > 250). Notably, the ACT was measured after the initial bolus as well as at the end of the procedure. Several studies have emphasized significant interindividual variability in the amount of heparin required during PTCA (24,25). Twelve to twenty-three percent of patients required heparin in excess of the standard 10,000-unit bolus to achieve an adequate ACT.

Finally, several studies have evaluated the role of heparinization *after* PTCA in preventing postprocedural vessel closure. Each trial enrolled patients undergoing elective PTCA (26–28), and one trial specifically excluded patients with significant coronary dissection (27). Saenz et al. demonstrated no reduction in the incidence of vessel occlusion in the post-PTCA period, although there was an increase in significant bleeding in patients randomized to (18–24 hr of) heparin (26). Ellis et al. (27) similarly failed to demonstrate a reduction in postprocedural occlusion among 469 patients randomized to heparin (2.2%) compared to control patients (2.8%). McGarry et al. analyzed 336 patients receiving postprocedural heparin according to the level of the partial thromboplastin time (PTT) measured 6–18 hr following PTCA (28). The group with a greater degree of anticoagulation (mean PTT 150 sec) had a lower incidence of post-PTCA myocardial infarction (2.6%) and prolonged ischemia (1.5%) compared to patients with less intense anticoagulation (mean PTT 62 sec; 10.7% incidence of myocardial infarction and 9.2% incidence of prolonged ischemia). Notably, there was no greater need for transfusion (2.9% versus 4.6%, respectively).

It should be clear, however, given the persistent occurrence of occlusive complications of PTCA, particularly in patients with unstable angina, that even "adequate" heparinization may be ineffective in the prevention of these events. There is cogent evidence in the experimental literature that, in spite of heparin administration, platelet-dependent thrombus formation is unchecked, but that concomitant administration of specific thrombin inhibitors substantially halts this process (29). Furthermore, thrombin inhibition via mechanisms distinct from the action of heparin, i.e., anti-thrombin-III-independent, has led to the synthesis of quite specific thrombin inhibitors (30). The recent experimental application of this approach to the PTCA setting (31) represents an opportunity to study the limitations of heparin therapy and the utility of adjunctive approaches designed to inhibit thrombin formation and activity.

In summary, whether analyzing patients based on clinical presentation, i.e., unstable angina, or the presence of intracoronary thrombus, several days of heparinization prior to PTCA promotes a greater likelihood of angiographic success and less frequent vessel occlusion. The relatively poor immediate and long-term clinical outcome of abrupt vessel occlusion has recently been documented (8). The ideal ACT that should be attained *during* PTCA has not been specifically determined although preliminary data suggest that levels > 250 sec are desirable. Finally, the difficulty in demonstrating a benefit of prolonged anticoagulation following PTCA in low-risk patients does not invalidate the use of heparin post-PTCA in patients with unstable coronary syndromes, intraluminal clot, or large dissections. Further study is needed to establish the ideal intensity and duration of anticoagulation in this setting.

Antiplatelet Therapy

The five studies summarized in Table 2 compare antiplatelet therapy administered before PTCA to placebo. None of the trials was limited to patients with unstable angina, and only two (32,33) reported on the fraction of patients who presented with unstable angina. These studies evaluated the effectiveness of antiplatelet therapy by assessing either the impact on intracoronary thrombus formation (32), complication rates (32–37), or success rate of PTCA (34). For each of these end-points, antiplatelet therapy exhibited a beneficial effect. Barnathan et al. reported that aspirin administered in any dose, alone or in combination with dipyridamole, reduced the frequency of intracoronary throm-

Table 2 Adjunctive Antiplatelet Therapy

Study	n	Prospective?	Agent and dose	Patients with unstable angina (%)	Event rate	
					Treated patients	Control patients
Barnathan (32)	300	No	ASA and/or dipyridamole, any dose	54	0–1.8% IC Th 0–2.7% CABG	10.7% IC Th 9.9% CABG
White (33)	333	Yes	ASA, 325 mg b.i.d. Ticlopidine, 250 mg t.i.d.	42	5% complication 2% complication	14% complication
Chesebro (34)	407	Yes	ASA, 975 mg/day		11% complication	20% complication
Kent (35)	500	No	ASA, 65 mg/day		92% success 3% CABG or MI	80% success 18% CABG or MI
Bertrand (36)	244	Yes	Ticlopidine, 250 mg b.i.d.		5.1% acute closure	16.2% acute closure
Bourassa (37)	376	Yes	ASA, 330 t.i.d., and dipyridamole, 75 mg t.i.d.		1.6% MI 4.8% CABG/re-PTCA	6.9% MI 4.8% CABG/re-PTCA

ASA = aspirin; CABG = coronary artery bypass graft; IC Th = intracoronary thrombus; MI = myocardial infarction.

bus formation and the need for emergency bypass surgery (32). White et al. found that either aspirin (325 mg b.i.d.) or ticlopidine (250 mg t.i.d.) reduced the incidence of immediate complications (defined as abrupt occlusion, thrombus, and major dissection) from 14% to 5% and 2% for the two treatment arms (33). Chesebro et al. evaluated the effectiveness of a combination of aspirin (975 mg/day) and dipyridamole (225 mg/day) and reported a reduction in acute complications (occlusion, myocardial infarction, repeat PTCA, or urgent surgical revascularization) from 20% to 11% (34). Kent et al. administered low-dose aspirin (65 mg/day), which facilitated more frequent success in PTCA (92% versus 80% in patients receiving placebo) and reduced the rate of complications (emergency bypass or myocardial infarction) from 18% to 3% (35). Bertrand et al. evaluated ticlopidine (250 mg b.i.d.) and reported a reduction in acute closure from 16.2% to 5.1% (36). Finally, Bourassa et al. compared a combination of aspirin (330 mg t.i.d.) and dipyridamole (75 mg t.i.d.) to placebo. They reported a reduction in procedural-related myocardial infarction from 6.9% to 1.6% (37).

Two groups of investigators have evaluated the relative merits of different antiplatelet regimens. Mufson et al. randomized 495 patients to receive either low-dose (80 mg/day) or high-dose (1500 mg/day) aspirin on the day prior to PTCA (38). The rates of myocardial infarction (3.6% versus 3.9%), emergency bypass surgery (3.6% versus 3.7%), successful angioplasty (94% versus 95%), and death did not differ between the two groups (38). Lembo et al. evaluated the benefit of adding dipyridamole (75 mg t.i.d.) to a standardized dose of aspirin (325 mg t.i.d.) in 268 patients (39). Patients receiving dipyridamole did not fare better than those receiving aspirin alone in terms of myocardial infarction, emergency bypass, or death.

The hope of reducing thrombotic complications of PTCA has prompted the evaluation of novel antiplatelet treatments. These efforts reflect the narrow therapeutic scope of cyclo-oxygenase inhibition by aspirin or nonsteroidal anti-inflammatory drugs (40) and the increasing recognition of a full spectrum of "antiplatelet" agents that act on various aspects of adhesion or aggregation. Ellis and colleagues administered an antibody to patients undergoing PTCA, which binds to the platelet glycoprotein complex IIb/IIIa, thereby inhibiting platelet aggregation. They demonstrated a prolongation of the bleeding time and a reduction in ex vivo platelet aggregation (41). Timmermans et al. administered ridogrel, a combined thromboxane synthetase inhibitor and thromboxane receptor blocker, to 32 patients during PTCA and reported no acute occlusions while documenting elimination of thromboxane B2 generation during angioplasty (42). Neither of these agents has been evaluated in a controlled clinical trial.

Implicit in these latter approaches is the hypothesis that the final common pathway for platelet aggregation (and thrombus formation and propagation) is the interaction of the platelet IIb/IIIa glycoprotein complex with fibrinogen. Thus, there is great potential for the development of highly specific antiplatelet agents such as monoclonal antibodies or natural or synthetic peptides with the arginine-glycine-aspartic acid sequence (43). The efficacy of each of these agents in inhibiting platelet aggregation and preventing thrombotic complications must, of course, be weighed against the increased risk of hemorrhage.

In summary, the reported clinical data support a role for available antiplatelet drugs in the prevention of thrombotic complications of PTCA. No regimen has been demonstrated to have improved efficacy or safety over another. Once-daily aspirin has the advantage of ease of administration and low cost. Such therapy prior to PTCA, particularly for patients with unstable angina, should be considered standard. However, because occlusive and thrombotic complications occur with higher frequency in patients with unstable angina in spite of concomitant ASA therapy, the development and testing of more specific and safe forms of platelet inhibition is mandatory.

Fibrinolytic Therapy

Fibrinolytic therapy as an adjunct to PTCA has been applied in three ways: (a) it has been administered in the clinical setting of unstable angina with subsequent PTCA, (b) it has been administered at the beginning of the PTCA procedure to prevent occlusion, and (c) it has been administered after coronary thrombosis or occlusion has occurred as a complication of PTCA.

Several groups of investigators have administered fibrinolytic therapy to patients with unstable angina prior to the performance of PTCA (44–47). Hurley et al. administered 100 mg of intravenous tissue plasminogen activator (tPA) in three patients with unstable angina and intraluminal thrombus (44). After an additional 24–72 hr of heparin, aspirin, and dipyridamole therapy, the patients returned to the catheterization laboratory, where the thrombi were demonstrated to have resolved and uncomplicated PTCA was performed.

In a similar fashion, Grill and Brinker administered either intracoronary streptokinase (80–500,000 units) or intravenous tPA (100 mg) to 14 patients with unstable angina and large (>2 cm long) intracoronary thrombi followed by heparin, aspirin, and dipyridamole (45). After 0.3–4 days (mean 1.6 days) the patients returned to the catheterization laboratory. Eight demonstrated considerable or complete resolution of clot, and all eight underwent successful PTCA. Of the six patients with no demonstrated thrombolysis, two underwent successful PTCA, one had an unsuccessful attempt at PTCA and required surgery, one underwent bypass surgery without attempted PTCA, and two were treated conservatively (with one subsequent death).

Chapekis et al. administered 24 hr of intracoronary urokinase (100–120,000 unit bolus followed by 80–100,000 unit/hr infusion) to 10 patients with intracoronary thrombus (46). Eight of ten patients demonstrated complete resolution of thrombus, and all 10 underwent successful PTCA.

In the only controlled trial to date, Topol and colleagues randomized 40 patients with unstable angina to receive 150 mg of tPA intravenously or placebo

(47). All patients received aspirin and heparin. Subsequent PTCA was attempted in eight tPA patients and 11 control patients. None of the tPA patients and three of the controls experienced abrupt closure ($p = 0.11$). Successful PTCA was achieved in seven of the tPA (88%) and eight of the control (73%) patients ($p = 0.44$). In this regard, in a recently completed randomized, placebo-controlled trial of intravenous tPA in patients with unstable angina (prior to any further intervention), there were no important changes in stenosis severity following tPA in comparison to patients treated with aspirin and heparin (48).

Several groups have reported on the administration of thrombolytic therapy at the beginning of the PTCA procedure (47–49). Gulker and Heuer gave 100 patients undergoing PTCA 100,000 units of urokinase 10 min prior to balloon dilatation (49). The clinical status of the patients and the presence or absence of intracoronary thrombus were not delineated and no control patients were provided. Only 1 of the 100 patients developed an acute occlusion.

Ambrose and colleagues randomized 72 patients with unstable angina to either 150,000 units of intracoronary urokinase or placebo before PTCA (50). The rate of thrombus complicating PTCA was reduced from 32% to 12% ($p < 0.05$), but acute closures still occurred in three of the patients receiving urokinase and one patient who received placebo.

Finally, Zeiher et al. randomized 251 patients to receive either continuous intracoronary urokinase (5000 units/min) or intracoronary heparin (250 units/min) during PTCA (51). The prevalence of unstable angina in this group of patients was not specified. The rate of intracoronary thrombus formation, angiographic success, myocardial infarction, and vessel occlusion did not differ between the two groups.

Five published series have addressed the role of fibrinolytic therapy in managing thrombotic complications during PTCA (52–55). Suryapranata et al. administered 250,000 units of intracoronary streptokinase to 12 patients who developed acute closure (52). Nine of these patients underwent successful PTCA after thrombolysis, one suffered an infarction despite repeat PTCA, and the two remaining patients underwent urgent bypass surgery.

Haft and colleagues administered either 150–600,000 units of intracoronary streptokinase or 60–80 mg of intracoronary tPA to 36 patients who developed acute occlusion despite attempts to maintain patency with repeat dilatation (53). Twenty-six (72%) were successfully recanalized with thrombolysis. No analysis of the relative merits of streptokinase and tPA was provided.

Goudreau et al. administered intracoronary streptokinase (250–500,000 units) to 23 patients who had developed extensive intracoronary thrombus ($n = 12$), distal embolization ($n = 7$), or abrupt closure ($n = 4$) (54). Angiographic success was achieved in 22 (96%) of these patients. Four of these patients, however, developed enzymatic evidence of myocardial infarction.

Gulba et al. performed thrombolysis with 70 mg of intracoronary tPA in 27 patients with acute occlusion after PTCA (55). Antegrade blood flow was reestablished in 22 patients (81%), but follow-up angiography 24 hr later documented reocclusion in 12 (54.5%). All patients received adequate heparin therapy following fibrinolysis. The group with reocclusion had significantly higher levels of thrombin–antithrombin III complex, suggesting that continued thrombin production predisposes these patients to rethrombosis.

A recent carefully designed, retrospective study analyzed the angiographic and clinical outcome in 48 patients with an occlusive complication of PTCA treated with intracoronary urokinase (mean dose 141,000; range 100,000–250,000) (56). Eighteen subjects underwent PTCA in the setting of an acute myocardial infarction. Thrombolytic therapy reestablished antegrade flow in 90% of these subjects, and there were no procedure-related deaths or infarctions. Notably, no patient had evidence of reocclusion on follow-up angiography.

In summary, definitive evidence from a randomized, controlled clinical trial of the benefits of fibrinolysis preceding PTCA in patients with unstable angina is lacking. TIMI 3B is a large multicenter trial that will address this issue among others. The administration of fibrinolytic therapy at the beginning of the PTCA has been evaluated primarily in select patients, and therefore the proper role of this strategy in most patients with unstable angina is undefined. Finally, in patients who develop thrombotic occlusion during the course of PTCA, fibrinolysis is effective in reestablishing flow in the majority of patients. Many of these arteries, however, may reocclude within 24 hr. Insufficient data preclude the recommendation of any one agent or dosing regimen in these settings.

ANTI-ISCHEMIC THERAPY

Calcium Channel Blockers

Many studies have examined the ability of various calcium channel blockers to ameliorate the effects of ischemia during PTCA (57–70). As summarized in Table 3, varying doses of currently available agents were administered by the intracoronary, intravenous, or sublingual route. With few exceptions, these drugs were shown to reduce the degree of electrocardiographic (ECG) perturbation during balloon inflation (57,60,61,65,68), prolong the time to onset of angina (64,67), prolong the time to onset of ECG changes (58,64–67,70), decrease lactate production (59–61,63,64,68,70), and ameliorate left ventricular dysfunction (63,66). Five studies examining the impact of calcium channel blockers on collateral flow as assessed by great cardiac vein or coronary sinus blood flow during PTCA have yielded conflicting results (59,61–63,70).

In examining the most clinically relevant issue, available studies present conflicting data as to whether calcium channel blockers allow for longer balloon inflation. Five studies demonstrated that adjunctive intracoronary or intravenous calcium channel blockers facilitated longer balloon inflation (58,60,64,67,68). However, two studies failed to demonstrate a benefit in this regard with intra-

Table 3 Adjunctive Calcium-Channel-Blocker Therapy

Study	n	Agent	Dose, route	Lactate extraction	Time to angina	Time to ECG changes	Degree of ECG changes	Time to WMA	Degree of LV dysfunction	CSF	Inflation time	Angiographic outcome
Hombach (57)	12	Nifedipine	0.2 mg IC				+					
Erbel (58)	20	Nifedipine	20 mg SL			+ (8)					+ (18)	
Hanet (59)	12	Nicardipine	0.2 mg IC	+						0		
Horiuchi (60)	15	Nicardipine	0.1 mg IC	+			+				+ (11)	
Pop (61)	12	Nifedipine	0.2 mg IC	+			+					
Kern (62)	9	Nifedipine	10 mg SL			0				0		0
Perry (63)	12	Nifedipine	0.2 mg IC	+						+		
Werner (64)	20	Verapamil	0.1 mg IC		+	+ (40)			+		+ (25)	
Amende (65)	18	Nifedipine	0.1 mg IC			+ (10)	+					
Kern (66)	17	Diltiazem	10 mg and 0.5 mg/min IV			+ (14)		+ (12)	+			
Piessens (67)	42	Diltiazem	25 mg and 15 mg/hr IV		+ (24)	+ (15)						
Werner (68)	30	Verapamil	2 mg IC / 5 mg IV	+ / 0			+ / 0				+ (29) / 0	
Bonnier (69)	26	Diltiazem	0.4 mg/kg and 15 mg/hr IV				0				0	0
Feldman (70)	10	Nicardipine	2 mg and 25–50 µg/min IC		+					+		

IC = intracoronary; IV = iontravenous; SL = sublingual; CSF = coronary sinus flow; WMA = wall-motion abnormalities. Numbers in parentheses indicate change, in seconds.

348

venous diltiazem or verapamil (68,69). In the studies reporting a longer inflation time with calcium channel blocker therapy, the increase in inflation time ranged from 14 to 29 sec (58,60,64,67,68).

In the two studies reporting on angiographic outcome, neither study demonstrated improved results in treated patients compared to controls (61,69). It is important to note that none of the calcium channel blocker studies was undertaken in patients who had unstable angina. Furthermore, none of the studies enrolled patients who would likely experience deleterious hemodynamic consequences during PTCA. Therefore, the potential benefit of calcium channel blockers in ameliorating myocardial ischemia during PTCA, thereby preserving left ventricular function in patients with unstable angina, remains unproven.

Nitrates

As summarized in Table 4, 10 studies have evaluated the effects of nitrates in ameliorating ischemia during PTCA (60,62,63,65,71–76). Despite comparable regimens of nitroglycerin administration, the impact on lactate extraction (60,63), frequency or intensity of angina (75,76), time to onset of ischemic electrocardiographic changes (60,62,65,72,74), or degree of ischemic electrocardiographic changes (60,65) has been inconsistent. Only one study has reported a prolongation of inflation time (by 15 sec) with nitroglycerin (71). Similarly, evaluation of regional or global left ventricular systolic function has yielded mixed results (63,72,74). Each of the studies that has examined the impact of nitroglycerin on the degree or rapidity of elevation in left ventricular filling pressure during PTCA has reported a benefit (65,72–74). Only one study presented data on angiographic outcome and was unable to demonstrate a beneficial effect of buccal nitroglycerin (75). One study evaluated the relative merits of sublingual and intracoronary administration of nitrates as adjunctive therapy to PTCA (77). The primary success rates and the occurrence of major complications did not differ between these two routes of administration.

The ability of nitrates to prevent or reverse coronary vasospasm occurring in the course of PTCA has also been evaluated. Several studies have demonstrated the ability of intravenous nitroglycerin to prevent coronary artery vasoconstriction during PTCA (78,79). Furthermore, intracoronary nitroglycerin is generally successful in reversing vasoconstriction complicating PTCA (78,80). Several reports in the literature have described patients with intense coronary artery spasm unresponsive to intracoronary nitroglycerin (81,82). Such spasm has occurred in the setting of PTCA undertaken in patients with complex coronary artery lesions (81) or intracoronary thrombus (82), suggesting that humoral factors released from the thrombus may play a role in coronary vasoconstriction. In these cases the intracoronary administration of verapamil appeared to be effective in reversing vasospasm (81).

Table 4 Adjunctive Nitroglycerin Therapy

Study	n	Dose	Route	Time to angina	Degree of angina	Time to ECG changes	Degree of ECG changes	Degree of WMA	Time to or degree of ↑ LVEDP	Inflation time	Angiographic outcome
Horiuchi (60)	12	0.1 mg	IC	+		+ (8)	+				
Kern (62)	17	0.2 mg	IC			0					
Perry (63)	12	0.2 mg	IC					0			
Amende (65)	20	0.2 mg	IC/IV			0	0		+		
Schreiner (71)	33	0.2 mg	IC							+ (15)	
Doorey (72)	10	0.2 mg	IV	+ (29)		+ (32)		+	+		
Herrmann (73)	66	0.2 mg	IV/IC					+	+		
Darius (74)	24	0.2 mg	IC			+ (16)		+	+		
Johansson (75)	86	5 mg	B		+					0	
Feldman (76)	21	25 µg/min	IV		0						0

B = buccal; IC = intracoronary; IV = intravenous; LVEDP = left-ventricular end-diastolic pressure; WMA = wall motion abnormalities. Numbers in parentheses indicate change, in seconds.

350

Beta-Blockers

Two studies have examined the utility of beta-blockers as an adjunct to PTCA. Zalewski et al. administered 0.5–2.0 mg of intracoronary propranolol (83), and Feldman et al. administered 0.1 mg/kg intravenous propranolol (84). Propranolol was effective in prolonging the time to the development of ischemic electrocardiographic changes and reduced the intensity of angina as well as the degree of electrocardiographic changes. However, these results were not seen uniformly in all patients (84) and angiographic outcome was not improved (83). There are no data reporting the effects of adjunctive beta-blockade during PTCA in patients with unstable angina.

Perfluorochemicals

Eight studies, summarized in Table 5, have investigated the use of oxygenated perfluorochemical (Fluosol) infusion during PTCA (85–92). These studies uniformly used an intracoronary infusion rate of 60 ml/min. Fluosol infusion was associated with a delayed and diminished degree of anginal symptoms and ischemic electrocardiographic changes (85,90,92). Improved myocardial metabolic parameters could not be demonstrated (88), but the degree of regional left ventricular dysfunction during PTCA was diminished in most of the studies that examined this question (86,87,90–92). Two studies reported on the impact of Fluosol on balloon inflation time. One showed no benefit of Fluosol (90) whereas the other showed that inflation was 12 sec longer with Fluosol (85). In the only study reporting on angiographic outcome, Fluosol did not improve the result of PTCA (90).

Many of the studies evaluating the role of anti-ischemic therapy as an adjunct to PTCA share a common flaw in trial design. They compare the ischemic manifestations during a first "control" inflation to subsequent inflations during which the therapy is administered. It has been demonstrated in animals (93) and recently in humans (94) that a preconditioning effect may occur whereby even brief inflations lessen the deleterious effects of subsequent inflations. This is an important confounding variable. The very modest apparent benefits of anti-ischemic therapy may reflect the effects of preconditioning. Appropriate trial design should involve randomization to treatment and control groups before any inflations are performed or use a crossover design in which the sequence of control and drug inflations are randomly assigned. Several of the studies reviewed here have adhered to such protocols.

Another important issue—the effect of procedural success itself—must be noted in any discussion of approaches to the amelioration of ischemia in the setting of unstable angina. No better example exists of the risk/benefit profile of PTCA than the experience reported in patients with unstable angina and regional or global left ventricular dysfunction (95,96). The demonstrated immediate improvement in regional and global ventricular function in the subset of patients

Table 5 Adjunctive Perfluorochemical Therapy

Study	n	Dose	Lactate extraction	Time to angina	Intensity of angina	Time to ECG changes	Intensity of ECG changes	Degree of LV dysfunction	Degree of ↑ LVEDP	Inflation time	Angiographic outcome
Anderson (85)	34	60 ml/min		+ (8)	+		+			+ (12)	
Cleman (86)	20	60 ml/min						+			
Jaffe (87)	42	60 ml/min						+			
Young (88)	8	60 ml/min	0								
Bell (89)	10	60 ml/min							0		
Kent (90)	215	60 ml/min			+	+ (12)	+	+	0	0	
Young (91)	12	60 ml/min						+			
Cowley (92)	38	60 ml/min		0	0	+ (10)	+	+		0	0

LVEDP = left-ventricular end-diastolic pressure. Numbers in parentheses indicate change, in seconds.

with unstable angina undergoing PTCA, albeit with many of the adjunctive pharmacological agents described (calcium channel blockers, nitroglycerin, heparin, etc.), indicates the importance of restoration of normal coronary flow patterns in the ischemic segment. The prompt normalization of systolic function and reduction in end-diastolic and end-systolic dimensions consequent to improved function will of themselves lower myocardial oxygen requirements. However, failure to restore a normalized distribution of coronary flow and improved pump performance in these high-risk patients may have serious consequences (97), which emphasizes the importance of mechanical as well as pharmacological support of PTCA in this setting.

In summary, nitrates, calcium blockers, beta-blockers, and Fluosol administered during PTCA each uniquely mitigates measures of myocardial ischemia during balloon inflation. The benefits are modest and allow for small increases in balloon inflation time and no definitive evidence of improved angiographic outcome. Consequently, no regimen or agent can be recommended as superior to any other. The beneficial effects of nitroglycerin, whether administered intravenously or via the intracoronary route, in preventing or ameliorating vasospasm during PTCA are well established. The limited data on anti-ischemic pharmacological adjuncts to PTCA in patients with unstable angina support the intuitive notion that preservation of ischemic myocardium in these clinically and hemodynamically tenuous patients is beneficial. However, appropriate identification of these patients and optimal treatment agents remain the subject of further study.

In this discussion we have, of necessity, separated the pharmacological support of PTCA in patients with unstable angina into those components that represent the potential for procedural failure. It should be clear from the foregoing that anticoagulant, antiplatelet, fibrinolytic, and anti-ischemic agents are all necessary, although perhaps not sufficient, to provide optimal angiographic, hemodynamic, and clinical end-points. It should also be clear from this review that although many studies have examined these procedural components in populations of patients with unstable angina, there are not only important prognostic differences within this general category (98), but also scant data on underlying left ventricular function in these patients. Thus, the focus of future investigations should be directed toward the optimal means of providing clinically successful revascularization in high-risk subgroups. These issues become even more acute given the increasing proportion of patients with unstable angina who have multivessel disease and left ventricular dysfunction. Supported PTCA (pharmacological and mechanical-hemodynamic) in this latter setting approaches a complex level of strategic planning (99).

Given this increasing level of complexity (and risk), it is appropriate to consider the need for a randomized trial of surgical versus mechanical (PTCA) revascularization, if not in a clinically uniform population, then certainly in a well-defined and recognized high-risk subgroup with precise, clearly defined inclusion criteria and end-points. For example, attention to stratification of patients with reversibly injured (such as might occur after a non-Q-wave myocardial infarction) versus normally functioning myocardium would provide important insights into the mechanisms whereby ventricular function (and survival) improve with intervention. Similarly, the effect of providing revascularization to only the "culprit" region (provided the latter can be precisely defined) or region at highest risk of infarction leading to significant hemodynamic deterioration, versus providing revascularization to all potentially ischemic zones, could also be explored in such a study. Finally, the opportunity provided by such a study for the relation between structure (coronary anatomy) and function (myocardial function and metabolic activity) would enable investigators to more completely understand how ventricular myocardium adapts to varying degrees of ischemia and reperfusion.

REFERENCES

1. Falk E. Unstable angina with fatal outcome: Dynamic coronary thrombosis leading to infarction and/or sudden death. Circulation 1985; 71:699–708.
2. Ambrose JA, Winters SL, Stern A, et al. Angiographic morphology and the pathogenesis of unstable angina pectoris. J. Am Coll Cardiol 1985; 5:609–16.
3. Sherman CT, Litvack F, Grundfest W, et al. Coronary angioscopy in patients with unstable angina pectoris. N Engl J Med 1986; 315:913–9.
4. Fitzgerald DJ, Roy L, Catella F, Fitzgerald G. Platelet activation in unstable coronary disease. N Engl J Med 1986; 315:983–9.
5. Grande P, Grauholt AM, Madsen JK. Unstable angina pectoris: Platelet behavior and prognosis in progressive angina and intermediate coronary syndrome. Circulation 1990; 81(Suppl I):I16–9.
6. Ellis SG, Roubin GS, King SB, Douglas JS, Weintraub WS, Thomas RG, Cox WR. Angiographic and clinical predictors of acute vessel closure after native vessel coronary angioplasty. Circulation 1988; 77:372–9.
7. Myler RN, Shaw RE, Stertzer SH, Gashour TT, Ryan C, Hecht HS, Cumberland DC. Unstable angina and coronary angioplasty. Circulation 1990; 82(Suppl II):II88–95.
8. de Feyter PJ, Suryapranata H, Serruys PW, et al. Coronary angioplasty for unstable angina: Immediate and late results in 200 consecutive patients with identification of risk factors for unfavorable early and late outcome. J Am Coll Cardiol 1988; 12:324–33.
9. Detre K, Holubkov R, Kelsey S, et al. One year follow-up results of the 1985–86 National Heart, Lung, and Blood Institute's Percutaneous Transluminal Coronary Angioplasty Registry. Circulation 1989; 80:421–8.
10. Detre KM, Holmes DR, Holubkov R, et al. Incidence and consequences of periprocedural occlusion. The 1985–1986 National Heart, Lung, and Blood Institute Percutaneous Transluminal Coronary Angioplasty Registry. Circulation 1990; 82:739–50.
11. Laskey MA, Deutsch E, Hirshfeld JW, Kussmaul WG, Barnathan E, Laskey WK.

Influence of heparin therapy on percutaneous transluminal coronary angioplasty outcome in patients with coronary arterial thrombosis. Am J Cardiol 1990; 65:179–82.

12. Sugrue DD, Holmes DR, Smith HC, et al. Coronary artery thrombus as a risk factor for acute vessel occlusion during percutaneous coronary angioplasty. Improving results. Br Heart J 1986; 56:62–6.

13. VanHoutte PM, Houstin DS. Platelets, endothelium, and vasospasm. Circulation 1985; 72:728–34.

14. Davies MJ, Thomas AC. Plaque fissuring: Cause of acute myocardial infarction, sudden ischaemic death, and crescendo angina. Br Heart J 1985; 53:363–73.

15. Fischell TA, Derby G, Cse Tse, Stadius ML. Coronary artery vasoconstriction routinely occurs after percutaneous transluminal coronary angioplasty. A quantitative arteriographic analysis. Circulation 1988; 78:1323–34.

16. Lam JY, Chesebro JA, Fuster V. Platelets, vasoconstriction and nitroglycerin during arterial wall injury. A new antithrombotic role for an old drug. Circulation 1988; 78:712–6.

17. Douglas JS, Lutz JS, Clements SD, Robinson PH, Roubin GS, Lembo NJ, King SB. Therapy of large intracoronary thrombi in candidates for percutaneous transluminal coronary angioplasty. J Am Coll Cardiol 1988; 11(Suppl A):238A.

18. Pow TK, Varricchione TR, Jacobs AK, Ruocco NA, Ryan TJ, Christelis EM, Faxon DP. Does pretreatment with heparin prevent abrupt closure following PTCA? J Am Coll Cardiol 1988; 11(Suppl A):238A.

19. Hartman D, Wolf NM, Schechter JA, Sokil AB, Capone G, Meister SG. Effect of heparin on intracoronary thrombi in unstable ischemic syndromes. J Am Coll Cardiol 1986; 7(Suppl A):107A.

20. Hettleman BD, Aplin RL, Sullivan PR, Lemal H, O'Connor GT. Three days of heparin pretreatment reduces major complications of coronary angioplasty in patients with unstable angina. J Am Coll Cardiol 1990; 15(Suppl A):154A.

21. Laskey MA, Deutsch E, Barnathan E, Laskey WK. Influence of heparin therapy on percutaneous transluminal coronary angioplasty outcome in unstable angina pectoris. Am J Cardiol 1990; 65:1425–9.

22. Dean LS, Anderson JC, Garrahy PJ, Bulle TM, Baxley WA. Do standard heparin doses adequately protect patients during coronary angioplasty. Circulation 1989; 80(Suppl I):II-373.

23. Dougherty KG, Marsh KC, Edelman SK, Gaos CM, Ferguson JJ, Leachman DR. Relationship between procedural activated clotting time and in-hospital post PTCA outcome. Circulation 1990; 83(Suppl III):III-189.

24. Ogilby JD, Kopelman HA, Kline LW, Agarwal JB. Adequate heparinization during PTCA: Assessment using activated clotting time. J Am Coll Cardiol 1988; 11(Suppl A):237A.

25. Rath B, Bennett DH. Monitoring the effect of heparin by measurement of activated clotting time during and after percutaneous transluminal coronary angioplasty. Br Heart J 1990; 63:18–21.

26. Saenz CB, Baxley WA, Bulle TM, Cherre JM, Dean LS. Early and late effective heparin infusion following elective angioplasty. Circulation 1988; 78(Suppl II):II-98.

27. Ellis SG, Roubin GS, Wilentz J, Lin S, Douglas JS, King SB. Results of a

randomized trial of heparin and aspirin vs aspirin alone for prevention of acute closure and restenosis after angioplasty. Circulation 1987; 78(Suppl IV):IV-213.

28. McGarry T, Gottlieb R, Zelenkofske S, Duca P, Kasparian H, Kreulen T, Morganroth J. Relationship of anticoagulation level and complications after successful percutaneous transluminal coronary angioplasty. Circulation 1990; 82(Suppl III):III-189.

29. Heras M, Chesebro JH, Penny WJ, Bailey KR, Badimon L, Fuster V. Effects of thrombin inhibition on the development of acute platelet-thrombin deposition during angioplasty in pigs. Heparin versus hirudin, a specific thrombin inhibitor. Circulation 1989; 79:657–65.

30. Manson S, Marker L. Interception of acute platelet-dependent thrombosis by the synthetic anti-thrombin D-phenylalanyl-L-prolyl-L-arginyl chloromethyl ketone. Proc Natl Acad Sci USA 1988; 85:3184–8.

31. Leung WH, Kaplan AV, Grant GW, Leung LL, Fischell TA. Local delivery of anti-thrombin agent reduces platelet deposition at site of balloon angioplasty. Circulation 1990; 82(Suppl III):III-428.

32. Barnathan ES, Schwartz JS, Taylor L, Laskey WK, Kleaveland JP, Kussmaul WG, Hirshfeld JW. Aspirin and dipyridamole in the prevention of acute coronary thrombosis complicating coronary angioplasty. Circulation 1987; 76:125–34.

33. White CW, Chaitman B, Lassar TA, et al. Antiplatelet agents are effective in reducing the immediate complications of PTCA: Results from the Ticlopidine multicenter trial. Circulation 1987; 76(Suppl IV):IV-400.

34. Chesebro JH, Webster MW, Reeder GS., et al. Coronary angioplasty: Antiplatelet therapy reduces acute complications but not restenosis. Circulation 1989; 80(Suppl II):II-64.

35. Kent KM, Ewels CJ, Kehoe MK, Lavelle JP, Krucoff MW. Effect of aspirin on complications during transluminal coronary angioplasty. J Am Coll Cardiol 1988; 11(Suppl A):132A.

36. Bertrand ME, Allain H, Lablanche JM. Results of a randomized trial of Ticlopidine versus placebo for prevention of acute closure and restenosis after coronary angioplasty: The TACT study. Circulation 1990; 82(Suppl 3):III-190.

37. Bourassa MG, Schwartz L, David PR, et al. The role of antiplatelet agents in reducing periprocedural coronary angioplasty (PTCA) complications. J Am Coll Cardiol 1988; 11(Suppl A):238A.

38. Mufson L, Black A, Roubin G, et al. A randomized trial of aspirin in PTCA: Effect of high vs low dose aspirin on major complications and restenosis. J Am Coll Cardiol 1988; 11(Suppl A):236A.

39. Lembo NJ, Black AJ, Roubin GS, Mufson LH, Willentz JR, Douglas JS, King SB. Does addition of dipyridamole to aspirin decrease acute coronary angioplasty complications? The results of a prospective randomized clinical trial. J Am Coll Cardiol 1988; 11(Suppl A):237A.

40. Lam JY, Chesebro JH, Dewanjee MK, Badimon L, Fuster V. Ibuprofen: A potent anti-thrombotic agent for arterial injury after balloon angioplasty. J Am Coll Cardiol 1987; 9(Suppl A):64A.

41. Ellis SG, Navetta FI, Tcheng JT, Weisman HF, Wang AL, Pitt B, Topol EJ. Antiplatelet GP IIb/IIIa (7E3) antibody in elective PTCA: Safety and inhibition of platelet function. Circulation 1990; 82(Suppl III):III-191.

42. Timmermans C, Vanhaecke J, Vrolix M, Stammen F, Piessens J, DeGeest H. Ridogrel in the prevention of early acute reocclusion after coronary angioplasty. Circulation 1990; 82(Suppl III):III-190.

43. Runge MS. Prevention of thrombosis and rethrombosis. New approaches. Circulation 1990; 82:655–7.

44. Hurley DV, Bresnahan DR, Holmes DR. Staged thrombolysis and percutaneous transluminal coronary angioplasty for unstable and postinfarction angina. Cathet Cardiovasc Diagn 1989; 18:67–72.

45. Grill HP, Brinker JA. Nonacute thrombolytic therapy: An adjunct to coronary angioplasty in patients with large intravascular thrombi. Am Heart J 1989; 118: 662–7.

46. Chapekis AT, George BS, Candela RJ. Rapid thrombus dissolution by continuous infusion of urokinase through an intracoronary perfusion wire prior to PTCA: Results in native coronaries and patent saphenous vein grafts. J Am Coll Cardiol 1990; 15(Suppl A):154A.

47. Topol EJ, Nicklas JM, Kander NH, Walton JA, Ellis SG, Gorman L, Pitt B. Coronary revascularization after intravenous tissue plasminogen activator for unstable angina pectoris: results of a randomized, double-blind, placebo-controlled trial. Am J Cardiol 1988; 62:368–71.

48. Williams DO, Topol EJ, Califf RM, et al. Intravenous recombinant tissue-type plasminogen activator in patients with unstable angina pectoris. Results of a placebo-controlled, randomized trial. Circulation 1990; 82:376–83.

49. Gulker H, Heuer H. Prophylactic use of combined heparine-urokinase for the prevention of coronary artery occlusion following percutaneous transluminal coronary angioplasty. J Am Coll Cardiol 1988; 11(Suppl A):128A.

50. Ambrose JA, Torre SR, Sharma S, et al. A double blind randomized trial of low dose intracoronary urokinase during angioplasty in unstable angina. Circulation 1990; 82(Suppl III):III-190.

51. Zeiher AM, Kasper W, Gaissmaier C, Wollschlager H. Concomitant intracoronary treatment with urokinase during PTCA does not reduce acute complications during PTCA: A double blind randomized study. Circulation 1990; 82(Suppl III):III-189.

52. Suryapranata H, deFeyter PJ, Serruys PW. Coronary angioplasty in patients with unstable angina pectoris: is there a role for thrombolysis? J Am Coll Cardiol 1988; 12(Suppl A):69A–77A.

53. Haft JI, Goldstein JE, Homoud MK, Aaronoff M. PTCA following myocardial infarction: Use of bailout fibrinolysis to improve results. Am Heart J 1990; 120:243–7.

54. Goudreau E, DiSciascio G, Vetrovec GW, Nath A, Cowley MJ. The role of intracoronary urokinase in combination with coronary angioplasty in patients with complex lesion morphology. J Am Coll Cardiol 1990; 15(Suppl A):154A.

55. Gulba DC, Daniel WG, Simon R, et al. Role of thrombolysis and thrombin in patients with acute coronary occlusion during percutaneous transluminal coronary angioplasty. J Am Coll Cardiol 1990; 16:563–8.

56. Schieman G, Cohen BM, Kozina J, et al. Intracoronary urokinase for intracoronary thrombus accumulation complicating percutaneous transluminal coronary angioplasty in acute ischemic syndromes. Circulation 1990; 82:2052–60.

57. Hombach V, Hopp HW, Fuchs M, Behrenbech DW, Tauchert M, Hilger HH.

Beneficial effects of intracoronary nifedipine during percutaneous transluminal coronary angioplasty. Herz 1986; 11:232–6.

58. Erbel R, Huttemann M, Schreiner G, Darius N, Pop T, Meyer J. Ischamietoleranz des herzens wahrend perkutaner transluminaler koronarangioplastie. Herz 1987; 12:302–11.

59. Hanet C, Rousseau MF, Vincent MF, Lavenne-Pardonge E, Pouleur H. Myocardial protection by intracoronary Nicardipine during percutaneous transluminal coronary angioplasty. Am J Cardiol 1987; 59:1035–40.

60. Horiuchi K, Mizuno K, Matsuih, et al. Improved ischemic tolerance during percutaneous transluminal coronary angioplasty by antianginal agents. Circulation 1987; 76(Suppl IV):IV-275.

61. Pop G, Serruys PW, Piscione F, et al. Regional cardioprotection by sub-elective intracoronary nifedipine is not due to enhanced collateral flow during coronary angioplasty. Int J Cardiol 1987; 16:27–41.

62. Kern MJ, Deligonul U, Labovitz A, Gabliani G, Vandormael M, Kennedy HL. Effects of nitroglycerin and nifedipine on coronary and systemic hemodynamics during transient coronary artery occlusion. Am Heart J 1988; 115:1164–70.

63. Perry RA, Wankling PF, Seth A, Hunt AC, Shiu MF. The effects of intracoronary nitrate and nifedipine on regional wall motion, coronary flow and myocardial metabolism during angioplasty. Circulation 1988; 78(Suppl II):II-103.

64. Werner GS, Schmid M, Klein HH, Wiegand V, Kreuzer H, Tebbe U. Die kardioprotektive wirkung von verapamil bei perkutaner transluminaler koronarangioplastie. Z Kardiol 1988; 77:728–35.

65. Amende I, Herrmann G, Simon R, Lichtlen PR. Modification of myocardial ischemia and dysfunction by nifedipine and nitroglycerin during coronary occlusion. J Am Coll Cardiol 1989; 13(Suppl A):154A.

66. Kern MJ, Pearson A, Woodruff R, Deligonul U, Vandormael M, Labovitz A. Hemodynamic and echocardiographic assessment of the effects of Diltiazem during transient occlusion of the left anterior descending coronary artery during percutaneous transluminal coronary angioplasty. Am J Cardiol 1989; 64:849–55.

67. Piessens J, Brzostek T, Stammen F, Vanhaecke J, Vrolix M, DeGeest H. Effect of intravenous Diltiazem on myocardial ischemia occurring during percutaneous transluminal coronary angioplasty. Am J Cardiol 1989; 64:1103–7.

68. Werner GS, Schmid M, Kline HH, Wiegand V, Kreuzer H, Tebbe U. Verapamil as a potent cardioprotective agent for coronary angioplasty: First clinical experience. J Am Coll Cardiol 1989; 13(Suppl A):154A.

69. Bonnier JJ, Huizer T, Troquaer, van Es G, deJong JW. Myocardial protection by intravenous Diltiazem during angioplasty of single-vessel coronary artery disease. Am J Cardiol 1990; 66:145–50.

70. Feldman RL, MacDonald RG, Hill TA, Pepine CJ. Effect of nicardipine on determinants of myocardial ischemia occurring during acute coronary occlusion produced by percutaneous transluminal coronary angioplasty. Am J Cardiol 1987: 60:267–70.

71. Schreiner G, Erbel R, Henkel B, Pop T, Meyer J. Improved ischemic tolerance during percutaneous coronary angioplasty by antianginal drugs. Eur Heart J 1984; 5(Suppl I):39.

72. Doorey AJ, Mehmel HC, Schwarz FX, Kubler W. Amelioration by nitroglycerin of

left ventricular ischemia induced by percutaneous transluminal coronary angioplasty: Assessment by hemodynamic variables and left ventriculography. J Am Coll Cardiol 1985; 6:267–74.

73. Herrmann G, Simon R, Lichtlen PR. Intracoronary vs intravenous nitroglycerin during coronary angioplasty. Eur Heart J 1985; 6(Suppl I):24.

74. Darius H, Schmucker B. Antianginal agents administered intracoronarily ameliorate functional impairment and extend time to ischemia during PTCA. Circulation 1987; 76(Suppl IV):IV-275.

75. Johansson SR, Ekstrom L, Emanuelsson H. Buccal nitroglycerin decreases ischemic pain during coronary angioplasty: A double-blind, randomized, placebo-controlled study. Am Heart J 1990; 120:275–81.

76. Feldman RL, Joyal M, Conti CA, Pepine CJ. Effects of nitroglycerin on coronary collateral flow and pressure during acute coronary occlusion. Am J Cardiol 1984; 54:958–63.

77. Finci L, Meier B, Ruiz J, et al. Nitrates before coronary angioplasty: Sublingual versus intracoronary administration. Eur Heart J 1987; 8(Suppl I):76.

78. Fischell TA, Nellessen U, Johnson DE, Ginsburg R. Endothelium-dependent arterial vasoconstriction after balloon angioplasty. Circulation 1989; 79:899–910.

79. Fischell TA, Derby G, Tse TM, Stadius ML. Intravenous nitroglycerin prevents coronary artery vasoconstriction after PTCA. J Am Coll Cardiol 1989; 13(Suppl A):59A.

80. Margolis JR, Chen C. Coronary artery spasm complicating PTCA: Role of intracoronary nitroglycerin. Z Kardiol 1989; 78(Suppl II):41–4.

81. Babbitt DG, Perry JM, Forman MB. Intracoronary verapamil for reversal of refractory coronary vasospasm during percutaneous transluminal coronary angioplasty. J Am Coll Cardiol 1988; 12:1377–81.

82. Wilson RF, Laxson DD, Lesser JR, White CW. Intense microvascular constriction after angioplasty of acute thrombotic coronary arterial lesions. Lancet 1989; 1:807–11.

83. Zalewski A, Goldberg S, Dervan JP, Slysh S, Maroko PR. Myocardial protection during transient coronary artery occlusion in man: Beneficial effects of regional β-adrenergic blockade. Circulation 1986; 73:734–9.

84. Feldman RL, MacDonald RG, Hill JA, Limacher MC, Conti CR, Pepine CJ. Effect of propranolol on myocardial ischemia during acute coronary occlusion. Circulation 1986; 73:727–33.

85. Anderson HV, Leimgruber PT, Roubin GS, Nelson DL, Gruentzig AR. Distal coronary artery perfusion during percutaneous transluminal coronary angioplasty. Am Heart J 1985; 110:720–6.

86. Cleman N, Jaffee C, Wohlgelernter D. Prevention of ischemia during percutaneous transluminal coronary angioplasty by transcatheter infusion of oxygenated Fluosol DA 20%. Circulation 1986; 74:555–62.

87. Jaffe CC, Wohlgelernter D, Cabin H, Bowman L, Deckelbaum L, Remetz M, Cleman M. Presentation of left ventricular ejection fraction during percutaneous transluminal coronary angioplasty by distal transcatheter coronary perfusion of oxygenated Fluosol DA 20%. Am Heart J 1988; 115:1156–64.

88. Young LH, Bowman LK, Revkin JH, Jaffee CC, Barrett EJ, Cabin HS, Cleman M. Cardiac metabolism during coronary angioplasty with Fluosol protection: discor-

dance between LV systolic function and lactate metabolism. J Am Coll Cardiol 1988; 11(Suppl A):149A.

89. Bell MR, Nishimura RA, Holmes DR, Bailey KR, Schwartz RS, Vlietstra RE. Does intracoronary infusion of Fluosol-DA 20% prevent left ventricular diastolic dysfunction during coronary balloon angioplasty? J Am Coll Cardiol 1990; 16:959–66.

90. Kent KM, Cleman MW, Cowley MJ, et al. Reduction of myocardial ischemia during percutaneous transluminal coronary angioplasty with oxygenated Fluosol. Am J Cardiol 1990; 66:279–84.

91. Young LH, Jaffe CC, Revkin JH, McNulty PH, Cleman M. Metabolic and functional effects of perfluorocarbon distal perfusion during coronary angioplasty. Am J Cardiol 1990; 65:986–90.

92. Cowley MJ, Snow FR, DiSciascio G, Kelly K, Guard C, Nixon JV. Perfluorochemical perfusion during coronary angioplasty in unstable and high-risk patients. Circulation 1990; 81(Suppl IV):IV-27–34.

93. Murry CE, Jennings, RB, Reimer KA. Preconditioning with ischemia: A delay of lethal cell injury in ischemic myocardium. Circulation 1986; 74:1124–36.

94. Deutsch E, Berger M, Kussmaul WG, Hirshfeld JW, Herrmann HC, Laskey WK. Adaptation to ischemia during PTCA: Clinical, hemodynamic and metabolic features. Circulation 1990; 82:2044–51.

95. Carlson EB, Cowley MJ, Wolfgang TC, Vetrovec GW. Acute changes in global and regional rest left ventricular function after successful coronary angioplasty in stable and unstable angina. J Am Coll Cardiol 1989; 13:1262–9.

96. de Feyter PJ, Suryapranata H, Serruys PW, Beatt K, van den Brand M, Hugenholtz PG. Effects of successful percutaneous transluminal coronary angioplasty on global and regional left ventricular function in unstable angina pectoris. Am J Cardiol 1987; 60:993–7.

97. Kohli RS, DiSciascio G, Cowley MJ, Nath A, Goudreau E, Vetrovec GW. Coronary angioplasty in patients with severe left ventricular dysfunction. J Am Coll Cardiol 1990; 16:807–11.

98. Braunwald E. Unstable angina. A classification. Circulation 1989; 80:410–4.

99. Wohlgelernter D, Highman MA, Cleman M, Zaret BL. Percutaneous transluminal coronary angioplasty of the culprit lesion for management of unstable angina pectoris in patients with multivessel coronary disease. Am J Cardiol 1986; 58:460–4.

19

Bridging Techniques to Emergent Surgical Revascularization After Failed Angioplasty

David William Nelson

University of California, Davis
Sacramento, California

Alden H. Harken

University of Colorado Health Sciences Center
Denver, Colorado

INTRODUCTION

Percutaneous transluminal coronary angioplasty (PTCA) has developed from a technique used primarily for isolated, proximal stenoses in patients with stable angina, to wider applications, including multiple-vessel disease and clinical presentations of unstable angina. Lesions seen in patients with unstable angina are frequently more severe, longer, and more eccentric than lesions seen in stable patients. With the increasing use of coronary angioplasty in the more complex variants of coronary artery disease, techniques to stabilize the patient and optimize myocardial oxygenation prior to possible emergent surgical revascularization take on critical importance. Although PTCA is performed successfully in the vast majority of patients, the technique carries an inherent risk of coronary arterial injury or plaque disruption, with the consequent compromise of myocardial blood flow and ischemia. Urgent myocardial revascularization is the accepted therapy for the patient with acute ischemia following failed PTCA. A number of techniques are available to stabilize the patient, improve myocardial oxygenation, preserve cardiac muscle, and optimize the chances for a successful revascularization.

The purpose of this chapter is to examine available ''bridging techniques'' to emergent surgical revascularization after failed angioplasty. In so doing we propose: (a) to stratify the characteristics of patients at increased risk of angioplasty failure; (b) to explore the anatomical risks of PTCA; (c) to examine the opportunity to prevent PTCA complications in patients at high risk; (d) to review the mortality associated with attempted rescue of patients undergoing emergent surgical revascularization following failed PTCA; (e) to encourage early utilization of reperfusion "bailout" catheters in failed PTCA; (f) to examine the theoretical and clinical advantages of high-oxygen-avidity perfluorochemical perfusion of the acutely ischemic distal coronary circulation; (g) to catalogue the benefits of mechanical intra-aortic balloon support; (h) to describe the appeal of percutaneous cardiopulmonary bypass support; (i) to explain the rationale of mechanical ventricular assist devices; and (j) to explore the value of mechanically "supported" angioplasty in high-risk patients.

RISK STRATIFICATION

The potential complications of PTCA include coronary artery dissection, perforation, and occlusion, which can lead to myocardial infarction and death (1,2). Because of these risks, PTCA is usually performed with some form of cardiac surgical standby, although emergency surgery is infrequently necessary. In a recent review, 5.7% of PTCAs required emergent coronary artery bypass graft surgery (CABG). The mortality rate for the emergent surgical revascularizations was 5.9% (Table 1) (3). The National Heart, Lung, and Blood Institute Percutaneous Transluminal Coronary Angioplasty Registry reported that emergency CABG was performed in 6.6% of patients undergoing PTCA, and the mortality rate with emergency CABG was 6.4% (4). The incidence of perioperative myocardial infarction following PTCA is reported between 30 and 50% (5–7). It is believed that most patients who undergo CABG and exhibit a perioperative myocardial infarction have the infarction in the catheterization laboratory, and surgery is performed during evolving infarction (4). Although emergency operation for acute ischemia may not eliminate the development of myocardial damage in all patients, evidence suggests that prompt revascularization can avert irreversible ischemic injury in many patients who suffer substantial ischemic insults.

For the patient who undergoes PTCA and suffers a complication, the most frequent indication for emergency revascularization is coronary dissection. In clinical reviews (4,8,9), this appears to be the etiology in 45–60% of acute occlusions. Plaque disruption was seen in 15–20% and unrelieved spasm in 3–12%. Unknown or unidentified causes make up the remainder. The clinical presentation includes constant or recurrent angina in 80–95%, electrocardiographic (ECG) changes suggestive of ischemia in up to 80%, and development of hypotension with cardiogenic shock in 20–25% of patients who require emergent CABG (7,8,10). Murphy et al. at Emory University identify the indications for revascularization following PTCA in two groups of patients: (a) patients with coronary arterial injury resulting in ischemic pain associated with ECG changes of ischemia, and (b) patients with coronary arterial injury and

Table 1 Review of PTCA Failures and Emergent Surgical Revascularizations Reported in the Literature

First author[a]	PTCAs	Emergency operations		AMIs		Deaths	
Bredlau	3,502	92	(2.7%)	47	(51%)	2	(2.0%)
Acinapura	198	21	(10.0%)	8	(38.1%)	0	
Akins	125	11	(8.8%)	—[b]		0	
Brahos	323	68	(21.0%)	—[b]		3	(4.4%)
Cowley	3,079	202	(6.6%)	83	(41.1%)	13	(6.4%)
Killen	3,000	115	(3.8%)	46	(40.0%)	13	(11.3%)
Pelletier	265	35	(13.2%)	10	(28.6%)	0	
Reul	518	70	(13.5%)	23	(32.8%)	4	(5.7%)
Smith	510	48	(9.4%)	16	(33.3%)	2	(4.2%)
Norell	69	13	(19.0%)	3	(23.1%)	1	(8.0%)
Page	750	31	(4.1%)	13	(41.9%)	3	(10.0%)
Kabbani	600	38	(6.3%)	—[b]		—[b]	
Fournial	74	10	(13.5%)	2	(20.0%)	0	
Golding	1,831	81	(4.4%)	—[b]		2	(2.5%)
Parsonnet	958	67	(7.0%)	19	(28.3%)	8	(11.9%)
Totals	15,802	902	(5.7%)	170	(5.9%)	51	(18.8%)

[a] Only the latest reports from an institution were selected. For example, a detailed study of 866 PTCAs by Murphy and colleagues from Emory University was not tabulated because it was superseded by that of Bredlau and associates.
[b] No information given.
AMI = acute myocardial infarction.
Source: Parsonnet V, Fisch D, Gielchinsky I, et al. Emergency operation after failed angioplasty. J Thorac Cardiovasc Surg 1988; 96:198–203, with permission.

acute ischemic pain in the absence of ECG changes if the extent of myocardium in jeopardy is likely to be clinically significant (11). They state that both these groups are best served by urgent surgical revascularization.

The usual scenario for emergent revascularization following attempted PTCA is ischemic cardiac pain as a result of interruption of flow in the instrumented artery. Immediate approaches to this problem are somewhat limited. The arterial dissection or occlusion may have an element of coronary artery spasm. Administration of calcium channel blockers (nifedipine) and intracoronary nitroglycerin may alleviate coronary spasm in some cases, although the relief is usually transient. Intravenous thrombolytic therapy has been used in some cases, with variable success (12,13). The ischemia is usually unresponsive to these measures as thrombosis or spasm is not typically the principal cause of the abrupt closure. In most cases, the inciting event is an intimal tear (14). With the persistence of the ischemic process, emergency revascularization is undertaken.

RISKS OF EMERGENT SURGERY

Emergency surgical revascularization for the patient who suffers an acute isch-emic insult secondary to failed PTCA has a significantly greater risk of operative death and perioperative infarction than elective CABG (10). Various studies have compared elective CABG patients to similar patients who failed angioplasty and then required emergent CABG. Patient profiles were similar in age, sex, ejection fraction, and number of diseased vessels. Significant differences were seen in mortality (1–1.5% versus 11–12%) and perioperative myocardial infarc-tion rate (6–9% versus 22–28%) (3,10). Despite the relatively low-risk status of many patients before coronary angioplasty, the acute ischemic insult suffered during a failed PTCA may change the factors that portend a favorable outcome.

The group of patients undergoing emergent PTCA who are evolving a myo-cardial infraction present an even higher risk. Emergent CABG on patients after unsuccessful emergent PTCA is associated with several potential complicating factors. These adverse factors include prolonged ischemia prior to surgical revascularization, the frequent presence of systemic thrombolysis, and a less hemodynamically stable patient (15). The significant difference in mortality and morbidity in patients who undergo emergent CABG after failed PTCA compared to those who undergo elective CABG emphasizes the importance of techniques to minimize post-PTCA ischemia in patients who require emergent surgical revascularization.

PREVENTION

One possible way to decrease the mortality and morbidity of emergent CABG after PTCA is to identify and avoid patients at prohibitive risk of ischemic injury during PTCA. Factors that place patients at increased risk include: (a) absence of visible collateral circulation to the coronary artery involved, and (b) extent of the coronary disease, including increased lesion eccentricity (4,16). Murphy et al. also suggest that identification of the high-risk patient is aided by: (a) measure-ment via the PTCA catheter of low pressure in the artery distal to the stenosis prior to performance of angioplasty, and (b) occurrence of pain and ST-T signs of ischemia when the PTCA balloon is inflated and the artery is completely obstructed (11). Others have noted that previous CABG may be a significant predictor of operative death in patients requiring emergent surgical revasculariza-tion after failed angioplasty (7), and patients undergoing multivessel PTCA who subsequently require emergency CABG are at a higher risk for a myocardial infarction (17). In the National Heart, Lung, and Blood Institute Registry, procedural factors associated with an increased likelihood of emergency CABG were: (a) inability to pass the stenosis (39 versus 25%), and (b) inability to dilate the lesion once it was traversed (30 versus 8%) (4). With an increased awareness of the factors that place a patient at increased risk, the need for emergent surgical intervention may become gratifyingly rare.

Coronary angioplasty is successful in the majority of patients who undergo the procedure. In the instance of complicated PTCA failure, emergent surgical revascularization is the accepted treatment. The risk of emergency surgery is determined by several factors, including the hemodynamic stability of the patient prior to operation. The ischemic insult of failed PTCA may lead to angina, myocardial infarction, arrhythmias, hypotension with cardiovascular collapse, and ultimately death. The ability to stabilize the patient while minimizing the ischemic insult is pivotal to successful rescue. The optimal mode of stabilization must be individualized. A number of different "bridging" techniques to reduce the risk of emergency surgery for complications of PTCA will be reviewed.

REPERFUSION CATHETERS

The major complication of coronary artery occlusion during PTCA is usually a result of arterial dissection, coronary artery spasm, or thrombosis (4,8,9). Techniques to reestablish blood flow, and thereby improve the outcome of the emergent surgical revascularization, have been investigated. In 1985, Hinohara et al. (18) described a percutaneously introduced stenting perfusion catheter to reestablish blood flow prior to emergent bypass surgery. The catheter was a 3.5-Fr catheter with 36 sideholes, through which passive aortocoronary blood flow could be achieved if positioned across the lesion and if adequate systemic blood pressure was present. The current reperfusion catheter is similar to the original catheter, but it also has an angioplasty balloon which allows prolonged inflation. The catheter allows blood to flow through sideholes in the catheter proximal to the inflated angioplasty balloon, through a central lumen in the catheter, and to the myocardium distal to the inflated balloon via distal sideholes and an endhole (Fig. 1) (19). Thus, the reperfusion catheter is designed to achieve flow to myocardium distal to the obstruction. The catheter may also function as a stent by coapting the intimal flap against the vessel wall (20). As the occurrence of myocardial infarction and mortality during emergent surgical revascularization following failed PTCA may be dependent on the duration of ischemia, the use of the reperfusion catheter appears to have a positive influence on surgical outcome. A technique that can maintain adequate coronary blood flow may permit a more optimal revascularization by expanding the options for vascular conduits such as the internal mammary artery (IMA) (21).

Use of a reperfusion catheter should be considered in its proper sequence. Acute occlusion of a coronary artery during PTCA may be caused by dissection, spasm, or thrombosis at the angioplasty site. Treatment with repeat balloon dilatation, coronary vasodilators, or thrombolytic therapy may be successful (22,23). However, as acute occlusion is most often secondary to dissection,

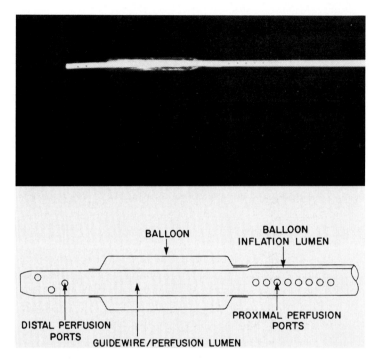

Figure 1 Photograph and schematic diagram of the distal end of an autoperfusion catheter. [*From* Turi et al. (19), by permission of the American Heart Association, Inc.]

refractory occlusion may occur despite the above-mentioned interventions. An attempt to insert a reperfusion catheter may be made at this time. Insertion should not be attempted unless the guidewire is clearly visualized in the true lumen distal to the obstruction (20).

The reperfusion catheter can be seen as a method for maintaining coronary blood flow and thus avoiding myocardial injury while the patient is prepared for emergency surgical revascularization. Studies have reported an approximate time from acute occlusion to surgical revascularization of 150 min (24,25). Successful use of the reperfusion catheter can reduce the ischemia time. In the series by Ferguson et al. (26), time from occlusion of the artery until catheter reperfusion was 20 min or less. Maintenance of blood flow after failed PTCA should reduce the morbidity and mortality of emergent revascularization and allow the performance of a more optimal procedure with the use of the IMA.

As with any invasive technique, there are complications associated with the use of a reperfusion catheter (14,18,20). In attempts to place the catheter, it may not be possible to recross the zone of occlusion with a wire. If the guidewire is secured across the obstruction, excessive tortuosity or angulation of the target vessel may not allow the catheter to be passed distally. If the catheter is successfully placed, adequate systemic blood pressure (>80 mm) is required for effective perfusion. Effective perfusion may not be achieved in instances of diffusely diseased vessels or small-caliber arteries because the catheter itself may be obstructive. The catheter may not function in patients with preexistent thrombus, and the catheter itself is predisposed to thrombotic occlusion most likely secondary to relative stagnation of flow. The risk of new thrombus formation increases with the length of time the catheter is in place. In addition, the placement of the catheter itself can damage the coronary artery and cause dissection or perforation. With these caveats in mind, the effectiveness of the reperfusion catheter has been studied.

The initial point to evaluate in ascertaining the efficacy of reperfusion catheters is the ability to successfully place them at the time of failed angioplasty. Successful catheter placement varies between 50 and 100% (26–28), with several series reporting rates > 90%. Successful catheter placement in patients has been shown to improve angina and normalize ST changes compared to matched controls who did not have the reperfusion catheter placed (27). In this study (27), however, no difference was seen in frequency of Q-wave infarction, and there were no catheter-related complications. The authors concluded that the catheters appeared to be safe and effective in reducing the signs and symptoms of myocardial ischemia, although the catheters may not prevent infarction in some patients and may be ineffective when systemic hypotension occurs. In another study (28), use of a reperfusion catheter was compared to intra-aortic balloon counterpulsation, and no therapy. The authors stated that the benefit of the catheter was evident in a significantly lower incidence of Q-wave infarctions (9 versus 75%) compared with patients managed with intra-aortic balloon counterpulsation alone. These results must be analyzed taking into account a catheter placement success rate of only 48%. These placement failures were then placed into the other treatment groups. The failure of catheter placement suggests a more severe lesion, which may have skewed the results by comparing mild disease (successful placement) versus more severe disease (other treatment). In the series by Hinohara et al., nine patients who failed PTCA all had successful catheter placement. In all patients, the restoration of blood flow was accompanied by resolution of ischemic symptoms and ECG changes. There were no catheter-related complications (26).

The reperfusion catheter is designed to achieve blood flow to myocardium distal to an obstruction. The catheter may also work as a stent by holding the intimal flap or dissection that is causing the acute occlusion against the vessel wall. If the catheter can be successfully placed, and adequate systemic blood pressure (>80 mm) is present, use of the reperfusion catheter can reduce the time during which acute ischemia is present. The reperfusion catheter appears to be safe and effective in reducing the signs and symptoms of myocardial ischemia, although the catheter may not prevent infarction in some patients and may be ineffective when systemic hypotension occurs. In cases where a catheter cannot be passed, or systemic hypotension is present, other "bridging" techniques should be utilized.

ALTERNATIVE OXYGEN CARRIERS

One of the limitations of the reperfusion catheter is that it is predisposed to thrombotic occlusion, secondary to relative stagnation of flow. Blood perfusion through the lumen of the balloon catheter is limited by this complication. Other oxygen carriers have been examined for various applications. Perfluorochemical emulsions have a uniquely high avidity for oxygen (29). This is beneficial in loading oxygen into the perfusate, but discourages oxygen release at the tissue level. Fluosol DA 20% is a specific oxygen-carrying fluorocarbon that has several favorable characteristics permitting its use during perfusion. These favorable characteristics include the following (27,30). (a) When oxygenated to a PO_2 of 600 mm Hg, it has an oxygen delivery capacity similar to that of whole blood at a HCT of 43%. (b) It has a CO_2 affinity comparable to whole blood, allowing it to efficiently remove CO_2 from ischemic regions. (c) The viscosity of Fluosol is approximately 50% of whole blood at body temperature. It also has a small particle size of 0.1–0.2 μm, approximately 1/70 the volume of a red blood cell. These features may allow delivery to small capillary beds not normally perfused.

The efficacy of Fluosol was initially examined in dog studies. Spears et al. have shown that distal infusion of oxygenated Fluosol during PTCA balloon occlusion for as long as 45 min in dogs could be performed safely and resulted in protection against myocardial ischemia (31). Cowley et al. performed a human study to assess the effects of Fluosol perfusion on amelioration of myocardial ischemia during coronary angioplasty in unstable and high-risk patients (32). In this study, patients received alternate 90-sec balloon inflations with and without distal perfusion of Fluosol at 60 ml/min. No adverse effects were encountered with Fluosol perfusion. Cardiac output decreased less with Fluosol perfusion than with routine inflation (-0.8 versus -1.2 L/min). The most pronounced beneficial effects of Fluosol perfusion were appreciated with 2-D echocardiographic evaluation of changes in global and regional left ventricular function. The authors concluded that distal coronary perfusion with Fluosol during PTCA in unstable and higher-risk patients was associated with reduction of balloon-induced myocardial ischemia determined by preservation of cardiac output and of global and regional left ventricular function. Other groups have reported only limited success with perfusion of Fluosol and have noted the complication of ventricular arrhythmias (33,34).

Another oxygen carrier that appears promising is stroma-free hemoglobin (SFH). SFH typically exists as a monomer that is rapidly cleared by the kidney. Gould, Moss, et al. have developed a polymerized SFH solution that achieves the goals of a normal hemoglobin concentration of 15 g/dl, a normal colloid

oncotic pressure of 20 torr, and is a sufficiently large molecule to avoid glomeru-
lar filtration (29,35). Poly SFH-P is an effective oxygen carrier and continues to
undergo evaluation.

Perfusion of Fluosol during PTCA reduces balloon-induced myocardial ischemia as determined by preservation of cardiac output and of global and regional
left ventricular function during balloon occlusion. A successfully placed reperfusion catheter, combined with distal perfusion of oxygenated Fluosol, may decrease the complication of thrombotic occlusion of the catheter when used in
failed PTCA. The use of Fluosol, with its high oxygen-carrying capacity, low
viscosity, and small particle size, may thus improve the chances of a successful
surgical outcome when used in this capacity. The combined use of the reperfusion catheter and distal Fluosol or polymerized SFH infusion in failed PTCA
deserves further clinical examination. There are no studies at this time.

INTRA-AORTIC BALLOON PUMP

For the patient who undergoes PTCA and suffers a complication, the most
frequent indication for emergency revascularization is coronary dissection. In
cases of acute coronary occlusion, placement of a reperfusion catheter may be
attempted with various rates of success. The clinical presentation includes the
development of hypotension with cardiogenic shock in 20–25% of patients, in
which case a reperfusion catheter would be ineffective. Other therapies are
needed to stabilize the patient, improve myocardial oxygenation, and limit the
ischemic insult. The intra-aortic balloon pump (IABP), which was introduced by
Moulopoulos and colleagues in 1962 (36), is the most widely used temporary
mechanical assist device. The IABP works by two complementary principles of
diastolic augmentation and presystolic unloading. Harken (37) and Kantrowitz
(38) initially demonstrated that the failing left ventricle could be positively
influenced by augmenting the diastolic pressure. The IABP is positioned in the
descending thoracic aorta (Fig. 2). The balloon is rapidly inflated during diastole, which is hemodynamically comparable to instantaneously infusing 40 ml
(the balloon volume) of blood. An augmented coronary perfusion pressure is
seen at the coronary ostiae (Fig. 3). Just prior to systole, the balloon is actively
deflated leaving a 40-ml void, allowing the forthcoming ventricular ejection to
pass unhindered. When the IABP is properly synchronized to the electrocardiogram, the balloon should both increase diastolic blood flow and reduce left
ventricular work (39). Thus, the IABP has several potential beneficial effects
(40–45): (a) augmentation of diastolic pressure (Fig. 4) can increase coronary
perfusion which may reduce the extent of myocardial necrosis, and (b) the
deflation of the balloon just prior to systole reduces left ventricular work (note
reduction in peak systolic pressure with use of IABP; Fig. 3). This reduction in
cardiac work and oxygen demand may be beneficial in preserving myocardium
distal to an acute coronary artery occlusion, even without an augmentation in

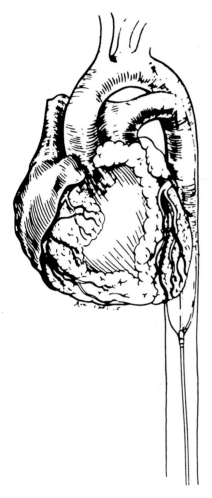

Figure 2 Placement of the intra-aortic balloon in the descending thoracic aorta, just distal to the left subclavian artery. [*From* Bregman and Kaskel (39), with permission.]

distal coronary perfusion. It has also been suggested that diastolic pressure augmentation may recruit coronary collaterals (46). In patients with cardiogenic shock from myocardial ischemia, IABP can raise *mean* arterial pressure and increase cardiac output 550–800 ml/min/m^2 (47–49). In cardiogenic shock, it is believed that the improved coronary perfusion by diastolic augmentation can prevent the extension of myocardial ischemia. Maintenance of coronary perfusion by diastolic augmentation stabilizes the patient during the induction of anesthesia (50).

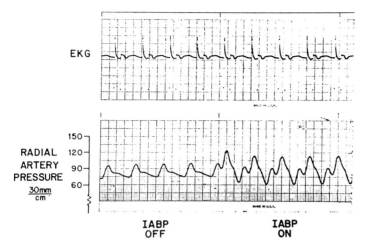

Figure 3 Radial artery pressure tracing demonstrating augmentation of pressure by IABP. [*From* Bregman and Kaskel (39), with permission.]

In the emergent situation of failed PTCA, percutaneous insertion of the balloon can be accomplished rapidly in the catheterization laboratory (39). This process can be expedited by passage of a guidewire into the opposite femoral artery while pharmacological and angioplastic attempts to reverse the acute ischemia are being made (11). A number of limitations and complications are associated with the use of the IABP (39,51,52). Percutaneous placement of the balloon is more difficult in a hypotensive patient. The more the patient needs the

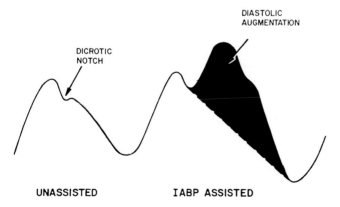

Figure 4 Schematic representation of IABP augmentation of diastolic pressure. [*From* Bregman and Kaskel (39), with permission.]

IABP, the tougher it is to gain arterial access and insert the device. Because of infra-aortic vascular disease and tortuosity, and IABP cannot be passed up either femoral artery in 10% of patients less than 70 years old and in 50% of patients older than 70 (53). Complication rates in the literature have ranged from 5% to as high as 36% (51,52). The most common complication is lower-leg ischemia, which can result from arterial dissection, thrombosis, plaque dislodgment, or obstruction of vessel lumen by the balloon catheter. The studies with low complication rates have stressed the experience of the operator, use of flexible guidewires, use of fluoroscopy, and early IABP removal.

Canine studies have demonstrated reduction in myocardial infarction size with IABP initiated within 3 hr of experimental coronary occlusion (42,44,54). Murphy and colleagues noted that patients with ECG changes immediately following failed PTCA had a higher incidence of perioperative myocardial infarction (55). In patients with refractory myocardial ischemia following failed PTCA, the authors found a 20% incidence of Q-wave infarction in 15 patients stabilized with IABP. This was in contrast to a 50% incidence of Q-wave infraction in six patients with ST-segment elevation who were not treated with IABP and a 42% incidence of infarction in a similar previously studied group (24,56). Interestingly, in a series studied by Lazar and Haan, use of IABP resulted in a lower rate of Q-wave infarctions, but no decrease in the incidence of perioperative myocardial infarction (defined by enzyme elevation) (17). Although in their study Murphy et al. were unable to demonstrate a statistical advantage with the use of IABP, the authors' clinical impression was that the IABP was instrumental in the successful management of the acutely ischemic patient with ST-segment elevation (55). The accumulated evidence indicates that the IABP may reduce the severity of myocardial ischemia through the mechanism of systolic afterload reduction and diastolic augmentation of coronary blood flow and thereby may contribute to greater myocardial salvage with subsequent surgical revascularization (40,57). The use of the IABP can also effectively stabilize the unstable patient until emergent revascularization can be performed. The extent of myocardial damage in patients with PTCA failure, chest pain, ST-T segment changes, and hemodynamic instability can be reduced by institution of the IABP prior to emergent surgical revascularization (9).

PERCUTANEOUS CARDIOPULMONARY BYPASS

The intra-aortic balloon pump has achieved popularity as a circulatory support technique not only because of its effectiveness, but also because of its relative ease of application in unstable patients. The traditional establishment of cardiopulmonary bypass requires surgical exposure of the femoral artery and vein. This requirement makes the implementation of cardiopulmonary bypass difficult in the unstable patient. The development of inexpensive, large-bore, thin-walled percutaneously inserted sheaths has allowed the development of a percutaneous cardiopulmonary support system utilizing the femoral vessels (Fig. 5) (58,59). Percutaneous cardiopulmonary bypass (PCB) utilizes external energy sources to support the failed circulation. Perfusion is usually established with a portable pump and oxygenator (60). This system can provide temporary cardiopulmonary support to a patient who cannot be supported by conventional resuscitative means, such as an IABP. Flow rates are dependent on cannula size, but with a 20-Fr cannula, flow rates of 3.0–5.2 L/min may be achieved (61). Placement of patients on PCB can be successfully completed in approximately 5–10 min and requires no special surgical instrumentation (59). PCB does, however, require some familiarity with tubing, connectors, and pump systems. With successful institution of PCB, systemic perfusion can be maintained, and unloading of the left ventricle may lead to a very low myocardial oxygen consumption (14). The complications associated with the short-term use of PCB are similar to those seen with the use of the IABP, with thrombotic complications and lower-extremity ischemia being the main concern.

The effectiveness of PCB has been investigated in patients in cardiogenic shock. Phillips et al. used PCB in 22 patients, including 11 patients in cardiac arrest due to acute myocardial infarction or failed angioplasty (60). All patients received good cardiopulmonary resuscitation, which included the use of the IABP in the majority of the myocardial infarction (MI) and failed angioplasty

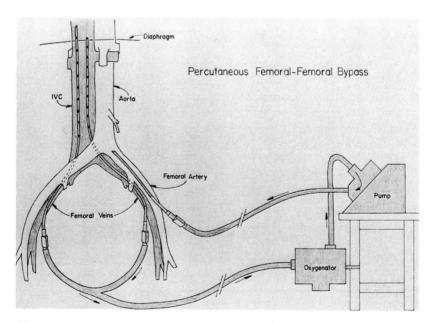

Figure 5 Schematic representation of percutaneous bypass. [*From* Phillips (59), with permission.]

patients. All patients except those with massive trauma were resuscitated with the use of PCB. Out of four failed angioplasty patients in cardiac arrest, there were two survivors. The authors concluded that PCB appears to be beneficial in resuscitating patients with refractory cardiac arrest or other forms of circulatory collapse except trauma. In the trauma patient, anticoagulation is contraindicated, thus excluding PCB as an alternative. Shawl et al. examined eight patients with post-MI cardiogenic shock (61). In their study, PCB provided flow rates of 3.5–5.2 L/min with mean blood pressures of 63–76 mmHg. There was one death, and the remaining seven patients underwent successful PTCA.

The concept of percutaneous cardiopulmonary bypass is a combination of percutaneous vascular access with cardiopulmonary bypass technology. The application of PCB generally takes 5–10 min and requires no special surgical instrumentation. In the case of failed PTCA, percutaneous cardiopulmonary bypass can provide a fairly simple means of circulatory support for the unstable patient with a failing circulation who has not improved with conventional therapy. PCB appears uniquely appropriate in patients exhibiting refractory cardiogenic shock.

VENTRICULAR ASSIST DEVICES

The IABP has been used as a form of mechanical assistance in patients with profound refractory heart failure. A large proportion of these patients die despite counterpulsation (62). The left ventricular assist device (LVAD) was developed in response to the need for a form of total mechanical circulatory support. Unlike the IABP, which augments existing cardiac output but is triggered off a regular ECG signal, the LVAD is a definitive blood pump, which can assume the entire cardiac output and can be activated either synchronously or asynchronously (63). The LVAD is an extracorporeally placed pneumatic pump with a polyurethane blood sac and two nonthrombogenic cannulae (Fig. 6) (64). The inflow cannula may be placed directly in the left ventricular apex, the left atrial appendage, or placed retrograde across the aortic valve. The return cannula usually consists of a 12-mm Dacron graft anastomosed to the ascending aorta (65). The LVAD is capable of flows as high as 7 L/min.

The LVAD is superior to the IABP in terms of left ventricular unloading and aortic pressure support (66). Because the LVAD requires surgical cardiac access, its use has been essentially limited to patients who cannot be weaned from cardiopulmonary bypass following cardiac surgery. There has been discussion concerning the application of the LVAD in post-MI patients with cardiogenic shock (64). The LVAD is more effective than the IABP in decreasing myocardial oxygen consumption (67), and it has also been shown to reduce infarct size (68,69). Because the placement of a LVAD requires a sternotomy or thoracotomy, the limitations of using the LVAD in cases of failed PTCA are prohibitive. This fact alone eliminates its use in the catheterization laboratory in the unstable

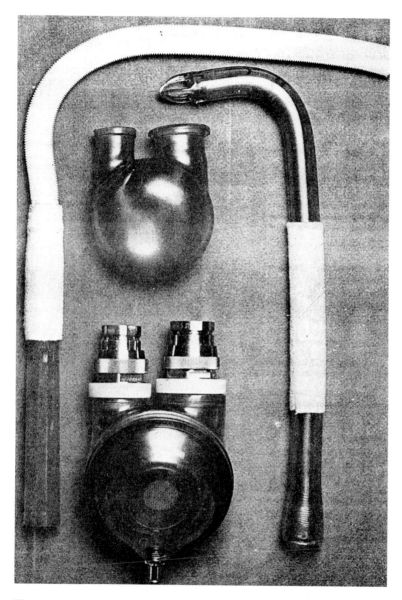

Figure 6   The left ventricular assist pump. Components include a polyurethane blood sac (top), composite segmented polyurethane woven Dacron outflow prosthesis (left), 51-Fr lighthouse-tip inflow cannula (right), and assembled assist device (bottom). [*From* Pennock et al. (65), with permission.]

patient who has an acute coronary occlusion secondary to failed PTCA. Following failed PTCA the patient can be better served by the institution of percutaneous cardiopulmonary bypass, which can be accomplished expediently in cases where the IABP proves inadequate.

Although the IABP is an accepted and effective modality for treatment of left ventricular failure, it may have only minimal effects on right ventricular failure. The IABP may lower left atrial pressure and, accordingly, pulmonary artery pressure. It may also improve right ventricular function by increasing coronary blood flow (65). Despite these beneficial effects, patients with acute right ventricular failure and hemodynamic instability may not be adequately salvaged by the use of an IABP alone.

Most attempts at right ventricular assist have applied a pulsatile assist counterpulsation device into the pulmonary artery through an open chest technique. An alternative method to treat right ventricular failure has been proposed by Phillips (59). In two patients with right ventricular infarctions, intravenous balloon pumping was initiated. A percutaneous balloon was inserted via the femoral vein and was positioned such that its tip was at the superior vena cava–right atrial junction. The intravenous balloon was synchronized with the aortic balloon to inflate during ventricular diastole and deflate during ventricular systole. With the placement of the intravenous balloon, the author believed the balloon assisted in pushing blood through the right ventricle. This "atrial kick" was seen to add up to 30% to the cardiac output and assisted in achieving hemodynamic stability in both patients. The cardiac output was increased by 700 ml/min in the patient with the venous balloon functioning compared with its being off. Intravenous balloon pumping may prove useful in cases of right ventricular infarction when supportive treatment with an IABP is ineffective and percutaneous cardiopulmonary bypass is not an option.

SUPPORTED ANGIOPLASTY

The IABP and percutaneous cardiopulmonary bypass have been successfully utilized to stabilize patients prior to emergent revascularization in the setting of failed PTCA. These techniques have also been examined as methods to support the circulation during coronary angioplasty in patients at risk for procedural death. Relative contraindications to PTCA include poor left ventricular function with low ejection fraction and a large area of remaining viable myocardium served by the target vessel (70,71). Acute coronary occlusion during PTCA can cause hemodynamic collapse in these vulnerable patients. In an effort to reduce the complications associated with high-risk PTCA and extend the use of this technique to patients with more advanced heart disease, patients have been prophylactically placed on circulatory support prior to the performance of PTCA. This "supported" angioplasty has consisted of the use of an IABP or institution of percutaneous cardiopulmonary bypass. It is believed that supported angioplasty may prevent possible hemodynamic collapse in the event of acute coronary occlusion. If vessel occlusion does occur, the hemodynamic support provided may permit more optimal surgical revascularization using the internal mammary artery (72).

In the various centers utilizing supported PTCA, indications for its use include: (a) the presence of severe or unstable angina pectoris, (b) at least one dilatable coronary stenosis, and (c) the presence of severe left ventricular dysfunction with ejection fraction less than 25%, or an extensive amount of the myocardium supplied by the target vessel (>50%), or both (71,73).

The National Registry of Elective Cardiopulmonary Bypass Supported Coronary Angioplasty has collated the data of 14 centers performing supported angioplasty (71). Percutaneous or semipercutaneous cardiopulmonary bypass was the method of support. In the Registry, there are 105 patients who underwent supported angioplasty, including 20 patients deemed surgically inoperable. The angioplasty success rate was 95%, and there has been a highly commendable mortality rate of 7.6%. Half the deaths have occurred in patients who were >75 years old and had left main coronary artery stenosis. Four patients subsequently underwent CABG. Blood transfusion was required in 43%, and there was a 39% rate of complications. The majority of these complications involved arterial, venous, or nerve injury at the cannulation site. The authors concluded that there was no advantage for supported angioplasty in patients with left main coronary artery disease, but that supported angioplasty can be utilized in certain subgroups of high-risk patients, including those with one patent vessel, low ejection fraction, and patients who are not surgical candidates. Kahn et al. studied 28 high-risk patients in whom IABP support was utilized in conjunction with PTCA (74). The patient profile included a mean left ventricular ejection fraction of 24%, three-vessel disease present in 93%, and significant left main coronary artery disease in 25%. The successful dilatation rate was 96%. There were no deaths or myocardial infarctions within 72 hr of the procedure, and there was an 11% rate of local vascular complications.

This initial experience has demonstrated that some type of circulatory support may permit successful PTCA intervention in certain high-risk patients. In comparing IABP- to PCB-supported angioplasty, PCB can provide flow rates of 3–5 L/min and is independent of intrinsic cardiac function and rhythm. The IABP augments cardiac output only 20–30% and is less effective in the face of arrhythmias. A major drawback of PCB is that the priming volume of the extracorporeal system necessitates blood transfusion. Vascular complications appear to be more frequent with PCB than with the IABP, although this is certainly related to cannula size (74). The initial experience has demonstrated that supported angioplasty can be successfully utilized in subgroups of high-risk patients, including those who are not surgical candidates. At this time, supported angioplasty has not yet been demonstrated to be superior to unsupported angioplasty or surgery in terms of clinical outcome.

SUMMARY

PTCA has developed into a technique with wide applications. Although PTCA is performed successfully in the vast majority of patients, potential complications, including coronary artery dissection, perforation, and occlusion, can occur. The ischemic insult of failed PTCA may lead to myocardial infarction, arrhythmias, hypotension with cardiovascular collapse, and ultimately death. Factors that place patients at increased risk of ischemic injury during PTCA include: (a) absence of collateral circulation to the coronary artery involved, and (b) more extensive coronary disease. Emergent surgical revascularization remains the accepted treatment for failed PTCA. Emergent surgery after failed PTCA is associated with an undeniably higher mortality and morbidity than elective CABG in similar patients stratified for preoperative risk. The ability to stabilize the patient, improve myocardial oxygenation, and decrease the ischemic insult favorably influences prognosis in emergent surgical revascularization following failed angioplasty.

The reperfusion "bailout" catheter is designed to achieve blood flow to myocardium distal to an acute obstruction. If the catheter can be successfully placed, and systemic blood pressure is adequate, this catheter can reduce the global ischemic insult. Successful use of the catheter may be effective in reducing myocardial ischemia, although the catheter may not prevent infarction in some patients and is ineffective in the face of systemic hypotension. The use of perfluorochemical perfusate solutions with their high oxygen-carrying capacity, low viscosity, and small particle size may minimize the complication of thrombotic occlusion. The use of the reperfusion bailout catheter in conjunction with distal Fluosol infusion needs to be further evaluated. Use of the reperfusion catheter remains an attractive initial intervention to be considered in the event of failed PTCA. In cases where a catheter cannot be passed, or systemic hypotension is present, an IABP is characteristically indicated.

The IABP is the most widely used temporary mechanical assist device. Its use may reduce the severity of myocardial ischemia by systolic afterload reduction and diastolic augmentation of coronary blood flow. In cardiogenic shock, the IABP can raise the mean arterial pressure and increase cardiac output 550–800 ml/min/m^2. There is evidence that institution of the IABP prior to surgical revascularization may decrease the extent of myocardial damage in many patients with ischemic changes after failed PTCA. The use of the IABP can also effectively stabilize the unstable patient until emergent surgical revascularization can be performed, especially in cases of unsuccessful placement of reperfusion catheters or systemic hypotension.

PCB combines percutaneous access with cardiopulmonary bypass technology. PCB can generate flow rates of 3.0–5.2 L/min and stabilize systemic perfusion. Patients can be placed on PCB fairly rapidly, and implementation requires no special surgical instrumentation. In the setting of failed PTCA, percutaneous cardiopulmonary bypass can provide a means of circulatory support for the unstable patient with a failing circulation who cannot be stabilized with an IABP.

The LVAD is superior to the IABP in terms of total left ventricular unloading and total support of aortic pressure. Its use has been essentially limited to patients who cannot be weaned from cardiopulmonary bypass following cardiac surgery. As placement of a LVAD requires major surgical access in the form of sternotomy or thoracotomy, it has rare application in cases of failed PTCA. In cases where support with an IABP proves inadequate, patients are better served by the institution of PCB.

Percutaneous insertion of an intravenous balloon, such that its tip is positioned at the superior vena cava–right atrium junction, provides a theoretical alternative in the treatment of right ventricular failure. The balloon assists in returning and pushing blood through the right ventricle, adding up to 30% to the cardiac output. Intravenous balloon pumping may prove useful in cases of right ventricular infarction following failed PTCA, when supportive treatment with an intra-aortic balloon pump is ineffective, and the institution of PCB is not an option.

Percutaneous cardiopulmonary bypass and the IABP have been used as methods to support the circulation during coronary angioplasty in high-risk patients. Indications for ''supported angioplasty'' include: (a) the presence of severe or unstable angina, (b) at least one dilatable coronary stenosis, and (c) the presence of severe left ventricular dysfunction, or an extensive amount of the myocardium supplied by the target vessel, or both. Initial experience has demonstrated that circulatory support may permit successful PTCA intervention in high-risk patients. Comparative trials may be necessary to better define the role of ''supported angioplasty'' in these high-risk patients.

REFERENCES

1. Dorros G, Cowley MJ, Simpson J, et al. Percutaneous transluminal coronary angioplasty: report of complications from the National Heart, Lung and Blood Institute PTCA registry. Circulation 1983; 67:723.
2. Holmes DR, Vlieststra RE, Kelsey S, Detre K. Comparison of current and earlier complications of angioplasty. NHLBI PTCA registry. J Am Coll Cardiol 1987; 9:19A.
3. Parsonnet V, Fisch D, Gielchinsky I, Hochberg M, Hussain M, Karanam R, Rothfeld L, Klapp L. Emergency operation after failed angioplasty. J Thorac Cardiovasc Surg. 1988; 96:198–203.
4. Cowley MJ, Dorros G, Kelsey SF, Van Raden M, Detre KM. Emergency coronary bypass surgery After Coronary Angioplasty: The National Heart, Lung, and Blood Institute's Percutaneous Transluminal Coronary Angioplasty Registry Experience. Am J. Cardiol 1984; 53:22C–26C.

5. Golding LAR, Loop FD, Hollman JL, et al. Early results of emergency surgery after coronary angioplasty. Circulation 1986; 74(Part 2):III-26–9.
6. Parsonnet V, Gielchinsky I, Hockberg M, Hussein SM, Fisch D, Rothfeld L. Emergency surgery after failed angioplasty. J Am Coll Cardiol 1987; 9:123A (Abstract).
7. Killen DA, Hamaker WR, Reed WA. Coronary artery bypass following percutaneous transluminal coronary angioplasty. Ann Thorac Surg 1985; 40(2):133–8.
8. Reul GJ, Cooley DA, Hallman GL, Duncan JM, Livesay JJ, Fraizer OH, Ott DA, Angelini P, Massumi A, Mathur VS. Coronary artery bypass for unsuccessful percutaneous transluminal coronary angioplasty. J. Thorac Cardiovasc Surg 1984; 88:685–94.
9. Jones EL, Murphy DA, Craver JM. Comparison of coronary artery bypass surgery and percutaneous transluminal coronary angioplasty including surgery for failed angioplasty. Am Heart J 1984; 107:830–5.
10. Naunheim KS, Fiore AC, Fagan DC, McBride LR, Barner HB, Pennington DG, Willman VL, Kern MJ, Deligonul U, Vandormael MC, Kaiser GC. Emergency coronary artery bypass grafting for failed angioplasty: Risk factors and outcome. Ann Thorac Surg 1989; 47:816–23.
11. Murphy DA, Craver JM, Jones EL, Gruentzig AR, King SB, Hatcher CR. Surgical revascularization following unsuccessful percutaneous transluminal coronary angioplasty. J Thorac Cardiovasc Surg 1982; 84:342–8.
12. Rentrop P, Blanke H, Karsch KR, Kaiser H, Kostering H, Leitz K. Selective intracoronary thrombolyses in acute myocardial infarction and unstable angina pectoris. Circulation 1981; 63:307–17.
13. Markis JE, Malagold M, Parker JA, Silverman KJ, Barry WH, Als AV, Paulin S, Grossman W, Braunwald E. Myocardial salvage after intracoronary thromboysis with streptokinase in acute myocardial infarction. Assessment by intracoronary thallium-201. N Eng J Med 1981; 305:777–82.
14. Topal EJ. Emerging strategies for failed percutaneous transluminal coronary angioplasty. Am J Cardiol 1989; 63:249–50.
15. Vanhaecke J, Flameng W, Sergent P, et al. Emergency bypass surgery: Late effects on size infarction and ventricular function. Circulation 1985; 72(Part 2):II179–84.
16. Pelletier LC, Pardini A, Renkin J, David PR, Hebert Y, Bourassa MG. Myocardial revascularization after failure of percutaneous transluminal coronary angioplasty. J. Thorac Cardiovasc Surg 1985; 90:265–71.
17. Lazar HL, Haan CK. Determinants of myocardial infarction following emergency coronary artery bypass for failed percutaneous coronary angioplasty. Ann Thorac Surg 1987; 44:646–50.
18. Hinohara T, Simpson JB, Phillips HR, Behar VS, Peter RH, Kong Y, Carlson EB, Stack RS. Transluminal catheter reprefusion: A new technique to reestablish blood flow after coronary occlusion during percutaneous transluminal coronary angioplasty. J Am Coll Cardiol 1988; 11:977–82.
19. Turi ZG, Campbell CA, Gottimukkala MV, Kloner RA. Preservation of distal coronary perfusion during prolonged balloon inflation with an autoperfusion angioplasty catheter. Circulation 1987; 75(6):1273–80.
20. Hinohara T, Simpson JB, Phillips HR, Stack RS. Transluminal intracoronary

reperfusion catheter: A device to maintain coronary perfusion between failed coronary angioplasty and emergency coronary bypass surgery. J Am Coll Cardiol 1988; 11(5):977–82.

21. Kereiakes DJ, Abbottsmith CW, Callard GM, Flege JB. Emergent internal mammary artery grafting following failed percutaneous transluminal coronary angioplasty: Use of transluminal catheter reperfusion. Am Heart J 1987; 113:1018–20.

22. Marquis JF, Schwartz L, Aldridge H, Majid P, Henderson M, Matushinsky E. Acute coronary artery occlusion during percutaneous transluminal coronary angioplasty treated by redilation of the occluded segment. J Am Coll Cardiol 1984; 4:1268–71.

23. Hollman J, Gruentzig AR, Douglas JS, King SB, Ischinger T, Meier B, Acute occusion after percutaneous transluminal coronary angioplasty: a new approach. Circulation 1983; 68:725–32.

24. Murphy DA, Craver JM, Jones EL, et al. Surgical management of acute myocardial ischemia following percutaneous transluminal coronary angioplasty: Role of the intra-aortic balloon pump. J Thorac Cardiovasc Surg 1984;87:332.

25. Reul GJ, Cooley DA, Hallman GL, et al. Coronary artery bypass for unsuccessful percutaneous transluminal angioplasty. J Thorac Cardiovasc Surg 1984; 88:685.

26. Ferguson TB, Hinohara T, Simpson J, Stack RS, Wechsler AS. Catheter reperfusion to allow optimal coronary bypass grafting following failed transluminal coronary angioplasty. Ann Thorac Surg 1986; 42:399–405.

27. Douglas JS, King SB, Roubin GS, Murphy DA, Namay DL, Anderson HV. Efficacy of coronary artery perfusion catheters in patients with failed angioplasty and acute myocardial ischemia. J Am Coll Cardiol 1987; 9(2):105A.

28. Sundram P, Harvey JR, Johnson RG, Schwartz MJ, Baim DS. Benefit of the perfusion catheter for emergency coronary artery grafting after failed percutaneous transluminal coronary angioplasty. Am J Cardiol 1989; 63:282–5.

29. Moss GS, Gould SA, Sehgal LR, Rosen AL, Sehgal HL. Polyhemoglobin and fluorocarbon as blood substitutes. Biomat Artif Cells Artif Org 1987; 15(2):333–6.

30. Cleman M, Jaffee CC, Wohlgelernter D. Prevention of ischemia during percutaneous transluminal coronary angioplasty by transcatheter infusion of oxygenated Fluosol DA 20%. Circulation 1986; 74(3):555–62.

31. Spears JR, Serur J, Baim DS, Grossman W, Paulin S. Myocardial protection with Fluosol-DA during prolonged coronary balloon occlusion in the dog. Circulation 1983; 68(Suppl III):III-80.

32. Cowley MJ, Snow FR, DiSciascio G, Kelly K, Guard C, Nixon JV. Perfluorochemical perfusion during coronary angioplasty in unstable and high-risk patients. Circulation 1990; 81(3):IV27–IV34.

33. Naito R, Yokoyama K. Perfluorochemical blood substitutes Fluosol-43, Fluosol-DA 20% and 35%. Technical Information Series #5. Green Cross Corp, June 30, 1978.

34. Mitsuno T, Ohyanagi H, Naito R. Clinical studies of a perfluorochemical whole blood substitute (Fluosol-DA). Ann Surg 1982; 195:60–9.

35. Gould SA, Moss G. Current perspectives on blood substitutes. Curr Surg 1987; July–August:279–81.

36. Moulopoulos SD, Topaz S, Kolff WJ. Diastolic balloon pumping (with carbon

dioxide) in the aorta-A mechanical assistance to the failing circulation. Am Heart J 1962; 63:669–75.

37. Harken DE. Presented at the International College of Cardiology Meeting, Brussels, Belgium, 1958.

38. Kantrowitz A. Experimental augmentation of coronary flow by retardation of arterial pressure pulse. Surgery 1953; 34:678–87.

39. Bregman D, Kaskel P. Advances in percutaneous intra-aortic balloon pumping. Crit Care Clin 1986; 2(2):221–36.

40. Gold HK, Leinbach RC, Sanders CA, Buckley MJ, Mundth ED, Austen WG. Intraaortic balloon pumping for control of recurrent myocardial ischemia. Circulation 1973; 47:1197–1203.

41. Leinbach RC, Buckley MJ, Austen WG, Petschek HE, Kantrowitz AR, Sanders CA. Effects of intra-aortic balloon pumping on coronary flow and metabolism in man. Circulation 1971; 43(Suppl 1):77–81.

42. Margolis JR. The role of the percutaneous intra-aortic balloon in emergency situations following percutaneous transluminal coronary angioplasty. In: Kaltenbach M, Gruentizig A, Rentrop K, Bussman WD, eds. Transluminal coronary angioplasty and intracoronary thrombolysis. New York: Springer-Verlag, 1982:144–50.

43. Goldfarb D, Friesinger GC, Conti CR, Brown BG, Gott VL. Preservation of myocardial viability by diastolic augmentation after ligation of the coronary artery in dogs. Surgery 1968; 63:320–7.

44. Sugg WL, Webb WR, Ecker RR. Reduction of extent of myocardial infarction by counterpulsation. Ann Thorac Surg 1969; 7:310–6.

45. Maroko PN, Bernstein EF, Lippy P, et al. Effects of intra-aortic balooncounterpulsation on the severity of myocardial ischemic injury following acute coronary occlusion. Circulation 1972; 45:1150–9.

46. Jacobey JA, Taylor WJ, Smith GT, Gorlin R, Harken DE. A new therapeutic approach to acute coronary occlusion. II. Opening dormant coronary collateral channels by counterpulsation. Am J Cardiol 1963; 11:218–27.

47. Dunkman WB, Leinbach RC, Buckley MJ, Mundth ED, Kantrowitz AR, Austen W G, Sanders CA. Clinical and hemodynamic results of intra-aortic balloon pumping and surgery for cardiogenic shock. Circulation 1972; 46:465–77.

48. Frazier OH, Painvin AG, Urrutia CO, Igo SR, Cooley DA. Medical circulatory support: clinical experience at the Texas Heart Institute. Heart Transplant 1983; 2(4):299–306.

49. Pierce WS, Bernhard WF, Golding LR, Norman JC, Pennington DG, Keilbach H, Wolner E. Cardiac support-panel conference. Trans Am Soc Artif Intern Org 1980; 16:625–8.

50. Kent KM, Bentivoglio LG, Block PC, Cowley MJ, Dorros G, Gosselin AJ, Gruntzig A, Myler RK, Simpson J, Stertzer S, Williams DO, Fisher L, Gillaspie MJ, Detre K, Kelsey S, Mullin SM, Mock MB. Percutaneous transluminal coronary angioplasty. Report from the registry of the National Heart, Lung and Blood Institute. Am J Cardiol 1982; 49:2011–20.

51. McCabe JC, Abel RM, Subramanian VA, Gay WA Jr. Complications of intra-aortic balloon insertion and counterpulsation. Circulation 1978; 57:769–73.

52. Alpert J, Bhaktan EK, Gielchinsky I, Gilbert L, Brener BJ, Brief DK, Parsonnet V. Vascular complications of intra-aortic balloon pumping. Arch Surg 1976; 111:1190–5.

53. Macoviak, J., Stephenson, LW, Edmunds, LH, Harken, AH, MacVaugh, H: The Intra-aortic balloon pump: An analysis of five years' experience. Ann Thorac Surg 1980; 29:451–8.

54. Maroko PR, Bernstein EF, Libby P, Delaria GA, Covell JW, Ross J, Braunwald E. Effects of Intra-aortic balloon counterpulsation on the severity of myocardial ischemic injury following acute coronary occlusion. Circulation 1972; 45:1150–9.

55. Quigley P, Erwin J, Maurer BJ, Walsh MJ, Gearty GF. Percutaneous transluminal angioplasty in unstable angina: comparison with stable angina. Br Heart J 1985; 55:227–30.

56. Murphy DA, Craver JM, Jones EL, Gruentzig AR, King SB III, Hatcher CR. Surgical revascularization following unsuccessful percutaneous transluminal coronary angioplasty. J Thorac Cardiovasc Surg 1982; 84:342–8.

57. Levine FH, Gold HK, Leinbach RC, et al. Management of acute myocardial ischemia with intraaortic balloon pumping and coronary bypass surgery. Circulation 1978; 58(Suppl 1):70–2.

58. Bregman D, Casarella WJ. Percutaneous intraaortic balloon pumping: initial clinical experience. Ann Thorac Surg 1980; 29:153–5.

59. Phillips SJ. Percutaneous cardiopulmonary bypass and innovations in clinical counterpulsation. Crit Care Clin 1986; 2(2):297–318.

60. Phillips SJ, Zeff RH, Kongtahworn C, Skinner JR, Toon RS, Grignon A, Kennerly RM, Wickemeyer W, Iannone LA. Percutaneous cardiopulmonary bypass: application and indication for use. Ann Thorac Surg 1989; 47:121–3.

61. Shawl FA, Domanski JM, Punja S, Hernandez TJ. Emergency percutaneous cardiopulmonary (bypass) support in cardiogenic shock. J Am Coll Cardiol 1989; 13(2):160A.

62. McEnany MT, Kay HR, Buckley MJ, et al. Clinical experience with intraaortic balloon pump support in 728 patients. Circulation 1978; 58(Suppl 1):I-124–32.

63. Pierce WS, Bernhard WF, Golding LR, Norman JC, Pennington DG, Keilbach H, Wolner E. Panel conference: Cardiac support. Trans Am Soc Artif Intern Org 1980; 26:625–9.

64. Jorge E, Pae WE, Pierce WS. Left heart and biventricular bypass. Crit Care Clin 1986; 2(2):267–75.

65. Pennock JL, Pierce WS, Wisman CB, Bull AP, Waldhausen JA. Survival and complications following ventricular assist pumping for cardiogenic shock. Ann Surg 1983; 198(4):469–76.

66. Smalling RW, Cassidy DB, Merhige M, Felli PR, Wise GM, Barrett RL, Wampler RD. Improved hemodynamic and left ventricular unloading during acute ischemia using the hemopump left ventricular assist device compared to intra aortic balloon counterpulsation. J Am Coll Cardiol 1989; (13)2:160A.

67. McDonnell MA, Kralior AC, Tsagarir TJ, et al. Comparative effect of counterpulsation and bypass on left ventricular myocardial oxygen consumption and dynamics before and after coronary occlusion. Am Heart J 1979; 97:78–88.

68. Grossi EA, Laschinger JC, Cunningham JN, et al. Time course of myocardial salvage with left heart assist in evolving myocardial infarction. Surg Forum 1984; 35:322–4.

69. Laschinger JC, Cunningham JN, Catinella FP, et al. "Pulsatile" left atrial–femoral artery bypass. A new method of preventing extension of myocardial infarction. Arch Surg 1983; 118:965–9.

70. Shawl FA, Domanski MJ, Punja S, Hernandez TJ. Percutaneous cardiopulmonary bypass to support high risk elective coronary angioplasty. J Am Coll Cardiol 1989; 13(2):160A.

71. Vogel RA, Shawl FA, Tommaso C, O'Neill W, Overlie P, O'Toole J, Vandormael M, Topol E, Tabari KK, Vogel J, Smith S, Freedmann R, White C , George B, Teirstein P. Initial report of the national registry of elective cardiopulmonary bypass supported coronary angioplasty. J Am Coll Cardiol 1990; 15(1):23–31.

72. Vogel RA. The Maryland experience: Angioplasty and valvuloplasty using percutaneous cardiopulmonary support. Am J Cardiol 1988; (62):11K–14K.

73. Tommaso CL, Gundry SR, Zoda AR, Stafford JL, Johnson RA, Vogel RA. Supported angioplasty: Initial experience with high risk patients. J Am Coll Cardiol 1989; 13(2):159A.

74. Kahn JK, Rutherford BD, McConahay DR, Johnson WL, Giorgi LV, Hartzler GO. Supported "high risk" coronary angioplasty using intraaortic balloon pump counterpulsation. J Am Coll Cardiol 1990; 15(4):1151–5.

20

Summary of "High Risk" and "Prohibitive Risk" for Surgery or Angioplasty in Unstable Angina

Douglass Andrew Morrison

Veterans Affairs Medical Center and
University of Colorado Health Sciences Center
Denver, Colorado

INTRODUCTION

The choice between angioplasty and surgery requires that one consider the benefits (likelihood of short- and long-term success in terms of patent arteries, relief of ischemia, relief of symptoms, etc.) and the risks (likelihood of death, acute infarction, morbidity, etc.). The fourth section of this book, "Surgical Therapy for Unstable Angina," addresses the benefit/risk profile of bypass surgery (CABG) in unstable angina. Updated reviews of the National Cooperative Study of medical versus surgical therapy for unstable angina (by Plotnick), the VA Cooperative Study of medical versus surgical therapy (by Scott), and the VA Surgical Registry (by Grover), as well as an up-to-date overview (by Hammermeister) all consider surgical benefit/risk in unstable angina.

Similarly, the fifth section, "Coronary Angioplasty for Unstable Angina," addresses the benefit/risk profile of coronary angioplasty in unstable ischemic syndromes. Bell and Holmes provide a description of the Mayo Clinic experience and discuss relevant risk/benefit issues as they effected the ongoing NIH Bypass Angioplasty Revascularization Investigation (BARI). de Feyter, Suryapranata, and Serruys review the experience worldwide with angioplasty for unstable angina.

Both in the design of trials, where inclusion and exclusion are critical issues, and in the decisions to use newer pharmacological and mechanical supports or bridges (the topic of the section "Bridge Techniques for Revascularization"), it is necessary to define "high-risk" and "prohibitive-risk" subsets. This chapter reviews available surgery and angioplasty literature in an effort to define high-risk and prohibitive-risk patient subsets for either of these interventions.

HIGH-RISK PATIENT SUBSETS FOR BYPASS SURGERY IN UNSTABLE ANGINA

The first study specifically addressing surgery for unstable angina (1971), or "impending myocardial infarction," reported two deaths in 18 patients, or 11%, considerably higher than the rate for stable patients (6). Similarly, Segal et al., in 1973, reported an operative mortality of 18% for "impending myocardial infarction" (7). Lambert et al., also in 1971, reported an operative mortality of 5.3% (12). (See Tables 1 and 2.)

The two large prospective randomized trials of surgery versus medical therapy were both reported in 1978 (9,11). Scott et al. (the VA Cooperative Study) reported a 5% operative mortality in unstable angina (9). Russell et al. (the National Cooperative Study) reported an overall operative mortality of 5% in unstable angina (11). Other randomized trials from this period, albeit with significantly smaller sample sizes, include those of Pugh et al., Bertolasi et al., Brown et al., and Jones et al. (10,14,15,21); those studies reported operative mortalities of 7.7%, 10%, 2%, and 1.2%, respectively. The conclusion that surgery on unstable patients carries a higher risk than surgery on stable patients seems clear.

High-Risk Subset for CABG: Medically Refractory

Wiles et al. reported an overall operative mortality of 4.8% for 124 patients with unstable angina (16). In contrast, the 71 patients within their total group who were deemed medically refractory had an operative mortality of 8.5% (16). Similarly, Langou et al. reported on a total series of 194 patients with unstable angina (18). Among their 64 medical responders mortality was 0, but among 130 medical nonresponders there were 12 deaths, a 9.2% mortality rate (18). They further subdivided the nonresponders into patients with and without intra-aortic balloon counterpulsation, arguing that this modality could reduce risk (18). This latter contention has been a point of controversy (44,45).

Cohn and co-workers also divided their series of 127 unstable angina patients into 54 medically controlled patients who had a 1.8% operative mortality and 73 medically refractory patients whose operative mortality was 5% (28). In the VA Cooperative Study of medicine versus surgery (Chapter 9), the overall operative mortality was 4.1%, but for medically refractory patients it was 10.3%.

In a more recent study (1989), Naunheim et al. used the need for IV nitroglycerin and/or intra-aortic balloon counterpulsation as indicative of particularly refractory subsets; the operative mortalities of these two groups were 6.2%

Table 1 Operative Mortality for Unstable Angina

First author	Ref.	Year	Operative mortality (%)	Definitional statement
Favolaro	6	1971	2/18 (11%)	Impending myocardial infarction
Segal	7	1973	3/17 (18%)	Impending myocardial infarction
Luchi (VA Coop)	8	1987	9/231 (4.1%)	Unstable angina
Scott (VA Coop)	9	1978	7/141 (5%)	Unstable angina
Bertolasi	10	1976	6/62 (10%)	Intermediate syndrome, progressive angina
Lambert	10	1971	3/57 (5.3%)	Impending infarction
Douglas	13	1978	6/92 (6.5%)	Unstable angina
Pugh	14	1978	1/13 (7.7%)	Unstable angina
Brown	15	1981	1/44 (2%)	Randomizable to surgery
Wiles	16	1977	6/124 (4.8%) 6/71 (8.5%)	Unstable angina, medically refractory
Hultgren	17	1977	1/52 (2%)	Unstable angina
Langou	18	1978	12/194 (6.1%)	Unstable angina
			0/64 (0)	Medical responders
			4/75 (5.3%)	Medical nonresponders with IABP
			8/55 (14.5%)	Medical nonresponders without IABP
Olinger	19	1978	1/95 (1%)	Unstable angina
			1/52 (2%)	"High risk"
			0/42 (0)	"Low risk"
Ahmed	20	1980	3/71 (4.2%)	Unstable angina
Jones	21	1982	1/78 (1.2%)	Unstable angina
Hultgren	22	1982	2/104 (2%)	Unstable angina
Cobanoglu	23	1984	/1163 (2%)	Unstable angina
Golding	24	1978	4/100 (4%)	Unstable angina
Rankin	25	1984	4/100 (4%)	Medically refractory unstable angina
Russell (Nat'l Coop)	11	1978		
Goldman	26	1985	/299 (5.4%)	Unstable angina
Edwards	27	1990	(14.5%)	"Emergency CABG"
Cohn	28	1978	1/54 (1.8%)	Medically controlled
			4/73 (5%)	Medically refractory
Hatcher	29	1978	/456 (3.5%)	Unstable angina
			(11.8%)	LVEF < 0.24
			(4.8%)	3-vessel disease
			(13%)	Left main
Branley	55	1980	/130 (7.7%)	Unstable angina
			(33%)	Unstable + age > 70
			(29%)	Unstable + LVEF < 0.40
Eugene	48	1985	8/207 (3.9%)	Unstable angina

Table 1   (*Continued*)

First author	Ref.	Year	Operative mortality (%)	Definitional statement
Christakis	56	1986	(2.8%)	Unstable angina
Naunheim	57	1989	8/129 (6.2%)	IV nitroglycerin for rest pain
			4/12 (33%)	IABP required
McCormick	58	1985	129/3,311 (3.9%)	Unstable angina
Grover (VA Registry)	59	1991	267/4404 (6.1%)	Rest angina
			201/2523 (8.0%)	NY Heart Class IV
			80/634 (12.6%)	Emergent surgery
			139/1477 (9.4%)	IV nitroglycerin
			44/279 (15.8%)	IABP
			111/1499 (7.4%)	Recent MI
			111/888 (12.5%)	Prior heart surgery
Williams	34	1983	2/103 (1.9%)	Post-MI angina
Baumgartner	35	1984	/34 (9%)	Post-MI angina
Gertler	36	1985	/44 (16%)	Post-MI angina
Singh	37	1985	/108 (1.8%)	Post-MI angina
Brower	38	1985	/34 (3%)	Post-MI angina
Breyer	39	1985	/75 (8%)	Post-MI angina
Stuart	40	1988	/225 (5.3%)	Post-MI angina
Bardet	41	1977		Post-MI angina
Jones	42	1981	0/116 (0%)	Post-MI angina
Madigan	43	1977	/28 (3.6%)	Post-MI angina
Brundage	44	1980		Post-MI angina
Weintraub	45	1979	1/60 (1.7%)	Post-MI angina
Feola	110	1977	8/23 (34.7%)	LVEF ≤ 0.30
			2/25 (8%)	LVEF ≤ 0.30 with IABP

and 33%, respectively (57). Edwards et al., reporting in 1990, described a particularly refractory group who required emergency surgery; their operative mortality was 14.5% (27). Their study specifically addresses the issues of resting ischemia with electrocardiographic confirmation and despite all available therapy (Ref. 27 and figures therein).

The largest and most recent series is the result of more than 8800 coronary bypass operations performed in 44 hospitals of the Veterans Administration system and reported by Grover et al. (59). In the subsets with rest angina, emergent surgery, preoperative intravenous nitroglycerin, and preoperative intra-aortic balloon counterpulsation, the operative (30 day) mortalities were 6.1%, 12.6%, 9.4%, and 15.8%, respectively; the denominators for these specific

Table 2 Risk Factors for Operative Mortality in Unstable Angina

	Ref.
Age > 70	(55,59)
LV dysfunction	(19,29,55)
Medically refractory	(16,18,25,27,28)
Require IV nitroglycerin	(57,59)
Require IABP	(18,57,59)
Myocardial infarction within 30 days	(59,34–45)

subsets were 4404 patients, 634 patients, 1477 patients, and 279 patients, respectively (59).

All these series are in agreement; patients who cannot be medically stabilized are at higher risk of operative death than patients who can be stabilized. By the same token, emergency surgery carries a higher risk than elective or semielective surgery. Finally, the more aggressive the therapy needed to define medically refractory (for example, intravenous nitroglycerin or intra-aortic balloon counterpulsation), the greater the operative mortality.

High-Risk Subset for CABG: Left Ventricular Dysfunction

A number of studies have looked at ventricular function and its impact on operative mortality for bypass surgery in unstable angina. Hatcher et al. reported an overall mortality of 3.5% for 456 unstable angina patients operated on before 1978 but a mortality of 11.8% for a subset with LVEF < 0.24 (29). Patients with left ventricular ejection fractions in that range were excluded from both the VA Cooperative and National Cooperative Studies (9,11). In 1980, Brawley et al. reported the Johns Hopkins University experience with 130 unstable angina patients (55). Their overall operative mortality was 7.7%, but for the subset with LVEF < 0.40, it was 29% (55). In the VA Surgical Registry reported by Grover et al., the LVEF was significantly higher in 6525 survivors than in 337 patients who died (0.54 ± 0.14 versus 0.50 ± 0.15, $p < 0.001$) (59).

In summary, left ventricular dysfunction appears to be a significant risk factor for operative mortality in bypass surgery for unstable angina.

High-Risk Subset for CABG: Recent (30 Days) Acute Infarction

A number of small series, listed in Table 1, have had wide variation in the operative mortality of CABG for postinfarct angina. Jones et al. reported 0 mortality in 116 patients (42). Williams et al. reported 1.3% mortality in 103 patients (34). Weintraub et al. attributed part of their 1.7% mortality in 60 patients on the aggressive use of intra-aortic balloon counterpulsation (45). Brundage et al. reported 0 mortality, in denying the need for IABP (44). Stuart et al. reported a 5.3% mortality in 225 patients (40). Breyer et al. reported 8% in 75 patients (39) and Baumgartner et al. reported 9% operative mortality in 34 patients (35). Gertler et al. had a 16% operative mortality in a 1985 series (36).

The 1990 report from the VA Surgical Registry included 1499 patients operated on within 30 days of an acute infarction, with a 30-day mortality in 111, or 7.4% (59).

The conclusion appears warranted that unstable patients who have had a recent infarct (30 days) are at higher risk than those who have not infarcted; how much higher risk is controversial. A number of these studies suggest that further division into <24 hr, 2–7 days, and 8–30 days further stratifies the risk (34–35). This conclusion is at least consistent with what we have learned about acute thrombosis and acute angioplasty in the peri-infarct period.

High-Risk Subset for CABG: Age > 70

Brawley's study (55) and the recent VA Registry (59) have specifically examined the elderly and concluded that age > 70 is a significant risk factor for operative mortality in CABG for unstable angina.

High-Risk Subset for CABG: Prior Heart Surgery

The VA Surgical Registry reported a 3.9% mortality in 7645 patients who had not had prior surgery compared to a 12.5% mortality in 888 patients who had prior surgery.

HIGH-RISK PATIENT SUBSETS FOR CORONARY ANGIOPLASTY IN UNSTABLE ANGINA

In the first NHLBI PTCA Registry, 2051 patients, or 67% of the total reported, had unstable angina. In a specific comparison of 330 unstable patients from the registry with 214 similar stable patients, the unstable patients had 0.9% hospital mortality and the stable group 0.47% hospital mortality (60). (See Tables 3 and 4.)

Similarly, in the large series from Emory University reported by Bredlau et al., 50% of the 3500 patients had unstable angina, which was not a predictor of major complication; nevertheless, most of the patients in this early series were patients with single-vessel disease and simple anatomy (70).

High-Risk Subset for PTCA: Medically Refractory

Several small series, notably the ones reported by Williams et al., de Feyter et al., and Steffenino et al., included patients with unstable angina who underwent PTCA after some degree of medical control without an acute mortality (61,64,65). The series of Quigley et al. (25 patients) had a 4% mortality (63).

Table 3 Angioplasty Mortality/Morbidity for Unstable Angina

First author	Ref.	Year	# of patients/ mortality	Definitional statement
Faxon	60	1983	330 (0.9%)	New onset; coronary insufficiency; changing pattern; rest or variant
Williams	61	1981	17 (0)	National Cooperative Study
Meyer	62	1983	40 ( )	Rest angina
Quigley	63	1986	25 (4%)	Unstable angina
deFeyter	64	1987	71 (0)	Unstable angina
Steffinino	65	1987	89 (0)	Unstable angina
deFeyter	66	1985	88 (0)	Refractory unstable
Plokker	67	1988	469 (1%)	Refractory unstable
Sharma	68	1988	40 (0)	Refractory unstable
Perry	69	1988	105 (2%)	Refractory unstable
deFeyter	71	1986	53 (0)	
Holt	72	1988	70 (2%)	Post-MI unstable
Gottlieb	73	1987	47 (2%)	Post-MI unstable
Safian	74	1987	68 (0)	Post-non-Q-MI unstable
Hopkins	75	1988	54 (0)	Post-MI unstable
Suryapranata	76	1988	60 (0)	Post-non-Q-MI unstable
Hartzler	82	1988	103 (3.9%)	Left main
			664 (2.7%)	LVEF < 0.40
			193 (1.5%)	Unstable
Vogel	108	1990	105 (7.6%)[a]	Bypass supported
Alcan	102	1983	9 (11%)	IABP supported
Vogel	103	1988		Bypass supported
Shawl	107	1989	51 (6%)	Bypass supported
Tommaso	109	1990	14 (14%)	Bypass supported
Morrison	91	1990	66 (3%)	Post-MI refractory rest angina
Morrison	92	1990	34 (0)	Unstable in post-CABG patients
Morrison	93	1990	56/18/3.6%/5.5%	IV nitroglycerin/IABP
Kahn	111	1990	28 (0)	IABP

[a] In hospital.

In contrast, medically refractory patients undergoing PTCA have had higher rates of infarction, emergency CABG, and death (65–68,90–92). In 88 refractory unstable patients, deFeyter reported 0 mortality (66). Plokker et al. reported a larger series of 469 patients who underwent angioplasty for medically refractory ischemia, and they had a 1% mortality (67). Perry et al. had a 2% mortality in 105 refractory unstable patients (69). Sharma et al. reported 0 mortality in 40 refractory patients (68). Morrison described a subset who required preprocedure intravenous nitroglycerin; in 56 patients there was a 3.6% mortality (93).

Table 4 Risk Factors for Angioplasty Mortality in Unstable Angina

	Ref.
Medically refractory	(67,69)
Recent myocardial infarction	(72,73,91)
Require IV nitroglycerin	(93)
Require IABP	(93,102)
Left main	(82,85)
Severe pump dysfunction	(102,107–109)
>50% muscle jeopardized	(102,107–109)

Intra-aortic balloon counterpulsation and percutaneous bypass have been used as bridge techniques for refractory ischemia patients undergoing angioplasty (92,101,102,106–108). In the series reported by Alcan et al. and Morrison, the IABP was inserted in most cases out of medical necessity; the procedural mortalities in these series were 11% and 5.5%, respectively (92,102). In Kahn's series the IABP was used prophylactically, and 0 mortality was reported (111).

Tommaso et al. reported a 14% mortality in 14 patients who required percutaneous bypass–assisted PTCA and 0 mortality in 13 patients who had standby only (109). Importantly, they could not predict which patients would need percutaneous bypass. In a series of 105 patients from a national registry experience with percutaneous bypass–assisted PTCA, Vogel et al. reported a 7.6% hospital mortality (108).

High-Risk Subset for PTCA: Impaired Pump Function

In one of the largest experiences with high-risk patients, Hartzler et al. compared 3501 low-risk procedures with a mortality of 0.2–0.3% to various high risk subsets (82). In this series, there were 664 patients with an LVEF < 0.40, and procedure-related mortality was 2.7% (82).

Similarly, some of the patients included in the percutaneous bypass series alluded to above had severely depressed pump function. For example, 90% of the 51 patients in Shawl et al.'s cohort had impaired left ventricular function; the hospital mortality in this group was 6% (107).

High-Risk Subset for PTCA: Sole Remaining Vessel

This issue, although well known clinically, has received scant attention in the literature. Some of these patients are found in nearly all the percutaneous bypass–assisted series, but not enough to tease out much specific information (102,106–108).

Table 5 Factors that Make Patient Prohibitive Risk for CABG

	Ref.
Diffuse distal vessel disease	(27)
Too small a territory to be revascularized	(27)
Uncontrolled cancer	(27)
Dementia	(27)
Serious neurological deficits	(27)
Incapacitating medical condition(s)	(27)
Severe pump dysfunction	(14)

"INOPERABLE" PATIENTS WITH UNSTABLE ANGINA

Each randomized trial of surgical therapy for unstable angina has reported some patients excluded from surgery (8–11,14–16). The same statement can be made about most retrospective series. Nevertheless, there appears to be scant literature about what constellation of factors makes a patient inoperable. One of the best listings is provided by Edwards et al. in their report of "emergency surgery" (27). In general, patients who have diffuse distal disease or other medical conditions that are felt to limit their survival to the same or greater extent than their coronary disease are excluded from trials and from clinical practice (8–11). (See Table 5.)

ABSOLUTE CONTRAINDICATIONS TO ANGIOPLASTY IN UNSTABLE ANGINA

The ACP/ACC/AHA guidelines on lesion morphology are among the best in the literature regarding anatomical suitability for PTCA (111). Many consider type C lesions in unstable patients as absolute contraindications. We do not (91–93). At this point, we consider unprotected left main stenosis and/or only chronic total occlusions in unstable patients as absolute contraindications. There have been several case reports of successful (in terms of stabilizing patients for surgery) PTCA in both settings, but they are unusual. Patients with a sole remaining vessel have been a part of the population for supported PTCA (106–111). (See Table 6.)

Table 6 Factors that Make Patient Prohibitive Risk for PTCA

Unprotected left main
Only chronic total occlusions

SUMMARY

Although there are certain well-recognized high-risk groups, in a given patient it is difficult to know that he would not survive CABG or require cardiopulmonary bypass for PTCA (1–59,105–111). Similarly, there is no subgroup for which it can be categorically stated that CABG or PTCA is preferable in the unstable setting, with the exception of patients who have only chronic total occlusions and/or unprotected left main stenoses, for whom CABG is preferable. How, if at all, left ventricular assist devices or percutaneous bypass will change the CABG versus PTCA dynamic is a topic of strong opinion but little fact.

REFERENCES

1. Krauss KR, Hutter AM, DeSanctis RW. Acute coronary insufficiency. Arch Intern Med 1972; 129:808–13.
2. Wood P. Acute and subacute coronary insufficiency. Br Med J 1961; 1:1779.
3. Gazes PC, Mobley EM Jr, Faris HM Jr, Duncan RC, Humphries GB. Preinfarctional (unstable) angina—A prospective study—Ten year follow up. Circulation 1973; 48:331–7.
4. Conti CR, Brawley RK, Griffith LSC, Pitt B, Humphries JO, Gott VL, Ross RS. Unstable angina pectoris: morbidity and mortality in 57 consecutive patients evaluated angiographically. Am J Cardiol 1973; 32:745–50.
5. Roberts KB, Califf RM, Harrell FE, Lee KL, Pryor DB, Rosati RA. The prognosis for patients with new-onset angina who have undergone cardiac catheterization. Circulation 1983; 68:970–8.
6. Favaloro RG, Effler DB, Cheanvecha C, Quint RA, Sones FM, Jr. Acute coronary insufficiency (impending myocardial infarction). Am J Cardiol 1971; 28:598–607.
7. Segal BL, Likoff W, Van den Broek H, Kimbiris D, Najmi M, Linhardt JW. Saphenous vein bypass surgery for impending myocardial infarction. JAMA 1973; 223:767–72.
8. Luchi RJ, Scott SM, Deupree RH, and the Principal Investigators and Their Associates of Veterans Administration Cooperative Study No 28. Comparison of medical and surgical treatment for unstable angina pectoris. N Engl J Med 1987; 316:977–84.
9. Scott SM, Luchi RJ, Deupress RH, and the Veterans Administration Unstable Angina Cooperative Study Group. Veterans Administration Cooperative Study for Treatment of Patients with Unstable Angina. Circulation 1978; 78(Suppl I):I-113–121.
10. Bertolasi CA, Tronge JE, Riccitelli MA, Villamayor RM, Zuffardi E. Natural history of unstable angina with medical or surgical therapy. Chest 1976; 70:596–605.
11. Unstable Angina Pectoris Study Group. Unstable angina pectoris: National Cooperative Study Group to Compare Surgical and Medical Therapy. II. In-hospital experience and initial follow-up results in patients with one, two, or three vessel disease. Am J Cardiol 1978; 42:839.

12. Lambert CJ, Adam M, Geisler GF, et al. Emergency myocardial revascularization for impending infarctions and arrhythmias. J Thorac Cardiovasc Surg 1971; 62:522–8.
13. Douglas BC, Adelman AG, Huckell VF, et al. Unstable angina: A clinical, angiographic and surgical profile. Cardiovasc Med 1978; 167–76.
14. Pugh B, Platt MR, Mills LJ, et al. Unstable angina pectoris: A randomized study of patients treated medically and surgically. Am J Cardiol 1978; 41:1291–8.
15. Brown CA, Hutter AM, Jr., De Sanctis RW, et al. Prospective study of medical and urgent surgical therapy in randomizable patients with unstable angina pectoris: Results of in-hospital and chronic mortality and morbidity. Am Heart J 1981; 102:959–64.
16. Wiles JC, Peduzzi PN, Hammond GL, Cohen LS, Langou RA. Preoperative predictors of operative mortality for coronary artery bypass grafting in patients with unstable angina pectoris. Am J Cardiol 1977; 39:939–43.
17. Hultgren HN, Pfeiffer JF, Angell WW, Lipton MJ, Bilisoly S. Unstable angina: Comparison of medical and surgical management. Am J Cardiol 1977;39:734–40.
18. Langou RA, Geha AS, Hammond GL, Cohen LS. Surgical approach for patients with unstable angina pectoris: Role of the response to initial medical therapy and intraaortic balloon pumping and perioperative complications after aortocoronary bypass grafting. Am J Cardiol 1978; 42:629–32.
19. Olinger GN, Bonchek LI, Keelan MH, et al. Unstable angina: The case for operation. Am J Cardiol 1978; 42:634–40.
20. Ahmed M, Thompson R, Searbra-Gomes R, et al. Unstable angina: A clinical arteriographic correlation and long term results of early myocardial revascularization. J Thorac Cardiovasc Surg 1980; 79:609–16.
21. Jones EL, Waites TF, Craver JM, et al. Unstable angina pectoris: Comparison with the National Cooperative Study. Ann Thorac Surg 1982; 34:427–34.
22. Hultgren HN, Sheitigar UR, Miller DC. Medical versus surgical treatment of unstable angina. Am J Cardiol 1982; 50:663–70.
23. Cobanoglu A, Freimanis I, Grunkemeier G, et al. Enhanced late survival following coronary artery bypass graft operation for unstable versus chronic angina. Ann Thorac Surg 1984; 37:52–9.
24. Golding LAR, Loop FD, Sheldon WC, et al. Emergency revascularization for unstable angina. Circulation 1978; 58:1163–6.
25. Rankin JS, Newton JR, Jr., Califf RM, et al. Clinical characteristics and current management of medically refractory unstable angina. Ann Surg 1984; 200:457–64.
26. Goldman BS, Katz A, Christakis G, Weisel R. Determinants of risk for coronary artery bypass grafting in stable and unstable angina pectoris. Can J Surg 1985; 28:505–8.
27. Edwards FH, Bellamy R, Burge JR, et al. True emergency coronary artery bypass surgery. Ann Thorac Surg 1990; 49:603–11.
28. Cohn LH, Alpert J, Koster JK, Mee RBB, Collins JJ Jr. Changing indications for the surgical treatment of unstable angina. Arch Surg 1978; 113:1312–6.
29. Hatcher CR Jr, King SB III, Kaplan A. Surgical management of unstable angina. World J Surg 1978; 2:689–700.
30. Nunley DL, Grunkemeier GL, Teply JF, et al. Coronary bypass operation follow-

ing acute complicated myocardial infarction. J Thorac Cardiovasc Surg 1983; 85:485–91.

31. Levine FH, Gold HK, Leinbach RC, et al. Safe early revascularization for continuing ischemia after acute myocardial infarction. Circulation 1979; 60(Suppl I):5–8.

32. Jones RN, Pifarre R, Sullivan HJ, et al. Early myocardial revascularization for post-infarction angina. Ann Thorac Surg 1987; 44:159–63.

33. Midwal J, Ambrose J, Pickard A, Abedin Z, Herman MV. Angina pectoris before and after myocardial infarction. Angiographic correlations. Chest 1982; 81:681–6.

34. Williams DB, Ivey TD, Bailey WW, Ivey SS, Redeout JT, Stewart D. Post infarction angina: Results of early revascularization. J Am Coll Cardiol 1983; 2:859.

35. Baumgartner WA, Borkon AM, Zibulewsky J, Watkins L, Gardner TJ, Bulkley BH, Achuff SC, Baughman KL, Traill TA, Gott VL, Reitz RA. Operative intervention for postinfarction angina. Ann Thorac Surg 1984; 38:265.

36. Gertler JP, Elefteriades JA, Kopf GS, Hashim SW, Hammond GL, Geha AS. Predictors of outcome in early revascularization after acute myocardial infarction. Am J Surg 1985; 149:441.

37. Singh AK, Rivera R, Cooper GN, Karlson KE. Early myocardial revascularization for post infarction angina: Results and long term follow-up. J Am Coll Cardiol 1985; 6:1121.

38. Brower RW, Fioretti P, Simoons ML, Haalebos M, Ruff ENR, Hugenholtz PG. Surgical vs. non-surgical management of patients soon after myocardial infarction. Br Heart J 1985; 54:460.

39. Breyer RH, Engelman RM, Rousou JA, Lemeshow S. Post infarction angina: An expanding subset of patients undergoing bypass surgery. J Thorac Cardiovasc Surg 1985; 90:532.

40. Stuart RS, Baumgartner WA, Soule L, Borkion AM, Gardner TJ, Gott VL, Watkins SL, Reitz BA. Predictors of perioperative mortality in patients with unstable postinfarction angina. Circulation 1988; 78(Suppl I): I-163–I-165.

41. Bardet J, Rigand M, Kahn JC, et al. Treatment of post myocardial infarction angina by intraaortic balloon pumping and emergency revascularization. J Thorac Cardiovasc Surg 1977; 74:299–305.

42. Jones EL, Waites TF, Craver JM, et al. Coronary bypass for relief of persistent pain following acute myocardial infarction. Ann Thorac Surg 1981; 32:33–43.

43. Madigan NP, Rutherford BD, Barnhorst DA, Danielson GK. Early saphenous vein grafting after endocardial infarction. Circulation 1977; 56(Suppl 2):II-1–3.

44. Brundage BH, Ullyot DJ, Winokur S, Chatterjee K, Ports TA, Turley K. The role of aortic balloon pumping in postinfarction angina. Circulation 1980; 62(Suppl I):I-119–23.

45. Weintraub RM, Aroesty JM, Paulin S, et al. Medically refractory unstable angina pectoris. Long term follow-up of patients undergoing intraaortic balloon counterpulsation and operation. Am J Cardiol 1979; 43:877–82.

46. Takaro T, Hultgren HN, Lipton MJ, Detre K, et al. The VA cooperative randomized study of surgery for coronary arterial occlusive disease. Subgroup with significant left main lesions. (Circulation 1976; 54(Suppl III):107.

47. Trenouth RS, Rosch J, Antonovic R, Chaitman BR, Rahimtoola SH. Ven-

triculography and coronary arteriography in the acutely ill patient: Complications, extent of coronary artery disease and abnormalities of left ventricular function. Chest 1976; 69:647.

48. Eugene J, Ott RA, Piters KM, Stemmer EA. Operative risk factors associated with unstable angina pectoris. Arch Surg 1985; 120:279–82.

49. Sherman CT, Litvack F, Grundfest W, et al. Coronary angioscopy in patients with unstable angina pectoris. N Engl J Med 1986; 315:913–9.

50. Chaux A, Lee ME, Blanche C, et al. Intraoperative coronary angioscopy. Technique and results in 58 patients. J Thorac Cardiovasc Surg 1986; 92:972–6.

51. Shapira N, Kirsh M, Jochim K, Behrendt DM. Comparison of the effect of blood cardioplegia on myocardial contractility in man. J Thorac Cardiovasc Surg 1980; 80:647–55.

52. Singh AK, Farrugia R, Teplitz C, Karlson KE. Electrolyte versus blood cardioplegia: Randomized clinical and myocardial ultrastructural study. Ann Thorac Surg 1982; 33:218–27.

53. Iverson LIG, Young JN, Ennix CL Jr, Ecker RR, Moretti RL, Lee J, Hayes RL, Farrar MP, May RD, Masterson R, May IA. Myocardial protection: A comparison of cold blood and cold crystalloid cardioplegia. J Thorac Cardiovasc Surg 1984; 87:509–16.

54. Buttner EE, Karp RB, Reves JG, Oparil S, Brummett C, McDaniel HG, Smith LR, Kreusch G. A randomized comparison of crystalloid and blood-containing cardioplegic solutions in 60 patients. Circulation 1984; 69:973–82.

55. Brawley RK, Merril W, Gott VL, Donahoo JS, Watkins L, Gardner TJ. Unstable angina pectoris. Factors influencing operative risk. Ann Surg 1980; 191:745–50.

56. Christakis GT, Fremes SE, Weisel RD, et al. Reducing the risk of urgent revascularization for unstable angina: A randomized clinical trial. J Vasc Surg 1986; 3:764–72.

57. Naunheim KS, Fiore AC, Arango DC, et al. Coronary artery bypass grafting for unstable angina pectoris: Risk analysis. Ann Thorac Surg 1989; 47:569–74.

58. McCormick JR, Schick EC, McCabe CH, Krounmal RA, Ryan TJ. Determinants of operative mortality and long-term survival in patients with unstable angina. J Thorac Cardiovasc Surg 1985; 89:683–8.

59. Grover FL, Hammermeister KE, Burchfiel C, and cardiac surgeons of the Department of Veterans Affairs. Initial report of the Veterans Administration Preoperative Risk Assessment Study for Cardiac Surgery. Ann Thorac Surg 1990; 50: 12–28.

60. Faxon DP, Detre KM, McCabe CH, et al. Role of percutaneous transluminal coronary angioplasty in the treatment of unstable angina: Report from the Heart, Lung, and Blood Institute Percutaneous Transluminal Coronary Angioplasty and Coronary Artery Surgery Study Registries. Am J Cardiol 1983; 53:131C–135C.

61. Williams DO, Riley RS, Singh AK, Gewirtz H, Most AS. Evaluation of the role of coronary angioplasty in patients with unstable angina pectoris. Am Heart J 1981; 102:1–9.

62. Meyer J, Schmitz HJ, Kiesslich T, et al. Percutaneous transluminal coronary angioplasty in patients with unstable angina pectoris: Analysis of early and late results. Am Heart J 1983; 106:963-80.

63. Quigley PJ, Erwin J, Maurer BJ, Walsh MJ, Gearty GF. Percutaneous translumi-

nal coronary angioplasty in unstable angina; comparison with stable angina. Br Heart J 1986; 55:227–30.

64. de Feyter PJ, Serruys PW, Suryapranata H, Beatt K, van den Brand M. PTCA early after the diagnosis of unstable angina. Am Heart J 1987; 114:48–54.

65. Stefenino G, Meier B, Finci L, Rutishauser W. Follow-up results of treatment of unstable angina by coronary angioplasty. Br Heart J 1987; 57:416–9.

66. deFeyter PJ, Serruys PW, van den Brand M, Balakumaran K, Mochtar B, Soward AL, Arnold AER, Hugenholtz PG. Emergency coronary angioplasty in refractory unstable angina. N Engl J Med 1985; 313:342–7.

67. Plokker HWT, Ernst SMPG, Bal ET, van den Berg ECJM, Mast GEG, Feltz TA, Ascoop CAPL. Percutaneous transluminal coronary angioplasty in patients with unstable angina pectoris refractory to medical therapy. Cathet Cardiovasc Diag 1988; 14:15–8.

68. Sharma B, Wyeth RR, Kolath GS, Gimenez HJ, Franciosa JA. Percutaneous transluminal coronary angioplasty of one vessel for refractory unstable angina pectoris: Efficacy in single and multivessel disease. Br Heart J 1988; 59:280–6.

69. Perry RA, Seth A, Hunt A, Shiu MF. Coronary angioplasty in unstable angina and stable angina: A comparison of success and complications. Br Heart J 1988; 60:367–72.

70. Bredlau CE, Roubin GS, Leimgruber PP, Douglas JS, King SB, Gruentzig AR. In-hospital morbidity and mortality in patients undergoing elective coronary angioplasty. Circulation 1985; 72:1044–52.

71. deFeyter PJ, Serruys PW, Soward A, van den Brand M, Bos E, Hugenholtz PG. Coronary angioplast for early postinfarction unstable angina. Circulation 1986; 54:460–5.

72. Holt GW, Gersh BJ, Holmes DR, Vliestra RE, Reeder GS, Bresnahan JF, Smith HC. The results of percutaneous transluminal coronary angioplasty (PTCA) in post infarction angina pectoris. J Am Coll Cardiol 1986; 7:62A. (Abstract).

73. Gottlieb SO, Brim KP, Walford GD, McGaughey M, Riegel MB, Brinker JA. Initial and late results of coronary angioplasty for early postinfarction unstable angina. Cathet Cardiovasc Diag 1987; 13:93–9.

74. Safian RD, Snijder LD, Snyder BA, McKay RG, Lorrell BH, Aroesty M, Pasternak RC, Bradley AB, Monrad S, Baim DS. Usefulness of PTCA for unstable angina pectoris after non Q-wave myocardial infarction. Am J Cardiol 1987; 59:263–6.

75. Hopkins J, Savage M, Zaluwski A, Dervan JP, Goldberg S. Recurrent ischemia in the zone of prior myocardial infarction: Results of coronary angioplasty of the infarct related artery. Am Heart J 1988; 115:14–9.

76. Suryapranata H, Beatt K, deFeyter PJ, Verroste J, van den Brand M, Zijlstra F, Serruys PW. Percutaneous transluminal coronary angioplasty for angina pectoris after a non Q-wave acute myocardial infarction. Am J Cardiol 1988; 61:240–3.

77. deFeyter PJ, Serruys PW, Beatt K, van den Brand M, Hugenholtz P. Effects of successful percutaneous transluminal coronary angioplasty of the ''culprit lesion'' for management of unstable angina pectoris. Am J Cardiol 1987; 60:993–7.

78. Wohlgertner D, Cleman M, Highman HA, Zaret BL. Percutaneous transluminal coronary angioplasty of the ''culprit lesion'' for management of unstable angina pectoris.

79. deFeyter PJ, Serruys PW, Arnold A, et al. Coronary angioplasty of the unstable angina related vessel in patients with multivessel disease. Eur Heart J 1986; 7: 460–7.

80. deFeyter PJ, Suryapranata H, Serruys PW, Beatt K, van Domburg R, van den Brand M, Tijssen JJ, Azar AJ, Hugenholtz PG. Coronary angioplasty for unstable angina: Immediate and late results in 200 consecutive patients with identification of risk factors for unfavorable early and late outcome. J Am Coll Cardiol 1988; 12:324–33.

81. Myler RK, Topol EJ, Shaw RE, Stertzer SH, Clark DA. Multiple vessel coronary angioplasty: Classification, results and patterns of restenosis in 494 consecutive patients. Cathet Cadiovasc Diag 1987; 13:1–14.

82. Hartzler GO, Rutherford BD, McConahay DR, Johnson WL, Giorgi LV. "High-risk" percutaneous transluminal coronary angioplasty. Am J Cardiol 1988; 61:33G–37G.

83. Dorros G, Cowley MJ, Kanke L, Kelsey SF, Mullin SM, Van Raden M. In-hospital mortality rate in the National Heart, Lung, and Blood Institute Percutaneous Transluminal Coronary Angioplasty Registry. Am J Cardiol 1984; 53:17C–21C.

84. Mock MB, Holmes DR, Vliestra RE, Gersh BJ, Detre KM, Kelsey SF, Orszulak TA, Schaff HV, Piehler JM, Van Raden MJ, Passamani ER, Kent KM, Gruentzig AR. Percutaneous transluminal coronary angioplasty (PTCA) in the elderly patient: Experience in the National Heart, Lung, and Blood Institute PTCA Registry. Am J Cardiol 1984; 53:89C–91C.

85. Stertzer SH, Myler RK, Insel H, Wallsh E, Rossi P. Percutaneous transluminal coronary angioplasty in left main stem coronary stenosis: A five-year appraisal. Int J Cardiol 1985; 9:149–59.

86. Feldman RL, MacDonald RG, Hill JA, Limacher MC, Conti CR, Pepine CJ. Effect of propanolol on myocardial ischemia occurring during acute coronary occlusion. Circulation 1986; 73:727–33.

87. Feldman RL, MacDonald RG, Hill JA, Pepine CJ. Effect of nicardipine on determinants of myocardial ischemia occurring during acute coronary occlusion produced by percutaneous transluminal coronary angioplasty. Am J Cardiol 1987; 60:267–70.

88. Zalewski A, Goldberg S, Dervan JP, Slysh S, Maroko PR. Myocardial protection during transient coronary artery occlusion in man: Beneficial effects of regional beta-adrenergic blockade. Circulation 1986; 73:734–9.

89. Zalewski A, Savage M, Goldberg S. Protection of the ischemic myocardium during percutaneous transluminal coronary angioplasty. Am J Cardiol 1988; 61:54G–60G.

90. Serruys PW, van den Brand M, Brower RW. Regional cardioplegia and cardioprotection during transluminal angioplasty, which role for nifedipine. Eur Heart J 1983; 4:115–21.

91. Morrison DA. Coronary angioplasty for medically refractory unstable angina within 30 days of acute myocardial infarction. Am Heart J 1990; 120:256–61.

92. Morrison DA. Coronary angioplasty for medically refractory unstable angina in patients with prior coronary bypass. Cathet Cardiovasc Diag 1990; 20:174–81.

93. Morrison DA. Percutaneous transluminal coronary angioplasty for rest angina

pectoris requiring intravenous nitroglycerin and intraaortic balloon counterpulsation. Am J Cardiol 1990; 66:168–71.

94. Doorey AJ, Mehmel HC, Schwartz FX, Kubler W. Amelioration by nitroglycerin of left ventricular ischemia induced by percutaneous transluminal coronary angioplasty: Assessment by hemodynamic variables and left ventriculography. J Am Coll Cardiol 1985; 6:267–74.

95. Angelini P, Heibig J, Leachman R. Distal hemoperfusion during percutaneous transluminal coronary angioplasty. Am J Cardiol 1986; 58:252–5.

96. Hinohara T, Simpson JB, Phillips HR, Behar VS, Peter RH, King Y, Carlson EB, Stack RS. Transluminal catheter reperfusion: A new technique to reestablish blood flow after coronary occlusion during percutaneous transluminal coronary angioplasty. Am J Cardiol 1986; 57:684–6.

97. Stack RS, Quigley PJ, Collins G, Phillips HR. Reperfusion balloon catheter. Am J Cardiol 1988; 61:77G–80G.

98. Jaffe CC, Wohlgertner D, Cabin HS, Bowman L, Deckelbaum L, Rementz M, Cleman M. Preservation of left ventricular ejection fraction during percutaneous transluminal coronary angioplasty by distal transcatheter coronary perfusion of oxygenated Fluosol DA 20%. Am Heart J 1988; 115:1156–64.

99. Tokioka H, Miyazaki A, Fung P, Rajagopolan RE, Kar S, Meerbaum S, Corday E, Drury K. Effects of intracoronary infusion of arterial blood or Fluosol DA 20% on regional myocardial metabolism and function during brief coronary artery occlusion. Circulation 1987; 75:473–81.

100. Cleman M, Jaffe C, Wohlgelertner D. Prevention of ischemia during percutaneous transluminal coronary angioplasty by transcatheter infusion of oxygenated Fluosol DA 20%. Circulation 1986; 74:555–62.

101. Zalewski A, Goldberg S, Slysh S, Maroko RP. Myocardial protection via coronary sinus interventions: Superior effects of arterialization compared with intermittent occlusion. Circulation 1987; 71:1215–23.

102. Alcan KE, Stertzer SH, Wallsh E, DePasquale NP, Bruno MS. The role of intra-aortic balloon counterpulsation in patients undergoing percutaneous transluminal coronary angioplasty. Am Heart J 1983; 105:527–30.

103. Vogel RA. Maryland experience: Angioplasty and valvuloplasty using percutaneous cardiopulmonary support. Am J Cardiol 1988; 62:11K–14K.

104. Vogel RA, Tommaso CL, Gundry SR. Initial experience with coronary angioplasty and aortic valvuloplasty using elective semipercutaneous cardiopulmonary support. Am J Cardiol 1988; 62:811–3.

105. Kennedy JH. The role of assisted circulation in cardiac resuscitation. JAMA 1988; 197:615–8.

106. Tomasso CL, Vogel RA, Stafford JL. Alikhan M, Gundry SR. Use of prophylactic semi-percutaneous cardiopulmonary bypass during aortic balloon valvuloplasty. Clin Res 1988; 36:867A.

107. Shawl FA, Domanski MJ, Punja S, Hernandez TJ. Percutaneous cardiopulmonary bypass support in high risk patients undergoing percutaneous transluminal coronary angioplasty. Am J Cardiol 1989; 64:1258–63.

108. Vogel RA, Shawl F, Tommaso CL, et al. Initial report of the National Registry of

elective cardiopulmonary bypass supported coronary angioplasty. J Am Coll Cardiol 1990; 15:23–9.

109. Tommaso CL, Johnson RA, Stafford JL, Roda AR, Vogel RA. Supported coronary angioplasty and stand-by supported coronary angioplasty for high-risk coronary artery disease. Am J Cardiol 1990; 66:1255–7.

110. Feola M, Weiner L, Walinsky P, et al. Improved survival after coronary bypass surgery in patients with poor left ventricular function: Role of intraaortic balloon counterpulsation. Am J Cardiol 1977; 39:1021–6.

111. Kahn JK, Rutherford BD, McConahay Dr, et al. Supported high-risk coronary angioplasty using intraaortic balloon pump counterpulsation. J Am Coll Cardiol 1990; 15:1151–5.

112. ACP/ACC/AHA Task Force. Competence in percutaneous transluminal coronary angioplasty.

VII
SUMMARY AND THE CASE FOR A RANDOMIZED TRIAL

21

The Internal Mammary Artery Experience
Can Nonrandomized Observational Studies Substitute for the Randomized, Controlled Clinical Trial?

William G. Henderson

Veterans Affairs Hospital
Hines, Illinois

INTRODUCTION

Several designs are possible to compare the efficacy of angioplasty therapy (PTCA) and surgical therapy (CABG) for patients with medically refractory rest angina. Retrospective data on patient risk factors, treatment, and outcomes could be collected for a cohort of patients receiving either PTCA or CABG in a defined period of time, in which treatment assignment was at the discretion of the physician and patient. Similar data could be collected in a prospective manner to reduce incompleteness and inaccuracy of the data, which might be a problem with the retrospective study. Or a randomized, controlled clinical trial could be conducted, in which patients are randomly assigned to PTCA or CABG and followed in a prospective manner. The complexity and cost of the latter designs are greater, but potential biases are reduced considerably.

Chalmers et al. (1) published a review article that poignantly showed the potential pitfalls of nonrandomized, observational studies. They reviewed 145 articles reporting studies of the treatment of acute myocardial infarction between 1946 and 1981. Fifty-seven studies used blinded randomization (e.g., envelopes or calls to a coordinating center), 45 studies used unblinded randomization (e.g., random number tables, date of birth, or chart number), and 43 studies used nonrandom assignment. In the blind randomized studies, there was imbalance in 3.5% of patient baseline characteristics, with 56.1% of these in favor of the treated patients having better risk. This is close to the 5% of the baseline patient characteristics expected to be unbalanced by chance alone. In the unblinded randomized studies, 7.0% of the patient baseline characteristics were unbalanced, with 77.6% of these favoring the treated groups. In the nonrandomized studies, 34.4% of the patient baseline characteristics were unbalanced, with 81.4% of these favoring the treated groups.

Furthermore, these findings correlated with the results of the 145 studies. Only 8.8% of the blinded randomized studies reached a statistically significant conclusion, and the case fatality rate in the treated group was on average 0.3% below that of the control group (not significant). Twenty-four percent of the unblinded randomized studies reached statistical significance, and the mean difference in case fatality rate was 5.2% lower in the treated group ($p < 0.001$). In contrast, 58.1% of the nonrandomized studies reached statistical significance, and the mean difference in case fatality was 10.5% lower in the treated group ($p < 0.001$). The authors concluded that as the studies became more rigidly controlled, fewer statistically significant results were found.

Could this same phenomenon be operating in other areas of cardiac research? In this chapter, I will review the literature comparing the efficacy of the internal mammary artery graft (IMAG) versus the saphenous vein graft (SVG) for post-CABG graft patency and survival. I will explain the deficiencies of these studies and emphasize the importance of conducting definitive randomized controlled clinical trials of new therapy as quickly as possible after the new therapies have been introduced and before unsubstantiated opinions have been formed. Implications will be drawn about establishing the comparative efficacy of PTCA versus CABG in medically refractory rest angina.

CRITIQUE OF THE LITERATURE COMPARING IMAG AND SVG

The IMAG was first used to revascularize the human heart by Vineberg in 1950. In this operation the IMA was dissected free and its open distal end implanted directly into the left ventricular wall.

The Vineberg operation was replaced in the 1960s by direct revascularization using saphenous vein grafts. The IMAG was first used for direct coronary artery bypass in 1968 by Green, who reported superior early patency of the IMAG compared to the SVG (2).

During the 1970s the IMA graft was used infrequently. However, following reports from the Montreal Heart Institute and the Cleveland Clinic that the long-term patency of the IMAG was superior to that of the SVG, there was an exponential increase in the use of the IMAG. A survey in 1976 by Miller revealed that only 6% of surgeons in the United States were using the IMAG. Within 5 years, this percentage increased to 13% and by 1986 to almost 95% (3). We have also noticed a significant increase in the use of the IMAG in our Veterans Affairs (VA) cooperative studies on antiplatelet drugs to prevent graft occlusion following CABG (4,5). In VA cooperative studies #207 and #297, patients requiring only an IMAG were excluded. However, patients requiring both IMAGs and SVGs were included in these studies. In study #207, involving patients operated on between 1983 and 1986, 20% of all patients received an IMAG. In study #297, involving patients operated on between 1986 and 1988, this percentage increased to 70%.

The IMAGs are used in various configurations to revascularize the heart, including single IMAGs, bilateral IMAGs, sequential anastomoses, and free grafts. However, by far the most common configuration is a single anastomosis of the left IMA to the left anterior descending (LAD) coronary artery.

In an editorial in the *New England Journal of Medicine* (6), Spencer observed that a study by Loop and others (7) indicated that longevity is increased when the IMAG rather than the SVG is used for bypass grafts. The 10-year patency rate of the IMAG was reported to be about 95%. Spencer also stated that although the series was nonrandomized, it represented the largest collection of data in the world on this issue, and retrospective application of modern statistical techniques supports the validity of the conclusions. He was referring to the use of Cox regression analysis to adjust for important baseline differences in the nonrandomized groups.

It is important that the use of the IMAG be based on solid clinical evidence of its superiority, because it is a more involved surgical procedure causing more morbidity and patient discomfort compared to using the SVG. In VA cooperative studies #207 and #297, we found that aortic crossclamp time, cardiopulmonary bypass duration, operative time, and 35-hr chest tube drainage were significantly greater in patients with IMA grafts compared with vein grafts to the LAD (8). (In spite of these differences, however, there were no significant differences between the two groups in operative mortality rate, the amount of blood and blood products received, the reoperation rate for control of postoperative bleeding, or the incidence of wound complications.)

Table 1 presents characteristics of 12 studies published between 1980 and 1989 comparing the efficacy of the IMAG to the SVG (3,7,9–18). All 12 studies were observational, nonrandomized studies. (To our knowledge, no randomized studies exist comparing the efficacy of the IMAG to the SVG.) Most were retrospective. The operations were performed mainly in the 1970s. Follow-up of patients ranged from 5 to 11 years. Most of the sample sizes were large (in the hundreds or thousands). Four of the studies compared the IMAG to the SVG in the same patients, while eight made the comparison using different patient groups. On the basis of these studies, the IMAG is now considered the conduit of choice for coronary artery bypass surgery.

Table 2 summarizes the results of these 12 studies. Some studies reported both patency rates and survival, while other studies reported patency rates only or survival rates only. Most of the comparisons between the IMAG and SVG were statistically significant; those that were not are designated with the symbol (N.S.).

408

Table 1 Characteristics of 12 IMAG Versus SVG Studies

First author	Journal, year	Period of operations	Average follow-up (years)	No. IMAG patients	No. SVG patients	Differences in patient baseline characteristics	Postop cath completion rates	IMAG vs SVG comparison using same or different patients
Tyras	JTCS, 1980	1972–77	5	765	694	SVG older, more LMCA, more UAP	60–70%	Different
Tector	JAMA, 1981	1972–74	7–9	298[a]	298[a]	—	29.5%	Same
Barner	ATS, 1982	1972–77	5.3	472[a]	472[a]	—	19.7%	Same
Singh	JTCS, 1983	1971–unk.	6.8	Unk.	Unk.		34(Unk.%)	Same
Grondin	CIRC, 1984	1969–72 SVG 1972–73 IMAG	10	40	238	SVG operated earlier	IMAG, 50% SVG, 24%	Different
Okies	CIRC, 1984	1969–82	5–6	1619	927	Unk., noncardiac deaths higher in SVG	IMAG, 16% SVG, 15%	Different
Lytle	JTCS, 1985	Prior to 1977	7.3	Unk.	Unk.	SVG patients had more grafts	IMAG, 137(unk.%) SVG, 364(unk.%)	Diff. and same
Loop	NEJM, 1986	1971–79	8–9	2306	3625	SVG had higher op. mortality, LV	IMAG, 37% SVG, 40%	Different

Cameron	CIRC, 1986	1970–73	10.3	532	216	SVG had more females, LMCA, LV dysfunction, less revascularization, operated earlier	—	Different
Cameron	CIRC, 1988	1974–82	5.5	950	6027	SVG older, more LMCA, worse LV function	—	Different
Ivert	JTCS, 1988	1972–74	10.8	99[a]	99[a]		37%	Same
Acinapura	ATS, 1989	1978–86	7.6	2100	1753	SVG operated earlier, older, had more grafts	IMAG, 29.8% SVG, 31.7%	Different

[a] Same patients had both IMAG and SVG.

JTCS = *Journal of Thoracic and Cardiovascular Surgery*; ATS = *Annals of Thoracic Surgery*; CIRC = *Circulation*; JAMA = *Journal of the American Medical Association*; NEJM = *New England Journal of Medicine*; LMCA = left main coronary artery disease; UAP = unstable angina pectoris.

Table 2 Comparison of IMAG Versus SVG Patency Rates and Survival in the 12 Studies

First author	Follow-up period (years)	IMAG patency (%)	SVG patency (%)	Follow-up period (years)	IMAG survival (%)	SVG survival (%)
Tyras	5	90	82	5	88	89(N.S.)
Tector	5–9	94	64	—	—	—
Barner	5	100	81	—	—	—
Singh	6.8	94	52	—	—	—
Grondin	1	88	76	10	84	70
	10	84	53			
Okies	5	81	64	5 (all grafts)	92	87
	10	69	45	10	82	69
				5 (LAD only)	95	91(N.S.)
				10	82	79(N.S.)
Lytle	1–2	97	87	—	—	—
	7–8	95	64			
Loop	8–9	96	81	10(1-vessel)	93	88
				10(2-vessel)	90	80
				10(3-vessel)	83	71
Cameron	—	—	—	5	91	86
				10	82	72
				14	72	57
Cameron	—	—	—	5	93	89
Ivert	11	88	61	—	—	—
Acinapura	7–8	86	72	9	90	78

(N.S.) = comparison is not statistically significant.

All the comparisons of the patency rates were statistically significant in favor of the IMAG. The patency rates ranged from 69% to 100% for the IMAG and from 45% to 87% for the SVG.

Only the studies comparing the IMAG to the SVG in different patients contribute to the survival analyses. Most of the studies found statistically significantly better survival for the IMAG patients compared to the SVG patients, with the exception of the first study and the sixth study in grafts to the LAD. There appears to be a trend toward increasing IMAG versus SVG differences in patency rates and survival with increasing follow-up time (Figs. 1 and 2).

Do these studies conclusively prove that the IMAG is superior to the SVG? Is a prospective, randomized clinical trial necessary to answer this question? Most cardiac surgeons and cardiologists probably now believe that the question has been answered and that a randomized trial would be unethical.

There are at least eight identifiable problems with these studies.

1. As previously mentioned, all 12 studies were observational and nonrandomized. As shown in Table 1, in the studies where patient characteristics were compared, the SVG patients tended to be operated on in an earlier period and tended to be sicker than the IMAG patients. The surgeons probably chose the healthier patients for the IMAG procedure because it is a more involved operation.
2. In most studies the data collection was retrospective. It is well known that retrospective studies can lead to nonuniform and incomplete data.

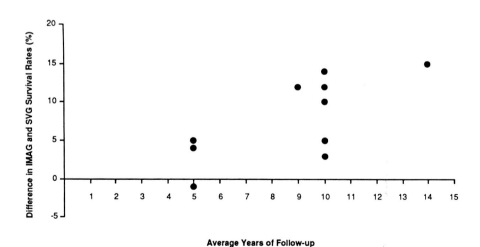

Figure 1 Relationship between follow-up time and difference in IMAG versus SVG survival rates.

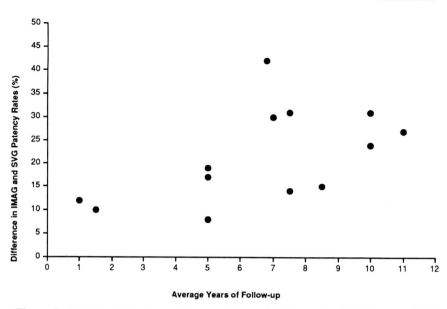

Figure 2   Relationship between follow-up time and difference in IMAG versus SVG patency rates.

3. The postoperative catheterization rates ranged from 15% to 70%, with an average of about 35%. In two studies these rates were not even reported. Also, the postoperative catheterizations were done mainly on symptomatic patients. Since most patients had several vein grafts to every one IMA graft placed, even if the patency rates were truly equal between the IMAG and SVG, catheterizing only symptomatic patients would tend to bias the results against the SVG.

4. Six of the twelve studies (3,7,9,15,16,17) compared the IMAG to SVG patients for relief of angina. Although relief of angina is perhaps a "softer" measurement than graft patency from an angiogram, it is a more complete measurement because it can be collected on all patients noninvasively. It was interesting to observe that in all but one study (3) there were no significant differences between the IMAG and SVG patients for relief of angina. One would expect the IMAG patients to experience more relief of angina if the IMA grafts had better patency.

5. Five of the twelve studies (10,11,12,15,18) compared the IMAG grafted to the LAD coronary artery to the SVG grafted to other coronary arteries. However, it is well established that the patency of grafts to the LAD in general is better than the patency of grafts to other coronary arteries. These comparisons would bias the results in favor of the IMAG.

6. The very long-term IMAG patency rates of 10 or more years are based on very small and selected samples—in one study 23 out of an initial 2306 patients (7), in another study 20 out of an initial 40 patients (13), and in a third study 37 out of an initial 99 patients (18). Estimates of long-term patency based on such small and selected samples are ''shaky'' at best.

7. All the studies precede the widespread use of antiplatelet therapy after CABG. It is now well established that antiplatelet treatment significantly improves SVG patency (4,19–22). It might be that SVG plus one aspirin daily has the same or better long-term patency and survival than the IMAG procedure.

8. Although the studies comparing IMAG and SVG *patency* have problems related to the incompleteness and selectivity of the postoperative catheterization, there are other studies that show improved *survival* of patients who receive the IMAG. However, these studies are also observational and nonrandomized. The selection of sicker patients for the SVG procedure and the fact that these patients were operated in an earlier time period might bias the survival results against the SVG. In some of the studies (e.g., 16), baseline differences in the IMAG and SVG groups were corrected for using Cox regression analysis, and the type of graft used (IMAG versus SVG) remained statistically significant. The problem with this type of analysis is that some (known or unknown) important baseline differences might not have been accounted for. In this author's opinion, use of covariate analysis in observational studies can never replace the randomized controlled clinical trial (RCT).

OBSTACLES TO THE RCT AND IMPLICATIONS ON THE DESIGN OF AN RCT OF PTCA VERSUS CABG IN MEDICALLY REFRACTORY REST ANGINA

Several criticisms of the randomized clinical trial methodology have been made over the past 30–40 years in which large-scale cooperative trials have become increasingly used: (a) physicians are not willing to randomize patients to alternative therapies because they already know which therapy is best; (b) RCTs exclude so many patients for various reasons that the sample of patients studied is not representative of the larger population of patients who need treatment; (c) RCTs take too long to conduct and are too expensive; and (d) treatment methods are changing so rapidly that the results of the RCT will be obsolete when they become available. These criticisms will be addressed one by one, and implications on the design of an RCT of PTCA versus CABG in medically refractory rest angina will be considered.

Sometimes physicians develop an expertise at providing a certain therapy, obtain good results, and are unwilling or unable to consider alternative therapies even when objective evidence comparing the various therapies does not exit.

Furthermore, if the treatments under consideration for an RCT are very different, and particularly when they involve different medical specialties, there can be "turf" problems. It is almost human nature that one physician would believe that the treatment he or she provides is as good as or better than the treatment provided by the next person. Economics could also play a role, although often one does not want to admit this. In order to be able to conduct an RCT, the physician investigator must have an open mind and truly believe that the correct answer is unknown. Hopefully, the earlier discussions about the pitfalls of observational studies might lead the reader to have a more open mind about the importance of randomized clinical trials. In a clinical trial comparing PTCA and CABG in medically refractory rest angina, it would be imperative that the team of cardiologist and surgeon at each center have a cooperative working relationship and open minds about the comparative efficacy of the two therapies.

It is true that many trials have so many exclusion criteria that the percentage of screened patients who are actually randomized is very low. In some trials this information is not even collected or reported. This situation does lead to problems in the generalizability of the trial. However, there should be relatively few exclusion criteria in the well-planned clinical trial. These exclusion criteria should relate to one of four situations: (a) the patient has a condition that is a serious contraindication to one of the treatments (e.g., a patient who cannot receive an anticoagulant in a randomized trial of a mechanical versus a tissue prosthetic heart valve); (b) the patient has a condition that would obscure the measurement of the primary outcome variable (e.g., a patient has a terminal illness with life expectancy less than 6 months); (c) the patient refuses to be in a study or to be randomized, in spite of an honest effort by the physician to explain that the best treatment is truly not known; or (d) the patient is unable to give informed consent (e.g., because of dementia). This author has found many physician trial planners to be too liberal in excluding patients from trials. In a trial of PTCA versus CABG for medically refractory rest angina, other than defining "medically refractory rest angina" and excluding some patients for whom there is clear evidence that CABG or PTCA is the better treatment, no other exclusion criteria should be allowed (e.g., limits on age, ejection fraction or single- versus multiple-vessel disease).

Clinical trials can be done faster and less expensively if more centers participate and exclude fewer patients and if a "low tech" approach to the data collection is taken. There is always the temptation to add one additional "interesting" data item because it is a large effort to initiate the trial and a similar trial will probably never be attempted again. Clinical trial planners often forget that each data item must be entered, edited, and "cleaned" by a number of people before it is used in the analysis (if ever!). Perhaps some trials are better designed with few and focused hypotheses, few exclusion criteria, and with data collection only related to the primary hypothesis. The largest expense of a trial are funds to pay the personnel at the participating centers. In a study in which the treatment is a one-time occurrence (e.g., PTCA versus CABG) and the primary outcome of interest is a major event (e.g., death or an event requiring hospitalization), personnel could be employed at the participating centers only for the enrollment period, and long-term follow-up could be accomplished less expensively through centralization in the chairman's office or coordinating center (e.g., by mail or telephone questionnaire, medical record review, and centralized computer databases).

In planning clinical trials, the inclusion of more centers and more patients and a short trial duration is probably always a desirable goal, provided the funding is available. Therapies do change, and most trials are in danger of being obsolete when their results become available. Some attempts can be made in the planning of the trial to choose those therapies that are likely to still be in widespread use at the end of the trial.

SUMMARY

Observational studies, even though carefully conducted and analyzed by advanced statistical methods, probably cannot replace the randomized clinical trial in providing definitive evidence to support use of a therapy for a given disease. Although it requires much effort and cost, after 30–40 years of application the RCT remains the "gold standard" for clinical research. Prospective clinical registries can provide interesting and useful data on different treatment methods for patients with different risk characteristics having different treatment outcomes. However, rather than providing definitive answers themselves, they should probably be used more as a tool to develop important hypotheses to be tested definitively by the RCT. Various design features can sometimes be built into the RCT to make them more focused, of shorter duration, and less costly.

REFERENCES

1. Chalmers TC, Celano P, Sacks HS, Smith H Jr. Bias in treatment assignment in controlled clinical trials. N Engl J Med 1983; 309:1358–61.
2. Green GE. Internal mammary artery to coronary artery anastomosis: Three years' experience with 165 patients. Ann Thorac Surg 1972; 14:260–71.
3. Acinapura AJ, Rose DM, Jacobowitz IJ, Kramer MD, Robertazzi RR, Feldman J, Zisbrod Z, Cunningham JN. Internal mammary artery bypass grafting: Influence on recurrent angina and survival in 2,100 patients. Ann Thoracic Surg 1989; 48:186–91.
4. Goldman S, Copeland J, Moritz T, Henderson W, Zadina K, Ovitt T, Doherty J, Read R, Chesler E, Sako Y, Lancaster L, Emery R, Sharma GVRK, Josa M, Pacold I, Montoya A, Parikh D, Sethi G, Holt J, Kirklin J, Shabetai R, Moores W, Aldridge J, Masud Z, DeMots H, Floten S, Haakenson C, Harker L. Improvement in early saphenous vein graft patency after coronary artery bypass surgery with

antiplatelet therapy: Results of a Veterans Administration Cooperative Study. Circulation 1988; 77:1324–32.

5. Goldman S, Copeland J, Moritz T, Henderson W, Zadina K, Ovitt T, Kern KB, Sethi G, Sharma GVRK, Khuri S, Richards K, Grover F, Morrison D, Whitman G, Chesler E, Sako Y, Pacold I, Montoya A, DeMots H, Floten S, Doherty J, Read R, Scott S, Spooner T, Masud Z, Haakenson C, Harker LA. Starting aspirin after operation: Effects on early graft patency. Circulation 1991; 84:520–6.

6. Spencer FC. The internal mammary artery: The ideal coronary bypass graft. N Engl J Med 1986; 314:50–1.

7. Loop FD, Lytle BW, Cosgrove DM, Stewart RW, Goormastic M, Williams GW, Golding LAR, Gill CC, Taylor PC, Sheldon WC, Proudfit WL. Influence of the internal-mammary-artery graft on 10-year survival and other cardiac events. N Eng J Med 1986; 314:1–6.

8. Sethi GK, Copeland JG, Moritz T, Henderson W, Zadina K, Goldman S. Comparison of postoperative complications between saphenous vein and IMA grafts to LAD. Ann Thoracic Surg 1991; 733–8.

9. Tyras DH, Barner HB, Kaiser GC, Codd JE, Pennington DG, Willman VL. Bypass grafts to the left anterior descending coronary artery. Saphenous vein versus internal mammary artery. J Thorac Cardiovasc Surg 1980; 80:327–33.

10. Tector AJ, Schmahl TM, Janson B, Kallies JR, Johnson G. The internal mammary artery graft. Its longevity after coronary bypass. JAMA 1981; 246:2181–3.

11. Barner HB, Swartz MT, Mudd JG, Tyras DH. Late patency of the internal mammary artery as a coronary bypass conduit. Ann Thoracic Surg 1982; 34:408–12.

12. Singh RN, Sosa JA, Green GE. Long-term fate of the internal mammary artery and saphenous vein grafts. J Thorac Cardiovasc Surg 1983; 86:359–63.

13. Grondin CM, Campeau L, Lesperance J, Enjalbert M, Bourassa MG. Comparison of late changes in internal mammary artery and saphenous vein grafts in two consecutive series of patients 10 years after operation. Circulation 1984; 70(Suppl I):I-208–I-212.

14. Okies JE, Page US, Bigelow JC, Krause AH, Salomon NW. The left internal mammary artery: the grafts of choice. Circulation 1984; 70(Suppl I):I-213–I-221.

15. Lytle BW, Loop FD, Cosgrove DM, Ratliff NB, Easley K, Taylor PC. Long-term (5 to 12 years) serial studies of internal mammary artery and saphenous vein coronary bypass grafts. J Thorac Cardiovasc Surg 1985; 89:248–58.

16. Cameron A, Kemp HG, Green GE. Bypass surgery with the internal mammary artery graft: 15 year follow-up. Circulation 1986; 74(Suppl III):III-30–III-36.

17. Cameron A, Davis KB, Green GE, Myers WO, Pettinger M. Clinical implications of internal mammary artery bypass grafts: The Coronary Artery Surgery Study experience. Circulation 1988; 77:815–9.

18. Ivert T, Huttunen K, Landou C, Bjork VO. Angiographic studies of internal mammary artery grafts 11 years after coronary artery bypass grafting. J Thorac Cardiovasc Surg 1988; 96:1–12.

19. Goldman S, Copeland J, Moritz T, Henderson W, Zadina K, Ovitt T, Doherty J, Read R, Chesler E, Sako Y, Lancaster L, Emery R, Sharma GVRK, Josa M, Pacold I, Montoya A, Parikh D, Sethi G, Holt J, Kirklin J, Shabetai R, Moores W, Aldridge J, Masud Z, DeMots H, Flotin S, Haakenson C, Harker LA. Saphenous

vein graft patency 1 year after coronary artery bypass surgery and effects of antiplatelet therapy. Results of a Veterans Administration Cooperative Study. Circulation 1989; 80:1190–7.

20. Chesebro JH, Clements IP, Fuster V, Elveback LR, Smith HC, Bardsley WT, Frye RL, Holmes DR Jr, Vliestra RE, Pluth JR, Wallace RB, Puga FJ, Orszulak TA, Piehler JM, Schaff HV, Danielson GK. A platelet-inhibitor drug trial in coronary artery bypass operations: Benefits of perioperative dipyridamole and aspirin therapy on early postoperative vein-graft patency. N Engl J Med 1982; 307:73–8.

21. Chesbro JH, Fuster V, Elveback LR, Clements IP, Smith HC, Holmes DR Jr, Bardsley WT, Pluth JR, Wallace RB, Puga FJ, Orszulak TA, Piehler JM, Danielson GK, Schaff HV, Frye RL. Effect of dipyridamole and aspirin on late vein-graft patency after coronary bypass operations. N Engl J Med 1984; 310:209–14.

22. Henderson WG, Goldman S, Copeland JG, Moritz TE, Harker LA. Antiplatelet or anticoagulant therapy after coronary artery bypass surgery. A meta-analysis of clinical trials. Ann Intern Med 1989; 111:743–50.

22

New Methods of Catheterization Assessment Will They Change PTCA Practice in Unstable Angina Patients?

Douglass Andrew Morrison

Veterans Affairs Medical Center and
University of Colorado Health Sciences Center
Denver, Colorado

ASSESSMENT OF ANGIOPLASTY RESULTS

Coronary angioplasty is an effective means of increasing coronary blood flow and relieving myocardial ischemia in selected patients with coronary artery disease (1–3). The most widely used criterion for assessing the results of angioplasty is the angiographer's visual determination of the percent (%) diameter stenosis (1–6). However, it is well known that the visual assessment of % diameter stenosis from even a high-quality angiogram (a) is not very reproducible, (b) does not take the geometry of the stenosis into account, and (c) correlates poorly with the physiological significance of the stenosis (7–15). Accordingly, a more reproducible, geometrically accurate, and physiological assessment of coronary artery disease is needed for coronary angioplasty.

In order to be useful for making decisions during the angioplasty procedure (such as whether to do more inflations or size up to a larger balloon), assessments must be available on-line (4–6). To have relevance for angioplasty in unstable patients, an assessment method cannot involve major interventions. For example, tests of flow reserve require a vasodilator, such as intracoronary papaverine. Administration of a vasodilator is not always safe for patients with refractory rest angina.

CURRENTLY AVAILABLE MEANS TO ASSESS ANGIOPLASTY RESULTS

Transstenotic Pressure Gradient

A number of early studies reported that the transstenotic pressure gradient was an important procedural predictor of both acute occlusion (which usually necessitates emergency surgery) and restenosis (which remains the major limitation of coronary angioplasty) (16–22). Anderson and co-workers at Emory University measured the translesional pressure gradient before and after angioplasty in 4263 patients (16); they found it to be predictive of the final angiographic outcome. Leimgruber et al., at the same institution, reviewed angioplasty data from 998 patients who underwent angioplasty of native coronary arteries (17). They found that a high (>15 mmHg) gradient after PTCA was predictive of restenosis (17). Hodgson and co-workers, at Brown University, reviewed the subsequent development of clinical events after percutaneous transluminal coronary angioplasty (PTCA) [repeat angioplasty, coronary artery bypass graft (CABG), recurrent angina or positive postangioplasty stress test] in 159 patients and found that the translesional pressure gradient was the only procedural variable that was predictive (18). Similarly, translesional gradients, both before and after PTCA, were found to be predictive of restenosis in the 3079 patients from the National Institutes of Health PTCA Registry of restenosis by Holmes et al. (19).

Ellis and co-workers compared 140 PTCA procedures that were complicated by acute closure of the angioplastied vessel with 311/4772 procedures that were not complicated and found that a postprocedure gradient > 20 mmHg was predictive of acute closure (20). Bredlau et al. reviewed the Emory University experience with 3500 consecutive PTCA procedures looking for predictors of major complications (emergency CABG, myocardial infarction, or death) (21). The strongest procedural predictor of major complication was the angiographic appearance of dissection (which should be identified with even greater accuracy using intracoronary ultrasound), but a high post-PTCA gradient was also important (21).

Clearly, the translesional pressure gradient may be influenced by the presence of collateral vessels (22). In that regard, Dervan et al. suggested that a downstream, or occluded pressure, of > 36 mmHg might be adequate to meet resting myocardial oxygen demands (22).

The pursuit of lower-profile balloons has come at the expense of the pressure-measuring lumen. For that reason, as well as technical artifacts of measurement (such as introduced by sharp bends), most laboratories rarely measure gradients.

Computer-Selected Digital Assessment

Studies from a number of centers have documented that computer selection of regions on digital angiograms is a highly reproducible method of measuring stenosis diameter and area (23–32). None of these studies, to date, has documented any *clinical advantage* from this enhanced reproducibility. This is important because a digital system is very expensive, and it takes extra dye injections to acquire the images (in addition to cine film) and extra time by a physician or technician to process the images to arrive at quantitative data. Processing can be done on-line, but it requires an additional person on the catheterization laboratory team that performs the angioplasty; in other words, processing orthogonal views before and after multiple dilatations is an additional full-time job during the procedure.

Beatt and co-workers demonstrated that visual assessment tended to underestimate angiographic restenosis relative to quantitative digital assessment (23). Katritsis and co-workers in London showed preangioplasty assessment of lesions by quantitative digital methods and videodensitometric means corresponded closely with each other but not with visual assessment (24). Problems developed in using postangioplasty images for videodensitometry (for example, densitometry of the same lesion from two views correlated poorly) (24).

Sanz and coauthors, at the University of Michigan, demonstrated that quantitative digital techniques were significantly more reproducible than visual assessment in 13 patients (25). These workers concluded that digital measurement of absolute (as opposed to %) diameter of stenosis was most reproducible, and they agreed with Katritsis et al. that densitometries of orthogonal views of the same lesion correspond poorly (25).

Serruys and co-workers also concluded (based on 138 patient studies) that visual interpretation overestimates lesion severity and is less reproducible than quantitative assessment (26). Interestingly, however, they have developed a complex densitometric method, which they favor over diameter measurements (26).

Mancini and co-workers developed a dog model by creating "stenoses" of known dimensions (27). They obtained excellent correlations between digital angiographic measurements and the known dimensions (27). Visual assessment of these known dimensions was not attempted.

Brown, another pioneer in the field of quantitative angiography, reviewed the theoretical advantages of quantitative techniques and the derivation (on a fluid mechanical basis) of a stenosis diameter > 1.3 mm or $> 50\%$ (28). Another study from the University of Washington, Seattle, which attempted to define "critical" stenosis, was reported by McMahon et al. (31). It reported that visual % diameter corresponded fairly well with measured % diameter for mild stenoses, but for severe stenoses visual % diameter corresponded more closely with measured % area (31).

Johnson and coauthors, at the University of Iowa, reviewed 23 patients undergoing PTCA using both digital diameter and videodensitometric methods (29). Although the quantitative methods were more reproducible, neither visual nor quantitative results predicted restenosis (29). It should be emphasized that it is not known whether restenosis can be reduced by achieving a more perfect angioplasty result or, alternatively, whether it is primarily a function of local biological factors related to the character of the lesion independent of the angioplasty result. Intracoronary ultrasound might be used to examine the lesion characteristics and assess the role of each in the development of restenosis.

Hodgson and co-workers compared measurements of coronary flow reserve using digital angiography with electromagnetic flow measurements in a dog model (32). Although this method appears practical for stable patients, the requirements for atrial pacing and multiple injections are not practical for unstable patients. Hodgson et al. then applied their technique to 20 patients in whom single-vessel angioplasty was performed; although flow reserve improved with successful PTCA, it did not become normal (33). Unstable patients were excluded from this study (33).

Vogel et al. reviewed digital techniques for coronary flow reserve and emphasized the importance of reproducibility relative to visual assessment (34). Specific clinical advantage was not demonstrated (34).

Coronary Doppler Flow Velocity (35–40)

Sibley et al. described a 3-Fr steerable Doppler catheter that could be used to assess coronary dynamics (35). This catheter was validated in an animal model against an external cuff-type Doppler probe, coronary sinus flow collections, and femoral artery flow calculations (35). The catheter was also tested in 28 patients in the catheterization laboratory; stable recordings were obtained in all 62 coronary artery cannulations and there were no complications (35).

Tadaoka and co-workers validated the Doppler coronary catheter against flows on a flow bench and obtained good correlations (36). Graham et al. compared coronary flow reserve measured simultaneously by Doppler flow velocity and digital angiographic methods as described by Hodgson et al. (33,37). There were reasonable correlations between the two methods, and the Doppler method was the most reproducible (37). Side- and end (Millar)-mounted crystals obtained comparable results (37).

Wilson et al. described animal and human validation of their 3-Fr Doppler catheter (side-mounted crystals) (38). They subsequently studied a group of patients with discrete single-vessel lesions and compared quantitative cross-sectional area of stenosis with translesional pressure gradient and coronary flow reserve in response to papaverine (41). These investigators obtained significant correlations between quantitative measures of stenosis severity and both the translesional pressure gradient and the coronary flow reserve (41).

Johnson and co-workers, in San Francisco, used the Millar 3-Fr Doppler catheter in a canine study (42). This catheter has an end-mounted crystal, and because it tracks over an angioplasty guidewire, it can be placed selectively in the arterial branch of interest, where it remains coaxial (42). Because the sample volume used by the authors was ~2 mm and flow interference occurred primarily within 1 mm of the tip, flow interference was not felt to be a problem (42). These investigators used a fast Fourier transform method (Meda Sonics) to obtain velocity ratios for the stenotic and reference arterial segments, using the continuity equation, such that the velocity ratio equals the ratio of cross-sectional areas between the stenotic and reference arterial segments (42). This use of fast Fourier transform spectral analysis is a significant advance over visual inspection for zero crossing (42).

Videodensitometry (43,44)

This is an area of some debate. Vogel's group has maintained that because videodensitometry of the same lesion in two views correlates so poorly, especially after angioplasty, the eccentric nature of most stenoses makes this an impractical method to even assess the pre versus post angioplasty results (25). Alternatively, by using a weighted average of two or more views, Serruys and colleagues, from Rotterdam, have suggested that this may be one of the best methods of quantitative angiography (26).

Tissue Characteristics and Intracoronary Ultrasound

Although ultrasound is still in its infancy, a number of intravascular systems have been described (45–48). Excellent correlation between histological specimens and ultrasound imaging was described by Gussenhoven et al. (47). In addition to excellent imaging of the intimal surfaces, like angiography, ultrasound provides for circumferential imaging of the arterial wall under the endothelial surface (45). Currently available systems should allow one to distinguish clot, calcified plaque, fibrolytic plaque, hypoechoic lipid plaque, fibromuscular plaque, and dissection (47). Hand-rotated, motor-driven, and phased array systems have all been used (45,46).

SUMMARY

Clearly, a number of new technologies are providing important pathophysiological insights (47–52). Several offer the potential of providing quantitative measures that are more reproducible than visual assessment of stenosis severity. At this point (1992), it is not a proven thesis that any can improve the procedural decision making during angioplasty, especially in unstable patients.

REFERENCES

1. Gruentzig AR, Senning A, Siegenthaler WE. Nonoperative dilatation of coronary artery stenosis, percutaneous transluminal coronary angioplasty. N Engl J Med 1979; 301:61–8.

2.   ACC/AHA Task Force Report. Guidelines for percutaneous transluminal coronary angioplasty: A report of the American College of Cardiology/American Heart Association Task Force on assessment of diagnostic and therapeutic cardiovascular procedures (Subcommittee on Percutaneous Transluminal Coronary Angioplasty). J Am Coll Cardiol 1988; 12:529–45.

3.   Detre K, Holubkov PH, Kelsey S, et al. Percutaneous transluminal coronary angioplasty in 1985–1986 and 1977–1981. N Engl J Med 1988; 318:265–70.

4.   Nichols AB, Smith R, Berke AD, Shlofmitz RA, Powers ER. Importance of balloon size in coronary angioplasty. J Am Coll Cardiol 1989; 13:1094–1100.

5.   Meier B, Gruentzig AR, King SB III, Douglas JS, Hollman J, Ischinger T, Galan K. Higher balloon dilatation pressure in coronary angioplasty. Am Heart J 1984; 107:619–22.

6.   Douglas JS Jr, King SB III, Roubin GS. Influence of the methodology of percutaneous transluminal coronary angioplasty on restenosis. Am J Cardiol 1987; 60:29B–33B.

7.   Marcus ML, Skorton DJ, Johnson MR, Collins SM, Harrison DG, Kerber RE. Editorial: Visual estimates of percent diameter coronary stenosis: A battered ''gold standard.'' J Am Coll Cardiol 1988; 11:882–5.

8.   Gould KL. Editorial: Percent coronary stenosis: Battered gold standard, pernicious relic or clinical practicality. J Am Coll Cardiol 1988; 11:886–8.

9.   Paulin S. Editorial: Assessing the severity of coronary lesions with angiography. N Engl J Med 1987; 316:1405–7.

10. Gould KL: Editorial: Assessing coronary stenosis severity: A recurrent clinical need. J Am Coll Cardiol 1986; 8:91–4.

11. White CW, Wright CB, Doty DB, Hiratza LF, Eastham CL, Harrison DG, Marcus ML. Does visual interpretation of the coronary arteriogram predict the physiologic importance of a coronary stenosis? N Engl J Med 1984; 310:819–24.

12. Deaver L, Gould KL, Kirkeeide R. Assessing stenosis severity: Coronary flow reserve, collateral function, quantitative coronary arteriography, positron imaging, and digital subtraction angiography. A review and analysis. Prog Cardiovasc Dis 1988; 30:307–22.

13. White CW, Wilson RF, Marcus ML. Methods of measuring myocardial blood flow in humans. Prog Cardiovasc Dis 1988; 31:79–94.

14. Wilson RF, Marcus ML, White CW. Effects of coronary bypass surgery and angioplasty on coronary blood flow and flow reserve. Prog Cardiovasc Dis 1988; 31:95–114.

15. Marcus ML, Harrison DG, White CW, McPherson DD, Wilson RF, Kerber RE. Assessing the physiologic significance of coronary obstructions in patients: Importance of diffuse undetected atherosclerosis. Prog Cardiovasc Dis 1988; 31:39–56.

16. Anderson HV, Roubin GS, Leimgruber PP, Cox WR, Douglas JS Jr, King SB III, Gruentzig AR. Measurement of transstenotic pressure gradient during transluminal coronary angioplasty. Circulation 1986; 73:1223–30.

17. Leimgruber PP, Roubin GS, Hollman J, et al. Restenosis after successful coronary angioplasty in patients with single-vessel disease. Circulation 1986; 73:710–7.

18. Hodgson JM, Reinert S, Most AS, Williams DO. Prediction of long-term clinical outcome with final translesional pressure gradient during coronary angioplasty. Circulation 1986; 74:563–6.

19. Holmes DR Jr, Vliestra RE, Smith HC, et al. Restenosis after percutaneous transluminal coronary angioplasty (PTCA): A report from the PTCA Registry of the National Heart, Lung, and Blood Institute. Am J Cardiol 1984; 53:77C–81C.

20. Ellis SG, Roubin GS, King SB III, et al. Angiographic and clinical predictors of acute closure after native vessel coronary angioplasty. Circulation 1988; 77:372–9.

21. Bredlau CE, Roubin GS, Leimgruber PP, Douglas JS, King SB, Gruentzig AR. In-hospital morbidity and mortality in patients undergoing elective coronary angioplasty. Circulation 1985; 72:1044–52.

22. Dervan JP, McKay RG, Baim DS. Assessment of the relationship between distal occluded pressure and angiographically evident collateral flow during coronary angioplasty. Am Heart J 1987; 114:491–7.

23. Beatt KJ, Lujiten HE, deFeyter PJ, van den Brand M, Reiber JHC, Serruys PW. Change in diameter of coronary artery segments adjacent to stenosis after percutaneous transluminal coronary angioplasty: Failure of percent diameter stenosis measurement to reflect morphologic changes induced by balloon dilatation. J Am Coll Cardiol 1988; 12:315–23.

24. Katritsis D, Lythall DA, Anderson MH, Cooper IC, Webb-Peploe MW. Assessment of coronary angioplasty by an automated digital angiographic method. Am Heart J 1988; 116:1181–7.

25. Sanz ML, Mancini J, LeFree MT, Mickelson JK, Starling MR, Vogel RA, Topol EJ. Variability of quantitative digital subtraction coronary angiography before and after percutaneous transluminal coronary angioplasty. Am J Cardiol 1987; 60:55–60.

26. Serruys PW, Reiber JHC, Wijns W, van den Brand M, Kooijman CJ, ten Katen HJ, Hugenholtz PG. Assessment of percutaneous transluminal coronary angioplasty by quantitative coronary angiography: Diameter versus densitometric area measurements. Am J Cardiol 1984; 54:482–8.

27. Mancini GBJ, Simon SB, McGillem MJ, LeFree MT, Friedman HZ, Vogel RA. Automated quantitative coronary arteriography: Morphologic and physiologic validation in vivo of a rapid digital angiographic method. Circulation 1987; 75:452–60.

28. Brown BG, Bolson EL, Dodge HT. Percutaneous transluminal coronary angioplasty and subsequent restenosis: Quantitative and qualitative methodology for their assessment. Am J Cardiol 1987; 60:34B–38B.

29. Johnson MR, Brayden GP, Ericksen EE, Collins SM, Skorton DJ, Harrison DG, Marcus ML, White CW. Changes in cross-sectional area of the coronary lumen in the six months after angioplasty: A quantitative analysis of the variable response to percutaneous transluminal angioplasty. Circulation 1986; 73:467–75.

30. Vogel RA. The radiographic assessment of coronary blood flow parameters. Circulation 1985; 72:445–60.

31. McMahon MM, Brown BG, Cukingnan R, Rolett EL, Bolson E, Frimer M, Dodge GT. Quantitative coronary angiography: measurement of the "critical" stenosis in patients with unstable angina and single vessel disease without collaterals. Circulation 1979; 60:106–13.

32. Hodgson J, LeGrand V, Bates ER, Mancini GBJ, Aueron FM, O'Neill WW, Simon SB, Beauman GJ, LeFree MT, Vogel RA. Validation in dogs of a rapid digital angiographic technique to measure relative coronary blood flow during routine cardiac catheterization. Am J Cardiol 1985; 55:188–93.

33. Hodgson J, Riley RS, Most AS, Williams DO. Assessment of coronary flow reserve using digital angiography before and after successful percutaneous transluminal coronary angioplasty. Am J Cardiol 1987; 60:61–5.
34. Vogel R, LeFree M, Bates E, O'Neill W, Foster R, Kirlin P, Smith D, Pitt B. Application of digital techniques to selective coronary ateriography: Use of myocardial contrast appearance time to measure coronary flow reserve. Am Heart J 1984; 107:153–64.
35. Sibley DH, Millar HD, Hartley CJ, Whitlow PL. Subselective measurement of coronary blood flow velocity using a steerable Doppler catheter. J Am Coll Cardiol 1986; 8:1332–40.
36. Tadaoka S, Kagiyama M, Osamu H, et al. Accuracy of 20-MHz Doppler catheter coronary artery velocimetry for measurement of coronary blood flow velocity. Cathet Cardiovasc Diag 1990; 19:205–13.
37. Graham SP, Cohen MD, Hodgson J. Estimation of coronary flow reserve by intracoronary Doppler flow probes and digital angiography. Cathet Cardiovasc Diag 1990; 9:214–21.
38. Wilson RF, Laughlin DE, Ackell PH, et al. Transluminal, subselective measurement of coronary artery blood flow velocity and vasodilator reserve in man. Circulation 1985; 72:82–92.
39. Kajiya F, Ogasawara Y, Tsujioka K, et al. Evaluation of human coronary blood flow with an 80 channel 20 MHz pulsed Doppler velocimeter and zero-cross and Fourier transform methods during cardiac surgery. Circulation 1986; 74(Suppl III):53–60.
40. Kajiya F, Tsujioka K, Ogasawara Y, et al. Analysis of flow characteristics in poststenotic regions of the human coronary artery during bypass graft surgery. Circulation 1987; 76:1092–1100.
41. Wilson RF, Marcus ML, White CW. Prediction of the physiologic significance of coronary arterial lesions by quantitative lesion geometry in patients with limited coronary artery disease. Circulation 1987; 75:723–32.
42. Johnson EL, Yock PG, Hargrave VK, Srebro JP, Manubens SM, Seitz W, Ports TA. Assessment of severity of coronary stenoses using a Doppler catheter. Circulation 1989; 80:526–35.
43. Nichols AB, Gabriel CFO, Fenoglio JJ, Esser PD. Quantification of relative coronary arterial stenosis by cinevideodensitometric analysis of coronary arteriograms. Circulation 1984; 69:512–22.
44. Ikeda H, Koga Y, Utsu F, Toshima H. Quantitative evaluation of regional myocardial blood flow by videodensitometric analysis of digital subtraction coronary arteriography in humans. J Am Coll Cardiol 1986; 8:809–16.
45. Roelandt J, Serruys PW. Intraluminal real-time ultrasonic imaging: Clinical perspectives. Int J Cardiac Imaging 1989; 4:89–97.
46. Yock PG, Linker DT. Catheter-based two-dimensional ultrasound imaging. In: Topol E. Textbook of interventional cardiology. Chapter 42. Philadelphia: Saunders, 1990:816–27.
47. Gussenhoven WJ, Essed CE, Frietman P, Mastik F, Lancee C, Slager C, Serruys P, Gerritsen P, Pieterman H, Bom N. Intraventricular echographic assessment of vessel wall characteristics: A correlation with histology. Int J Cardiac Imaging 1989; 4:105–16.

48. Hodgson J, Graham SP, Savakus AD, Dame SG, Stephens DN, Dhillon PS, Brands D, Sheehan H, Eberle MJ. Clinical percutaneous imaging of coronary anatomy using an over-the-wire ultrasound catheter system. Int J Cardiac Imaging 1989; 4:187–93.

49. Mabin TA, Holmes DR, Smith HC, et al. Intracoronary thrombus: role in coronary occlusion complicating percutaneous transluminal coronary angioplasty. J Am Coll Cardiol 1985; 5:198–202.

50. Ischinger T, Gruentzig AR, Meier B, Galan K. Coronary dissection and total coronary occlusion associated with percutaneous transluminal coronary angioplasty: Significance of initial angiographic morphology of coronary stenoses. Circulation 1986; 74:1371–8.

51. O'Neill WW, Walton JA, Bates ER, et al. Criteria for successful coronary angioplasty as assessed by alterations in coronary vasodilatory reserve. J Am Coll Cardiol 1984; 3:1382–90.

52. Wilson RF, Johnson MR, Marcus ML, et al. The effect of coronary angioplasty on coronary flow reserve. Circulation 1988; 77:873–85.

23

Summary of Contemporary Care of the Unstable Angina Patient and Proposal for a Prospective, Randomized Trial of PTCA Versus CABG in Rest Angina

Douglass Andrew Morrison

Veterans Affairs Medical Center and
University of Colorado Health Sciences Center
Denver, Colorado

Theme 1: Unstable angina is one of the most common and most difficult problems in contemporary cardiology (Chapter 1).

Admission to hospital intensive-care beds is as common for unstable angina as for ruling out myocardial infarction (1–12). Additionally, a significant proportion of "rule outs" do not have infarction and are subsequently reclassified as having unstable angina (1–16). Finally, among the most complicated myocardial infarction patients are those who have ongoing ischemia or "postinfarction angina" (17–31). For all these reasons, numerically, unstable angina is a larger problem than myocardial infarction.

Unstable angina is often a more difficult problem than myocardial infarction. More health care resources are spent on unstable angina than on myocardial infarction because most unstable angina patients require either coronary artery bypass graft surgery (CABG) or percutaneous transluminal coronary angioplasty (PTCA) and nearly all undergo coronary angiography. In contrast, the far largest subset of infarction patients to necessitate this degree of diagnostic/therapeutic intervention are the patients with postinfarction (unstable) angina (17–31).

At this time (1992), it is an unsolved question as to which unstable angina patient subsets are better served with PTCA or CABG (32–90). It is generally accepted that many unstable angina patients can be medically stabilized first, but patients who cannot be medically stabilized are in need of urgent revascularization (PTCA or CABG) (41–43). Similarly, although what constitutes "failure to stabilize medically" is subject to definitional problems, there is broad agreement that revascularization of such patients is done at higher risk than revascularization of stable patients (Chapters 7, 20) (41–43,49–59).

Theme 2: Some of the difficult clinical management problems with unstable angina arise from definitional imprecision or ambiguity.
What constitutes (a) unstable angina (Chapter 1) (1–17,119–126), (b) medically refractory (Chapter 7) (120–126), (c) high risk for CABG (Chapter 20) (41–43), and (d) high risk for PTCA (Chapter 20) (49–59) are among the definitional issues that make it difficult to design clinical studies or solve clinical management problems in unstable angina. To compare the situation of unstable angina with the situation of myocardial infarction:

(a) Myocardial infarction can be defined specifically by insisting on a specific value for measurable blood enzyme levels with or without readily defined electrocardiographic changes. No diagnostic blood tests are available for unstable angina. Although electrocardiographic (ECG) changes or nuclear scans (such as reversible thallium perfusion defect or reversible radionuclide ventriculographic wall motion abnormality) are relatively specific, they can be quite insensitive diagnostic tests for unstable angina.

(b) In contrast to medically refractory unstable angina, patients with myocardial infarction who have residual ischemia (silent or symptomatic) can be defined with relative precision by means of a low-level treadmill exercise test. Accordingly, this has become a relatively standard means of clinically subsetting patients. Medically refractory unstable angina can be defined by considering drug categories, drug dosages, and physiological end-points (Chapter 7) (127–144).

(c,d) It is reasonably well established that patients who are early (<7 days) after an infarct or have a low LVEF or are hemodynamically unstable after an infarct are high risk. These caveats, as well as extent of coronary disease (such as three-vessel disease), apply to unstable angina patients as well, albeit with less precision, because all studies of unstable angina involve less precisely defined patients than studies of myocardial infarction (1–12).

Theme 3: Some of the definitional ambiguity in unstable angina is soluble.
This theme is *the* point of Chapters 1, 7, and 20 and a major theme of this entire book. By establishing clinical definitions of reasonable precision, it should be possible to define and observe homogeneous patient subsets. In turn, it should be possible to intervene, first in an observational way and then in a prospective, randomized way, to determine which diagnostic and therapeutic options are best for specific, defined homogeneous patient subgroups.

We believe that rest chest syndromes with ECG confirmation of reversible ischemia in patients with angiographic narrowing ≥ 70% of one or more coronary epicardial arteries defines a large, homogeneous group of unstable angina patients. This group may be subdivided into those who have or have not had a recent (<7 days, <30 days) myocardial infarction (creatine phosphokinase

> 2 × control). In turn, refractory subsets, such as rest pain after a prescribed therapeutic algorithm or specifically requiring intravenous nitroglycerin or an intra-aortic balloon pump to stabilize, may be identified. Subsets based on coronary anatomy (number of vessels), left ventricular ejection fraction, and/or prior CABG or prior PTCA can also be objectively defined.

These definitional concepts applied prospectively should enable us to conduct more edifying observational studies or prospective, randomized trials.

Theme 4: The best method currently available to test the relative merits of multiple therapeutic options is the prospective, randomized clinical trials (Chapters 2, 6, 8, 9, and 21) (91–118).
Because of individual patient differences, varied disease natural history, and placebo effects of therapy, it is extremely difficult to objectively assess the merits of new therapies. Even seemingly well-controlled studies suffer from selection biases. For these and many other reasons, the prospective randomized trial has emerged as the best way to compare therapeutic alternatives.

Although the clinical stakes and logistic difficulties may be much greater in a trial of very sick/unstable patients than in a similar study of stable patients, it is not appropriate to generalize the results of a prospective trial to patients who would have been excluded from that trial (111–118). The patients described in this book (those with medically refractory rest angina) have been systematically excluded from most prospective trials of medical therapy versus CABG (87–118) and most trials of PTCA versus CABG currently ongoing (145).

Theme 5: As good as it is, there are limitations to and problems with prospective randomized trials.
Logistic, financial, and time constraints make it necessary for any trial, regardless of how well planned, to exclude some patients. In most trials in the medical literature, more than a simple majority of screened patients were excluded (91–118). This means that even most of the best trials apply to a minority of the general patient population with the disease entity being studied! It must be remembered that if a patient belongs to an excluded population, no matter how intuitive it may seem that the study results should apply to his group as well, it is possible that the results of the same study in his group would have been exactly opposite!

An additional point that deserves emphasis is that although "intention to treat" analyses may help to reduce the biases introduced by crossovers, and randomization is a tool to reduce selection biases, bias can still slip into the best-designed prospective, randomized trials (111–118). Adequate sample size to truly detect differences when they are present or truly exclude them when they are not is another major potential problem. For these and many other reasons, the prospective randomized trial should be viewed as a very powerful tool but not Holy Writ.

Theme 6: Three major therapeutic options are available for the treatment of patients with unstable angina: medical therapy, CABG, and/or PTCA.

There is no "cure" for coronary artery disease. For patients with symptomatic coronary disease, medicine, CABG, and PTCA are the only options. Chapters 6–7, 8–11, and 12–16, respectively, review the currently available observational data and prospective trial data on the application of these options to various unstable angina subsets. Although there is much strong opinion, there are relatively few well-established caveats regarding the choice between these options for any subset of unstable angina patients:

1. Patients with new rest angina are at high risk of death or infarction (1–12).
2. Patients with recent infarct are at high risk of death or infarction (1–12).
3. PTCA and CABG are higher-risk procedures in patients (a) with new rest angina, (b) with rest angina that is medically refractory, (c) with recent (>7 days, <30 days) myocardial infarction, (d) with prior CABG, (e) with impaired left ventricular pump function, (f) with requirement of intravenous nitroglycerin or intra-aortic balloon counterpulsation to stabilize (141–143).
4. Medical therapy that allows for stabilization of rest angina or delay from time of recent infarct (>7 days, >30 days) appears to reduce the risks of PTCA or CABG (120–126,141–143).
5. PTCA is not an option (or, at least, is significantly less favorable than CABG) in patients with left main stenosis > 50% that is unprotected or with only old total occlusions.
6. Whether PTCA is superior to CABG or CABG is superior to PTCA in almost any other unstable angina subsets is not known.

Theme 7: For patients with ischemia that is refractory to aggressive medical therapy, CABG and PTCA are the only therapeutic options (127–144).

In Chapter 7 we defined medically refractory in terms of categories of medications, target heart rates and blood pressure, and objectively confirmed ischemia (ECG changes, reversible perfusion, defects, and/or reversible wall motion abnormalities) at rest in an intensive-care setting (where bed rest, nasal oxygen, etc., allow the increased demand or medical noncompliance issues to be eliminated). Given the imperfect sensitivity of our tests for ischemia, it is likely these criteria would exclude some legitimately "refractory" patients. Nonetheless, those included would be homogeneous and well defined. For these patients only a CABG strategy or PTCA strategy remains as option.

Reviewing the current indications of the ISFC/WHO Task Force on Coronary Angioplasty, it is clear that a number of subsets of unstable angina, to which CABG has been effectively applied, albeit at increased risk, are often approached by PTCA as well. The situation where two very different forms of treatment have both been shown to be effective in a majority but associated with significant risk in a minority is precisely the setting where a prospective, randomized trial makes the most sense.

Nevertheless, as for CABG, PTCA is not without risk and unstable angina is associated with increased risk (25–30,49–59). Specific unstable angina subsets at high risk include:

1. LVEF < 0.40 (164,165)
2. Left main equivalent
3. Three-vessel disease
4. Sole remaining vessel
5. Hemodynamically unstable
6. Medically refractory

The use of supportive ''bridge'' devices such as intra-aortic balloon counter-pulsation or percutaneous bypass may make nearly *all* physiological subsets potential candidates for angioplasty (Chapters 17–20). Nevertheless, two relatively strong and anatomical contraindications are (a) significant unprotected left main stenosis and (b) only chronic total occlusions. (See characteristics of type A, B, and C lesions.)

Theme 8: Given the high risk of either PTCA or CABG in patients with medically refractory rest angina, a trial of PTCA versus CABG in this subset of unstable angina could likely have death and/or infarction as its end-point.
Of all the medical therapies tried for unstable angina, only aspirin and heparin have demonstrated benefit in reducing either myocardial infarction and/or death (119). As widespread as these are, and as obvious the symptomatic improvement, in many patients, neither of these benefits has been convincingly demonstrated for oral or intravenous nitroglycerin, oral or intravenous beta-blockers, or oral or intravenous calcium channel blockers (127–141).

Similarly, despite several excellent prospective, randomized trials comparing CABG to medical therapy, a clear-cut mortality benefit or reduction in myocardial infarction has been demonstrated for only a few subsets, such as critical (>50%) left main stenosis (120–126).

To date, no prospective, randomized trial data comparing PTCA versus CABG in unstable angina are available. Of the ongoing studies of PTCA versus CABG, none are focusing on unstable angina and one is specifically excluding this category (145). Similarly, most of the very high-risk subsets discussed in this book are being systematically excluded from these trials (145). Only BARI was designed to have a chance of detecting infarction or mortality differences (145). Given its rates of accrual, it is possible that BARI will not be able to detect these differences in any set of patients, much less subsets of unstable angina. Accordingly, a trial of PTCA versus CABG in high-risk unstable angina patients would likely be the only trial to have the potential for identifying mortality or infarction reduction from either PTCA or CABG.

Theme 9: Short-term and long-term outcomes may be very different. For example, PTCA may be more safe acutely in unstable patients whereas CABG may

confer more complete revascularization and more durable results (262–276).
Acute crossovers from PTCA to CABG (193–207) and long-term crossovers
from PTCA to CABG or repeat PTCAs (208–239,257–261) must be matched
against PTCA successes in high risk for CABG patients (25–30,160–174), acute
crossovers from CABG to PTCA, and long-term crossovers from CABG to
PTCA and/or repeat CABG (166–174,240–256).

*Theme 10: Given the numbers of patients with medically refractory rest angina
who receive care within the U.S. Department of Veterans Affairs system, and the
support veterans and the VA system have shown for Cooperative Studies, a VA
Cooperative prospective, randomized trial of PTCA versus CABG in unstable
angina is feasible, ethical, and should be seriously considered.*
The USVA system is the largest health care provider in the United States. It has
supported a cooperative studies program that has funded many of the most
important prospective clinical trials, including the VA Cooperative Aspirin
Study in Unstable Angina (Chapter 6) and the VA Cooperative Study of Medical
Versus Surgical Therapy of Unstable Angina (Chapter 8). Because of this
program and veterans' historic willingness to participate in clinical trials, the VA
is an ideal setting for large-scale clinical trials.

This book was organized, in part, to provide a literature review and a forum of
experts upon which to develop a proposal for a VA Cooperative Study of PTCA
versus CABG in unstable angina. In March 1991, the VA Cooperative Studies
Program approved funding of the planning meeting for VA Cooperative Study
385: PTCA Versus CABG in Unstable Angina. It is to that study and the U.S.
veteran patients, with whose voluntary participation it will become a reality, that
this book is now dedicated.

REFERENCES

1. Conti CR, Hill JA, Mayfield WR. Unstable angina pectoris: Pathogenesis and
   management. Curr Prob Cardiol 1989; 14:553–623.
2. Farhi JI, Cohen M, Fuster V. Editorial: The broad spectrum of unstable angina
   pectoris and its implications for future controlled trials. Am J Cardiol 1986;
   58:547–50.
3. Munger TM, Oh JK. Unstable angina. Mayo Clin Proc 1990; 65:384–406.
4. Scanlon PJ. The intermediate coronary syndrome. Prog Cardiovasc Dis 1981;
   23:351–64.
5. Cairns JA, Fantus IG, Klassen GA. Unstable angina pectoris. Am Heart J 1976;
   92:373–86.
6. Silverman KJ, Grossman W. Angina pectoris: Natural history and strategies for
   evaluation and management. N Engl J Med 1984; 310:1712–7.
7. Nichol ES, Fassett DW. An attempt to forestall acute coronary thrombosis. South
   Med J 1947; 40:631–7.

8. Beamish RE, Storrie VM. Impending myocardial infarction: Recognition and management. Circulation 1960; 21:1107–15.

9. Vakil RJ. Intermediate coronary syndrome. Circulation 1961; 24:557–71.

10. Vakil RJ. Preinfarction syndrome—Management and follow-up. Am J Cardiol 1964; 14:55–63.

11. Gazes PC, Mobley EM Jr, Faris HM Jr, Duncan RC, Humphries GB. Preinfarctional (unstable) angina—A prospective study—Ten year follow up. Circulation 1973; 48:331–7.

12. Bertolasi CA, Tronge JE, Riccitelli MA, Villamayor RM, Zuffardi E. Natural history of unstable angina with medical or surgical therapy. Chest 1976; 70:596–605.

13. Plotnick GD. Approach to the management of unstable angina. Am Heart J 1979; 98:243–55.

14. Russell RO, Rackley CE, Kouchoukos NT. Editorial: Unstable angina pectoris—do we know the best management? Am J Cardiol 1981; 48:590–1.

15. Brown BG, Dodge HT. Editorial: Unstable angina: Guidelines for therapy based on the last decade of clinical observations. Ann Intern Med 1982; 97:921–3.

16. Flaherty JT. Unstable angina: A rational approach to management. Am J Med 1984; 54:52–7.

17. Ambrose JA, Hjemdahl-Monsen CE, Borrico S, et al. Quantitative and qualitative effects of intracoronary streptokinase in unstable angina and non Q-wave infarction. J Am Coll Cardiol 1987; 9:1156–65.

18. Multicenter Diltiazem Postinfarction Trial Research Group. The effect of diltiazem and reinfarction after myocardial infarction. N Engl J Med 1988; 319:385–92.

19. Shapiro EP, Brinker JA, Gottlieb SO, Guzman PA, Bulkley BH. Intracoronary thrombolysis 3–13 days after acute myocardial infarction for postinfarction angina pectoris. Am J Cardiol 1985; 55:1453–8.

20. Rentrop P, Blanke H, Karsch KR, et al. Selective intracoronary thrombolysis in acute myocardial infarction and unstable angina pectoris. Circulation 1981; 63:307–17.

21. Vetrovec GW, Leinbach RC, Gold HK, Cowley MJ. Intracoronary thrombolysis in syndromes of unstable ischemia: Angiographic and clinical results. Am Heart J 1982; 104:946–92.

22. Nunley DL, Grunkemeier GL, Teply JF, et al. Coronary bypass operation following acute complicated myocardial infarction. J Thorac Cardiovasc Surg 1983; 85:485–91.

23. Levine FH, Gold HK, Leinbach RC, et al. Safe early revascularization for continuing ischemia after acute myocardial infarction. Circulation 1979; 60(Suppl I):5–8.

24. Jones RN, Pifarre R, Sullivan HJ, et al. Early myocardial revascularization for post-infarction angina. Ann Thorac Surg 1987; 44:159–63.

24. Gotoh K, Minamino T, Katoh O, et al. The role of intracoronary thrombus in unstable angina: Angiographic assessment of thrombolytic therapy during ongoing anginal attacks. Circulation 1988; 77:526–34.

25. Ouyang P, Brinker JA, Mellits ED, Weisfeldt ML, Gerstenblith G. Variables

predictive of successful medical therapy in patients with unstable angina. Selection by multivariate analysis from clinical, electrocardiographic and angiographic evaluations. Circulation 1984; 70:367–76.

26. Hopkins J, Savage M, Zalewski A, et al. Recurrent ischemia in the zone of prior myocardial infarction: Results of coronary angioplasty of the infarct related artery. Am Heart J 1988; 115:14–9.

27. Gottlieb SO, Walford GD, Ouyang P, et al. Initial and late results of coronary angioplasty for early postinfarction unstable angina. Cath Cardiovasc Diag 1987; 13:93–9.

28. Safian RD, Snyder LD, Snyder BA, et al. Usefulness of percutaneous transluminal coronary angioplasty for unstable angina pectoris after non Q-wave acute myocardial infarction. Am J Cardiol 1987; 59:263–6.

29. Suryapranata H, Beatt K, deFeyter PJ, et al. Percutaneous transluminal coronary angioplasty for angina pectoris after a non Q-wave myocardial infarction. Am J Cardiol 1988; 61:240–3.

30. Sabbah HN, Brymer JF, Gheorghiadez M, Stein PD, Kahaj A. Left ventricular function after successful percutaneous transluminal angioplasty for post-infarction angina pectoris. Am J Cardiol 1988; 62:358–62.

31. Campolo L, DeBaise AM, Cataldo MG, et al. Indications for surgical treatment in post infarction angina. Eur Heart J 1986; 7(Suppl):103–9.

32. Pugh B, Platt MR, Mills LJ, et al. Unstable angina pectoris: A randomized study of patients treated medically and surgically. Am J Cardiol 1978; 41:1291–8.

33. Brown CA, Hutter AM, Jr., DeSanctis RW, et al. Prospective study of medical and urgent surgical therapy in randomizable patients with unstable angina pectoris: Results of in-hospital and chronic mortality and morbidity. Am Heart J 1981; 102:959–64.

34. Hultgren HN, Pfeiffer JF, Angell WW, Lipton MJ, Bilisoly S. Unstable angina: Comparison of medical and surgical management. Am J Cardiol 1977; 39:734–40.

35. Langou RA, Geha AS, Hammond GL, Cohen LS. Surgical approach for patients with unstable angina pectoris: Role of the response to initial medical therapy and intraaortic balloon pumping and perioperative complications after aortocoronary bypass grafting. Am J Cardiol 1978; 42:629–32.

36. Olinger GN, Bonchek LI, Keelan MH, et al. Unstable angina: The case for operation. Am J Cardiol 1978; 42:634–40.

37. Ahmed M, Thompson R, Searbra-Gomes R, et al. Unstable angina: A clinical arteriographic correlation and long term results of early myocardial revascularization. J Thorac Cardiovasc Surg 1980; 79:609–16.

38. Jones EL, Waites TF, Craver JM, et al. Unstable angina pectoris: Comparison with the National Cooperative Study. Ann Thorac Surg 1982; 34:427–34.

39. Hultgren HN, Sheitigar UR, Miller DC. Medical versus surgical treatment of unstable angina. Am J Cardiol 1982; 50:663–70.

40. Cobanoglu A, Freimanis I, Grunkemeier G, et al. Enhanced late survival following coronary artery bypass graft operation for unstable versus chronic angina. Ann Thorac Surg 1984; 37:52–9.

41. Golding LAR, Loop FD, Sheldon WC, et al. Emergency revascularization for unstable angina. Circulation 1978; 58:1163–6.

42. Rankin JS, Newton JR Jr, Califf RM, et al. Clinical characteristics and current management of medically refractory unstable angina. Ann Surg 1984; 200:457–64.

43. Edwards FH, Bellamy R., Burge JR, et al. True emergency coronary artery bypass surgery. Ann Thorac Surg 1990; 49:603–11.

44. Cohn LH, Alpert J, Koster JK, Mee RBB, Collins JJ Jr. Changing indications for the surgical treatment of unstable angina. Arch Surg 1978; 113:1312–6.

45. Hatcher CR, Jr., King SB III, Kaplan A. Surgical management of unstable angina. World J Surg 1978; 2:689–700.

46. Firth BG, Hillis LD, Willerson JT. Unstable angina pectoris: Medical versus surgical treatment. Herz 1980; 5:16–24.

47. Mock MB, Smith HC, Mullaney CJ. The second generation NHLBI Percutaneous Transluminal Coronary Angioplasty Registry: Have we established the role for PTCA in treating coronary disease? Circulation 1989; 80:700–2.

48. Shawl FA, Velasco CE, Goldbaum TS, Forman MB. The effect of coronary angioplasty on electrocardiographic changes in patients with unstable angina secondary to left anterior descending coronary artery disease. J Am Coll Cardiol 1990; 16:325–31.

49. Williams DO, Riley RS, Singh AK, Gewirth H, Most AS. Evaluation of the role of coronary angioplasty in patients with unstable angina pectoris. Am Heart J 1981; 102:1–9.

50. Meyer J, Schmitz H, Erbel R, et al. Treatment of unstable angina pectoris with percutaneous transluminal coronary angioplasty (PTCA). Cathet Cardiovasc Diag 1981; 7:361–71.

51. Meyer J, Schmitz HJ, Kiesslich T, et al. Percutaneous transluminal coronary angioplasty in patients with stable and unstable angina pectoris: Analysis of early and late results. Am Heart J 1983; 106:973–80.

52. deFeyter PJ, Serruys PW, Suryapranata H, Beatt K, Van den Brand M. Coronary angioplasty early after diagnosis of unstable angina. Am Heart J 1987; 114:48–54.

53. Timmis AD, Griffin B, Crick CP, Sowton E. Early percutaneous transluminal coronary angioplasty in the management of unstable angina. Int J Cardiol 1987; 14:25–31.

54. Sharma B, Wyeth RP, Kolath GS, Gimenez HJ, Franciosa JA. Percutaneous transluminal coronary angioplasty of one vessel for refractory unstable angina pectoris: Efficacy and single and multi-vessel disease. Br Heart J 1988; 59:280–6.

55. DiMarco RF, McKeating JA, Pellegrin RV, et al. Contraindications for percutaneous transluminal coronary angioplasty in treatment of unstable angina pectoris. Texas Heart Inst J 1988; 15:152–4.

56. Hartzler GO, Rutherford BD, McConahay DR, et al. High risk percutaneous transluminal coronary angioplasty. Am J Cardiol 1988; 61:33G–37G.

57. ACC/AHA Task Force Report. Guidelines for percutaneous transluminal coronary angioplasty: A report of the American College of Cardiology/American Heart Association Task Force on assessment of diagnostic and therapeutic cardiovascular procedures (Subcommittee on Percutaneous Transluminal Coronary Angioplasty). J Am Coll Cardiol 1988; 12:529–45.

58. Ryan TJ, Faxon DP, Gunnar RM, et al. Guidelines for percutaneous transluminal

coronary angioplasty: A report of the American College of Cardiology/American Heart Association Task Force on Assessment of Diagnostic and Therapeutic Cardiovascular Procedures (Subcommittee on Percutaneous Transluminal Coronary Angioplasty). Circulation 1988; 78:486–502.

59. Bourassa MG, Alderman EL, Bertrand M, et al. Report of the Joint ISFC/WHO Task Force on coronary angioplasty. Circulation 1988; 78:780–9.

60. Hollman J. Coronary angioplasty: A procedure that has "come of age." Postgrad Med 1984; 75:137–51.

61. Kouchoukos NT. Percutaneous transluminal coronary angioplasty: A surgeon's view. Circulation 1985; 72:1144–7.

62. Holmes DR Jr, Vliestra RE. Percutaneous transluminal coronary angioplasty: current status and future trends. Mayo Clin Proc 1986; 61:865–76.

63. Scanlon PJ. The training for and practice of percutaneous transluminal coronary angioplasty: Results of two surveys. Cathet Cardiovasc Diag 1985; 11:561–70.

64. Kent KM. Coronary angioplasty: A decade of experience. N Engl J Med 1987; 316:1148–50.

65. King SB III. Percutaneous transluminal coronary angioplasty: The second decade. Am J Cardiol 1988; 62:2k–6k.

66. Higgins CB. Coronary angioplasty: A decade of advances. Am J Cardiol 1988: 62:7k–10k.

67. Chaissin MR, Park RE, Fink A, Rauchman S, Keesey J, Brook RH. Indications for selected medical and surgical procedures: A literature review and ratings of appropriateness of coronary artery bypass graft surgery. Santa Monica, CA: Rand Corp, 1986.

68. Braunwald E. Effects of coronary-artery bypass grafting on survival: Implications of the randomized Coronary Artery Surgery Study. N Engl J Med 1983; 309–1181–4.

69. Reeder GS, Krishan I, Nobrega FT, et al. Is percutaneous coronary angioplasty less expensive than bypass surgery? N Engl J Med 1984; 311:1157–62.

70. Loop FD, Christiansen EK, Lester JL, Cosgrove DM, Franco I, Golding LR. A strategy for cost containment in coronary surgery. JAMA 1983; 250:63–6.

71. Feinleib M, Havlik RJ, Gillum RF, Pokras R, McCarthy E, Molen M. Coronary heart disease and related procedures. National Hospital Discharge Survey Data. Circulation 1989; 79(Suppl I):13–118.

72. Hurst JW. Percutaneous transluminal coronary angioplasty: A word of caution. Circulation 1987; 75:902–5.

73. Ellis SG, Fisher L, Dushman-Ellis S, King SB III, Roubin GS, Alderman EL. Comparison of 3–5 year mortality and infarction rates after angioplasty (PTCA) or medical therapy for 1 or 2 vessel left anterior descending disease. Circulation 1987; 76(Suppl):IV392.

74. Fisher LD, Holmes DR Jr, Mock MB, et al. Design of comparative clinical studies of percutaneous transluminal coronary angioplasty using estimates from the Coronary Artery Surgery Study. Am J Cardiol 1984; 53:138C–146C.

75. Berreklouw E, Hoogsteen J, Van Wandelen R, et al. Bilateral mammary artery surgery or percutaneous transluminal coronary angioplasty for multivessel coronary artery disease? An analysis of effects and costs. Eur Heart J 1989; 10(Suppl H):61–70.

76. Kramer JR, Proudfit WL, Loop FD, et al. Late follow-up of 781 patients undergoing percutaneous transluminal coronary angioplasty or coronary artery bypass grafting for an isolated obstruction in the left anterior descending coronary artery. Am Heart J 1989; 118:1144–53.

77. Webb JG, Myler RK, Shaw RE, et al. Bidirectional crossover and late outcome after coronary angioplasty and bypass surgery: 8 to 11 year follow-up. J Am Coll Cardiol 1990; 16:57–65.

78. King SB III, Talley JD. Coronary arteriography and percutaneous transluminal coronary angioplasty: Changing patterns of use and results. Circulation 1989; 79:119–23.

79. Dimas AP, Healy B. Coronary artery bypass surgery versus coronary angioplasty: From antithesis to synthesis. Eur Heart J 1989; 10(Suppl H):85–91.

80. King SB III, Ivanhoe RJ. Has multivessel angioplasty displaced surgical revascularization? Cardiovasc Clin 1990; 21:123–37.

81. Henderson RA. The Randomised Intervention Treatment of Angina (RITA) Trial protocol: A long-term study of coronary angioplasty and coronary artery bypass surgery in patients with angina. Br Heart J 1989; 62:411–4.

82. Mock MB, Smith HC, Mullany CJ. The "second generation" NHLBI Percutaneous Transluminal Coronary Angioplasty Registry. Have we established the role for PTCA in treating coronary artery disease? Circulation 1989; 80:700–2.

83. Lee ME. How do you spell relief: PTCA or CABG? J Thorac Cardiovasc Surg 1989; 97:935–7 (Letter).

84. Hochberg MS, Gielchinsky I, Parsonnet V, Hussain SM, Mirsky E, Fisch D. Coronary angioplasty versus coronary bypass: three year follow-up of a matched series of 250 patients. J Thorac Cardiovasc Surg 1989; 97:496–503.

85. Dally PO. Early and five-year results for coronary artery bypass grafting: A benchmark for percutaneous transluminal coronary angioplasty. J Thorac Cardiovasc Surg 1989; 97:67–77.

86. Akins CW. Block PC, Palacios IF, Gold HK, Carroll DL, Grunkemeier GL. Comparison of coronary artery bypass grafting and percutaneous transluminal coronary angioplasty as initial treatment strategies. Ann Thorac Surg 1989; 47:507–16.

87. Kennedy JW, Kaiser GC, Fisher LD, et al. Multivariate discriminant analysis of the clinical and angiographic predictors of operative mortality from the Collaborative Study in Coronary Artery Surgery (CASS). J Thorac Cardiovasc Surg 1980; 80:876–87.

88. Myers WO, Davis K, Foster ED, Maynard C, Kaiser GC. Surgical survival in the Coronary Artery Surgery Study (CASS) registry. Ann Thorac Surg 1985; 40:245–60.

89. Myocardial infarction and mortality in the Coronary Artery Surgery Study (CASS) randomized trial. N Engl J Med 1984; 310:750–8.

90. Coronary Artery Surgery Study (CASS). A randomized trial of coronary artery bypass surgery. Survival data. Circulation 1983; 68:939–50.

91. Kaiser GC, Davis KB, Fisher LD, et al. Survival following coronary artery bypass grafting in patients with severe angina pectoris (CASS): An observational study. J Thorac Cardiovasc Surg 1985; 89:513–24.

92. The National Heart, Lung and Blood Institute Coronary Artery Surgery Study (CASS). Circulation 1981; 63(Suppl):1–39.

93. Kennedy JW, Kaiser GC, Fisher LD, et al. Clinical and angiographic predictors of operative mortality from the Collaborative Study in Coronary Artery Surgery (CASS). Circulation 1981; 63:793–802.

94. Killip T, Passamani E, Davis K. Coronary Artery Surgery Study (CASS): A randomized trial of coronary bypass surgery: Eight years follow-up and survival in patients with reduced ejection fraction. Circulation 1985; 72:V102–9.

95. Coronary Artery Surgery Study (CASS). A randomized trial of coronary artery bypass surgery. Quality of life in patients randomly assigned to treatment groups. Circulation 1983; 68:951–60.

96. Passamani E, Davis KB, Gillespie MH, Killip T. A randomized trial of coronary artery bypass surgery: Survival of patients with a low ejection fraction. N Engl J Med 1985; 312:1665–71.

97. Chaitman BR, Fisher LD, Bourassa MG, et al. Effect of coronary bypass surgery on survival patterns in subsets of patients with left main coronary artery disease: Report of the Collaborative Study in Coronary Artery Surgery (CASS). Am J Cardiol 1981; 48:765–77.

98. Lawrie GM, DeBakey ME. the Coronary Artery Surgery Study. JAMA 1984; 252:2609–11.

99. Weinstein GS, Levin B. The Coronary Artery Surgery Study (CASS): A critical appraisal. J Thorac Cardiovasc Surg 1985; 90:541–8.

100. Eaker ED, Kronmal R, Kennedy JW, Davis K. Comparison of the long-term, postsurgical survival of women and men in the Coronary Artery Surgery Study (CASS). Am Heart J 1989; 117:71–81.

101. Long-term results of prospective randomized study of coronary artery bypass surgery in stable angina pectoris. European Coronary Artery Surgery Study Group. Lancet 1982; 2:1173–80.

102. Prospective randomized study of coronary artery bypass surgery in stable angina pectoris. Lancet 1980; 2:491–5.

103. Coronary artery bypass surgery in stable angina pectoris: Survival at two years. Lancet 1979: 1:491–5.

104. Varnaiskas E. Twelve year follow-up of survival in the randomized European Coronary Surgery Study. N Engl J Med 1988; 319:332–7.

105. Varnaiskas E. Survival, myocardial infarction, and employment status in a prospective randomized study of coronary bypass surgery. Circulation 1985; 72:V90–101.

106. Prospective randomized study of coronary artery bypass surgery in stable angina pectoris: A progress report on survival. Circulation 1982; 65:67–71.

107. Murphy ML, Hultgren HN, Detre K, et al. Treatment of chronic stable angina: A preliminary report of survival data of the randomized Veterans Administration Cooperative Study. N Engl J Med 1977; 297–621–7.

108. Eleven-year survival in the Veterans Administration Randomized Trial of Coronary Artery Bypass Surgery Cooperative Study Group. N Engl J Med 1984; 311:1333–9.

109. Detre KM, Takaro T, Hultgren H, Peduzzi PL. Long-term mortality and mor-

bidity results of the Veterans Administration Randomized Trial of Coronary Artery Bypass Surgery. Circulation 1985; 72:V84–9.

110. Peduzzi P, Hultgren H, Miller C, Pfeifer J. Veterans Administration Cooperative Study of Medical Versus Surgical Treatment for Stable Angina—Progress report. Section 5. The five-year effect of coronary artery bypass surgery on relief of angina. Prog Cardiovasc Dis 1986; 28:267–72.

111. Varnauskas E. Lessons learned from the three randomized coronary bypass surgery trial. Cardiology 1986; 73:204–11.

112. Landolt CC, Guyton RA. Lessons learned from randomized trials of coronary bypass surgery: Viewpoint of the surgeon. Cardiology 1986; 73:212–22.

113. Killip T, Ryan TJ. Randomized trials in coronary bypass surgery. Circulation 1985; 71:418–21.

114. Hamptom JR. Coronary artery bypass grafting for the reduction of mortality: An analysis of the trails. Br Med J 1984; 289:1166–70.

115. Julian DG. The practical implications of the coronary artery surgery trials. Br Heart J 1985; 54:343–50.

116. Califf RM, Hlatky MA, Mark DB, et al. Randomized trials of coronary artery bypass surgery: Impact on clinical practice at Duke University Medical Center. Circulation 1985; 72:V136–44.

117. Davis KB, Fisher L, Pettinger M. The effects of clinical characteristics on the comparison of medical and surgical therapy in the Coronary Artery Surgery Study (CASS) and the Veterans Administration Cooperative trial. Circulation 1985; 72:V117–22.

118. Fisher LD, Davis KB. Design and study similarities and contrasts: The Veterans Administration, European, and CASS randomized trials of coronary artery bypass graft surgery. Circulation 1985; 72:V110–16.

119. Lewis, HD Jr., Davis JW, Archibald DG, Steinke WE, Smitherman TC, Doherty JE III, Schnaper HW, LeWinter MM, Linares E, Pouget JM, Sabharwal SC, Chesler E, DeMots H. Protective effects of aspirin against acute myocardial infarction and death in men with unstable angina. N Engl J Med 1983; 309:396–403.

120. Luchi RJ, Scott SM, Deupree RH, and the Principal Investigators and Their Associates of Veterans Administration Cooperative Study No 28. Comparison of Medical and Surgical Treatment for Unstable Angina Pectoris. N Engl J Med 1987; 316:977–84.

121. Scott SM, Luchi RJ, Deupree RH, and the Veterans Administration Unstable Angina Cooperative Study Group. Veterans Administration Cooperative Study for Treatment of Patients with Unstable Angina. Circulation 1988; 78:(Suppl I):I-113–I-121.

122. Parisi AF, Khuri S, Deupree RH, Sharma GVRK, Scott SM, Luchi RJ. Medical compared with surgical management of unstable angina 5 Year mortality and morbidity in the Veterans Administration Study. Circulation 1989; 80:1176–89.

123. Russell RO, Moraski RE, Kouchoukos N, et al. Unstable angina pectoris. National Cooperative Study Group to Compare Medical and Surgical Therapy. I. Report of protocol and patient population. Am J Cardiol 1976; 37:896–902.

124. Russell RO, Moraski RE, Kouchoukos N, et al. Unstable angina pectoris:

National Cooperative Study Group to Compare Surgical and Medical Therapy. II. In-hospital experience and initial follow-up results in patients with one, two, and three vessel disease. Am J Cardiol 1978; 42:839–48.

125. Russell RO, Moraski RE, Kouchoukos N, et al. Unstable angina pectoris: National Cooperative Study Group to Compare Surgical and Medical Therapy. III. Results in patients with S-T segment elevation during pain. Am J Cardiol 1980; 45:819–24.

126. Russell RO, Moraski RE, Kouchoukos N, et al. Unstable angina pectoris: National Cooperative Study Group to Compare Medical and Surgical Therapy. IV. Results in patients with left anterior descending artery disease. Am J Cardiol 1981; 48:517–24.

127. Roubin GS, Harris PJ, Eckhardt I, Hensley W, Kelly DT. Intravenous nitroglycerin in refractory unstable angina pectoris. Aust NZ J Med 1982; 12:598–602.

128. Squire A, Cantor R, Packer M. Abstract: Limitations of continuous intravenous nitroglycerin prophylaxis in patients with refractory angina at rest. Circulation 1982; 66(Suppl II):120.

129. Dauwe F, et al. Abstract: Intravenous nitroglycerin-refractory unstable angina. Am J Cardiol 1979; 43:416.

130. Brodsky SJ, et al. Abstract: Intravenous nitroglycerin-infusion in unstable angina. Clin Res 1980; 28:608A.

131. Curfman GD, Heinsimer JA, Lozner EC, Fung HL. Intravenous nitroglycerin in the treatment of spontaneous angina pectoris: A prospective randomized trial. Circulation 1983; 67:276–82.

132. McGregor M. Pathogenesis of angina pectoris and role of nitrates in relief of myocardial ischemia. Am J Med 1983; 56:21–7.

133. Parodi O, Maseri A, Simonetti I. Management of unstable angina at rest by verapamil. Br Heart J 1979; 41:167–74.

134. Mehta J, Pepine CJ, Day M, Guerrero JR, Conti CR. Short term efficacy of oral verapamil in rest angina. Am J Med 1981; 71:977–82.

135. Holland Interuniversity Nifedipine-Metoprolol Trial Research Group. Early treatment of unstable angina in the coronary care unit: A randomized double-blind placebo controlled comparison of recurrent ischemia in patients treated with nifedipine and metoprolol or both. Br Heart J 1986; 56:400–13.

136. Theroux P, Taeymans Y, Morrissette D, et al. A randomized study comparing propanolol and diltiazem in the treatment of unstable angina. J Am Coll Cardiol 1985; 5:717–22.

137. Gottlieb SO, Weisfeldt ML, Ouyang P, et al. The effect of the addition of propanolol to therapy with nifedipine for unstable angina pectoris: A randomized double-blind placebo controlled trial. Circulation 1986; 73:331–7.

138. Muller JE, Turi ZG, Pearl ED, et al. Nifedipine in conventional therapy for unstable angina pectoris: A randomized double-blind comparison. Circulation 1984; 69:728–39.

139. Gerstenblith G, Ouyang P, Achuff SC, et al. Nifedipine in unstable angina. N Engl J Med 1982; 306:885–9.

140. Norris RM, Sammel NL, Clark ED, Smith WN, Williams B. Protective effect of propanolol on impending myocardial infarction. Lancet 1978:907–9.

141. Yusuf S, Peto R, Bennett D, et al. Early intravenous atenolol treatment of suspected acute myocardial infarction. Lancet 1980:273–6.

142. Telford AM, Wilson C. Trial of heparin vs. atenolol in prevention of myocardial infarction in intermediate coronary syndrome. Lancet 1981:1225–8.

143. Ambrose JA, Alexopoulos D. Thrombolysis in unstable angina with a beneficial effect of thrombolytic therapy in myocardial infarction: The plight of patients with unstable angina. J Am Coll Cardiol 1989; 13:1666–70.

144. Gold HK, Johns JA, Leimbach RC, Yasuda T, Cohen D. Thrombolytic therapy for unstable angina pectoris: Rationale and results. J Am Coll Cardiol 1987; 10:91b–95b.

145. Gersh BJ, Robertson T. The efficacy of percutaneous transluminal coronary angioplasty (PTCA) is coronary artery disease—Why we need randomized trials. In: Topol EJ, ed. Textbook of interventional cardiology. Chapter 12. Philadelphia: Saunders 1990:240–53.

146. Anderson HV, Roubin GS, Leimgruber PP, Douglas JS Jr, King SB III, Gruentzig AR. Primary angiographic success rates of percutaneous transluminal coronary angioplasty. Am J Cardiol 1985; 56:712–7.

147. Detre KM, Myler RK, Kelsey SF, Van Raden M, To T, Mitchell H. Baseline characteristics of patients in the National Heart, Lung, and Blood Institute Percutaneous Transluminal Coronary Angioplasty Registry. Am J Cardiol 1984; 53:7C–11C.

148. Oakley GD. Coronary angioplasty—What can we reasonably expect? Br Heart J 1986; 55:221–2.

149. Detre KM, Holubkov R, Kelsey S, et al. Percutaneous transluminal coronary angioplasty in 1985–1986 and 1977–1981. The National Heart, Lung, and Blood Institute Registry. N Engl J Med 1988; 318:265–70.

150. Holmes DR Jr, Holubkov R, Vliestra RE, et al. Comparison of complications during percutaneous transluminal coronary angioplasty from 1977 to 1985 to 1986: The National Heart, Lung, and Blood Institute Percutaneous Transluminal Coronary Angioplasty Registry. J Am Coll Cardiol 1988; 12: 1149–55.

151. Vandormael MG, Chaitman BR, Ischinger T, et al. Immediate and short-term benefit of multilesion coronary angioplasty: Influence of degree of revascularization. J Am Coll Cardiol 1985; 6:983–91.

152. Thomas ES, Most AS, Williams DO. Coronary angioplasty for patients with multivessel coronary artery disease: Follow-up clinical status. Circulation 1988; 115:8–13.

153. Cowley MJ, Dorros G, Kelsey SF, Van Raden M, Detre KM. Acute coronary events associated with percutaneous transluminal coronary angioplasty. Am J Cardiol 1984; 53:12C–16C.

154. Meier B, Gruentzig AR, Hollman J, Ischinger T, Bradford JM. Does length or eccentricity of coronary stenoses influence the outcome of transluminal dilatation? Circulation 1983; 67:497–99.

155. Melchoir JP, Meier B, Urban P, et al. Percutaneous transluminal coronary angioplasty for chronic total coronary artery occlusion. Am J Cardiol 1987; 59:535–8.

156. Safian RD, Snyder LD, Snyder LD, et al. Long-term results and follow-up of

coronary angioplasty of totally occluded coronary arteries. Circulation 1985; 72(Suppl):141.

157. Kereiakes DJ, Selmon MR, McAuley BJ, Sheehan DJ, Simpson JB. Angioplasty in total coronary artery occlusion: experience in 76 consecutive patients. J Am Coll Cardiol 1985; 6:526–33.

158. Andrae GE, Myler RK, Clark DA, Shaw RE, Murphy MC. Acute complications following coronary angioplasty of totally occluded vessels. Circulation 1987; 76(Suppl):IV400.

159. Rentrop P, Cohen B, Hosat S, Cohen M. Technical factors resulting in decreased incidence of CABG after PTCA. Circulation 1985; 72(Suppl):399.

160. Dorros G, Janke L. Percutaneous transluminal coronary angioplasty in patients over the age of 70 years. Cathet Cardiovasc Diag 1986; 12:223–9.

161. Raizner AE, Hust RG, Lewis JM, Winters WL Jr, Batty JW, Roberts R. Transluminal coronary angioplasty in the elderly. Am J Cardiol 1986; 57:29–32.

162. Hust RG, Raizner AE, Lewis JM, Winters WL Jr, Batty JW. Transluminal coronary angioplasty in the elderly: An important therapeutic option. Circulation 1984; 70(Suppl):36.

163. Simpendorfer C, Raymond R, Schraider J, et al. Early and long-term results of percutaneous transluminal coronary angioplasty in patients 70 years of age and older with angina pectoris. Am J Cardiol 1988; 62:959–61.

164. Kohli RS, Vetrovec GW, DiSciascio G, Lewis SA, Nath A, Cowley MJ. Coronary angioplasty in patients with severe depression of left ventricular function. J Am Coll Cardiol 1989; 13:474–6 (Abstract).

165. Taylor GJ, Rabinovich E, Mikell FL, et al. Percutaneous transluminal coronary angioplasty as palliation for patients considered poor surgical candidates. Am Heart J 1986; 111:840–4.

166. Douglas JS Jr, King SB III, Roubin GS, et al. Native coronary artery angioplasty in patients with previous coronary bypass surgery: update of in-hospital and long-term results. Circulation 1987; 76(Suppl):IV465.

167. Ford WB, Wholey MH, Zikria EA, Somadani SR, Sullivan ME. Percutaneous transluminal dilation of aortocoronary saphenous vein bypass grafts. Chest 1981; 79:529–35.

168. El Gamal M, Bonnier H, Michels R, Heijman J, Stassen E. Percutaneous transluminal angioplasty of stenosed aortocoronary bypass grafts. Br Heart J 1984; 52:617–20.

169. Ford WB, Wholey MH, Zikria EA, et al. Percutaneous transluminal angioplasty in the management of occlusive disease involving the coronary arteries and saphenous vein bypass grafts: Preliminary results. J Thorac Cardiovasc Surg 1980; 79:1–11.

170. Jones EL, Douglas JS, Gruentzig AR, Craver JM, King SB III, Guyton RA. Percutaneous saphenous vein angioplasty to avoid reoperative bypass surgery. Ann Thorac Surg 1983; 36:389–95.

171. Reeder GS, Bresnahan JF, Holmes DR Jr, et al. Angioplasty for aortocoronary bypass graft stenosis. Mayo Clin Proc 1986; 61:14–9.

172. Douglas J, Robinson K, Schlumpf M, Gruentzig A. Percutaneous transluminal angioplasty in aortocoronary graft stenoses: Immediate results and complications. Circulation 1985; 74(Suppl):363.

173. Dorros G, Lewin RF, Janke L, Brenowitz JB, Johnson WD. Coronary angioplasty in patients with 2 or more prior bypass surgeries. Circulation 1986; 74(Suppl):363.

174. Cote G, Myler RK, Stertzer SH, et al. Percutaneous transluminal coronary angioplasty of stenotic coronary artery bypass grafts: 5 years' experience. J Am Coll Cardiol 1987; 9:8–17.

175. Hartzler GO. Coronary angioplasty is the treatment of choice for multivessel coronary artery disease. Chest 1986; 90:877–82.

176. Wohlgelernter D, Cleman M, Highman HA, Zaret BL. Percutaneous transluminal coronary angioplasty of the ''culprit lesion'' for a management of unstable angina in patients with multivessel coronary artery disease. Am J Cardiol 1986; 58: 460–4.

177. Vliestra RE, Holmes DR Jr, Reeder GS, et al. Balloon angioplasty in multivessel coronary artery disease. Mayo Clin Proc 1983; 58:563–7.

178. Cowley MJ, Vetrovec GW, DiSciascio G, Lewis SA, Hirsh PD, Wolfgang TC. Coronary angioplasty of multiple vessels: short-term outcome and long-term results. Circulation 1985; 72:1314–20.

179. Myler RK, Topol EJ, Shaw RE, et al. Multiple vessel coronary angioplasty: Classification, results, and patterns of restenosis in 494 consecutive patients. Cathet Cardiovasc Diag 1987; 13:1–15.

180. Dorros G, Stertzer SH, Cowley MJ, Myler RK. Complex coronary angioplasty: multiple coronary dilatations. Am J Cardiol 1984; 53:126C–130C.

181. Giorgi LV, Hartzler GO, Rutherford BD, McConahay DR, Johnson WL. Single-procedure PTCA for triple-vessel coronary disease: Results and long-term follow-up. Circulation 1987; 76(Suppl):IV399.

182. Knudtson ML, Hansen JL, Manyari DE, Roth DL, Flintoft VF. The role of incomplete revascularization by PTCA in patients with multivessel coronary artery disease. Circulation 1984; 70(Suppl):108.

183. Bredlau CE, Roubin GS, Leimgruber PP, Douglas JS Jr, King SB III, Gruentzig AR. In-hospital morbidity and mortality in patients undergoing elective coronary angioplasty. Circulation 1985; 72:1044–52.

184. Faxon DP, Detre KM, McCabe CH, et al. Role of percutaneous transluminal coronary angioplasty in the treatment of unstable angina. Report from the National Heart, Lung, and Blood Institute Percutaneous Transluminal Coronary Angioplasty and Coronary Artery Surgery Study Registries. Am J Cardiol 1984; 53:131C–135C.

185. Dorros G, Cowley MJ, Janke L, Kelsey SF, Mullin SM, Van Raden M. In-hospital mortality rate in the National Heart, Lung, and Blood Institute PTCA Registry. Am J Cardiol 1984; 53:17C–21C.

186. Sharma B, Baxley P, Bisset J, Franciosa J, Wyeth RP, Ferris E. Short-term efficacy of coronary angioplasty in unstable angina pectoris. Circulation 1985; 72(Suppl):370.

187. McAuley BJ, Selmon M, Sheehan DJ, Simpson JB. Coronary angioplasty of high risk patients in a combined catheterization laboratory-operating room setting. Circulation 1985; 72(Suppl):217.

188. Bentivoglio LG, Kelsey SF, Cowley MJ, Myler RK, Williams DO, Detre KM.

Outcome of PTCA in stable and unstable angina pectoris. Circulation 1986; 74(Suppl):II123.

189. Lorell BH, McCabe CH, Sipperly ME, Baim DS. Women and PTCA: No feminine mystique. Circulation 1987; 76(Suppl):IV400.

190. McEniery PT, Hollman J, Knezinek V, et al. Comparative safety and efficacy of percutaneous transluminal coronary angioplasty in men and in women. Cathet Cardiovasc Diag 1987; 13:364–71.

191. deFeyter P, van den Brand M, Suryapranata H. Predictors for unfavorable initial and late outcome of PTCA for unstable angina. Circulation 1987; 76(Suppl): IV466.

192. Delinogul U, Gabliani GI, Caralis DG, Kern MJ, Vandormael MG. Percutaneous transluminal coronary angioplasty in patients with coronary intracoronary thrombus. Am J Cardiol 1988; 62:474–6.

193. Simpendorfer C, Belardi J, Bellamy G, Galan K, Franco I, Hollman J. Frequency, management and follow-up of patients with acute coronary occlusions after percutaneous transluminal coronary angioplasty. Am J Cardiol 1987; 59:267–9.

194. Ellis SG, Roubin GS, King SB III, et al. Angiographic and clinical predictors of acute closure after native vessel coronary angioplasty. Circulation 1988; 77: 372–9.

195. Ellis SG, Roubin GS, King SB III, et al. In-hospital cardiac mortality after acute closure after coronary angioplasty: Analysis of risk factors from 8,207 procedures. J Am Coll Cardiol 1988; 11:211–6.

196. Hollman J, Gruentzig AR, Douglas JS Jr, King SB III, Ischinger T, Meier T. Acute occlusion after percutaneous transluminal coronary angioplasty—A new approach. Circulation 1983; 68:725–32.

197. Meyerovitz MF, Friedman PL, Ganz P, Selwyn AP, Levin DC. Acute occlusion developing during or immediately after percutaneous transluminal coronary angioplasty: Nonsurgical treatment. Radiology 1988; 169:491–4.

198. Talley JD, Jones EL, Weintraub WS, King SB III. Coronary artery bypass surgery after failed elective percutaneous transluminal coronary angioplasty: A status report. Circulation 1989; 13:230A.

199. Vliestra RE. Management of acute occlusion after percutaneous transluminal coronary angioplasty. Eur Heart J 1989; 10(Suppl):101–3.

200. Cowley MJ, Dorros G, Kelsey SF, Van Raden M, Detre KM. Emergency coronary bypass surgery after coronary angioplasty: The National Heart, Lung, and Blood Institute's Percutaneous Transluminal Coronary Angioplasty Registry experience. Am J Cardiol 1985; 53:22C–26C.

201. Golding LA, Loop FD, Hollman JL, et al. Early results of emergency surgery after coronary angioplasty. Circulation 1986; 74(Suppl):26–9.

202. Page US, Okies JE, Colburn LQ, Bigelow JC, Salomon NW, Krause AH. Percutaneous transluminal coronary angioplasty: a growing surgical problem. J Thorac Cardiovasc Surg 1986; 92:847–52.

203. Killen DA, Hamaker WR, Reed WA. Coronary artery bypass following percutaneous transluminal coronary angioplasty. Ann Thorac Surg 1985; 40:133–8.

204. Pelletier LC, Pardini A, Renkin J, David PR, Hebert Y, Bourassa MG. Myocardial revascularization after failure of percutaneous transluminal coronary angioplasty. J Thorac Cardiovac Surg 1985; 90:265–71.

205. Norell MS, Lyons J, Layton C, Balcon R. Outcome of early surgery after coronary angioplasty. Br Heart J 1986; 55:223–6.
206. Parsonnet V, Fisch D, Glelchinsky I, et al. Emergency operation after failed angioplasty. J Thorac Cardiovasc Surg 1988; 96:198–203.
207. Connor AR, Vliestra RE, Schaff HV, Ilstrup DM, Orszulak TA. Early and late results of coronary artery bypass after failed angioplasty: Actuarial analysis of late cardiac events and comparison with initially successful angioplasty. J Thorac Cardiovasc Surg 1988; 96:191–7.
208. Harker LA. Role of platelets and thrombosis in mechanisms of acute occlusion and restenosis after angioplasty. Am J Cardiol 1987; 60:20B–28B.
209. Chesbro JH, Lam JY, Badimon L, Fuster V. Restenosis after arterial angioplasty: A hemodynamic response to injury. Am J Cardiol 1987; 60:10B–16B.
210. Faxon DP, Sanborn TA, Haudenschild CC. Mechanisms of angioplasty and its relation to restenosis. Am J Cardiol 1987; 60:5B–9B.
211. McBride W, Lange RA, Hillis LD. Restenosis after successful coronary angioplasty: Pathophysiology and prevention. N Engl J Med 1988; 318:1734–7.
212. Roubin GS, King SB III, Douglas JS Jr. Restenosis after percutaneous transluminal coronary angioplasty: The Emory University Hospital experience. Am J Cardiol 1987; 60:39B–43B.
213. Blackshear JL, O'Callaghan WG, Califf RM. Medical approaches to prevention of restenosis after coronary angioplasty. Cardiology 1987; 9:834–48.
214. Serruys PW, Geuskens R, de Feyter PJ, van den Brand M, Lujiten HE. Incidence of restenosis at 1, 2, 3, and 4 months after successful coronary angioplasty: A quantitative angiographic follow-up study in 345 patients. J Am Coll Cardiol 1987; 9:63A (Abstract).
215. Holmes DR Jr, Vliestra RE, Smith HC, et al. Restenosis after percutaneous transluminal coronary angioplasty (PTCA): A report from the PTCA Registry of the National Heart, Lung, and Blood Institute. Am J Cardiol 1984; 53:77C–81C.
216. Leimgruber PP, Roubin GS, Hollman J, et al. Restenosis after successful coronary angioplasty in patients with single-vessel disease. Circulation 1986; 73: 710–7.
217. Hwang MH, Sihdu P, Pacold I, Johnson S, Scanlon PJ, Loeb HS. Progression of coronary artery disease after percutaneous transluminal coronary angioplasty. Am Heart J 1988; 115:297–301.
218. Black AJ, Anderson HV, Roubin GS, Powelson SW, Douglas JS Jr, King SB III. Repeat coronary angioplasty: correlates of a second restenosis. J Am Coll Cardiol 1988; 11:714–8.
219. Quigley PJ, Hlatky MA, Mark DB, Simonton CA, Hinohara T, Stack RS: Repeat coronary angioplasty: frequency and predictors of second restenosis. Circulation 1987; 76(Suppl):IV215.
219a. Tierstein PS, Hoover CA, Ligon RW, et al. Repeat coronary angioplasty: Efficacy of a third angioplasty for a second restenosis. J Am Coll Cardiol 1989; 13:191–6.
220. Quigley PJ, Hlatky MA, Hinohara T, et al. Repeat percutaneous transluminal coronary angioplasty and predictors of recurrent restenosis. Am J Cardiol 1989; 63:409–13.
220a. Hirzel HO, Eichhorn P, Kappenberger L, Gander MP, Schlumpf M, Gruentzig

AR. Percutaneous transluminal coronary angioplasty: Late results at 5 years following intervention. Am Heart J 1985; 109:575–81.

221. Leimgruber PP, Roubin GS, Anderson HV, et al. Influence of intimal dissection on restenosis after successful coronary angioplasty. Circulation 1987; 72:530–5.

222. Val PG, Bourassa MG, David PR, et al. Restenosis after successful percutaneous transluminal coronary angioplasty: the Montreal Heart Institute experience. Am J Cardiol 1987; 60:50B–55B.

223. Joelson JM, Most AS, Williams DO. Angiographic findings when chest pain recurs after successful percutaneous transluminal coronary angioplasty. Am J Cardiol 1987; 60:792–5.

223a. David PR, Waters DD, Scholl JM, et al. Percutaneous transluminal coronary angioplasty in patients with variant angina. Circulation 1982; 66:695–702.

224. Lambert M, Bonan R, Cote G, et al. Early results, complications, and restenosis rates after multilesion and multivessel percutaneous transluminal coronary angioplasty. Am J Cardiol 1987; 60:788–91.

224a. Henderson RA, Karani S, Bucknall CA, Dritsas A, Timmis AD, Sowton E. Clinical outcome of coronary angioplasty for single-vessel disease. Lancet 1989; 25:546–50.

225. Douglas JS Jr, King SB III, Roubin GS. Influence of the methodology of percutaneous transluminal coronary angioplasty on restenosis. Am J Cardiol 1987; 60:29B–33B.

225a. Shiu MF, Singh A. Spontaneous recanalization of side branches occluded during percutaneous transluminal coronary angioplasty. Br Heart J 1985; 54:215-7.

226. Whitworth HB, Roubin GS, Hollman J, et al. Effect of nifedipine on recurrent stenosis after percutaneous transluminal coronary angioplasty. J Am Coll Cardiol 1986; 8:1271–6.

227. Schwartz L, Bourassa MG, Lesperance J, et al. Aspirin and dipyridamole in the prevention of restenosis after percutaneous transluminal coronary angioplasty. N Engl J Med 1988; 318:1714–9.

228. Urban P, Buller N, Fox K, Shapiro L, Bayliss J, Rickards A. Lack of effect of warfarin on the restenosis rate or on clinical outcome after balloon coronary angioplasty. Br Heart J 1988; 60:485–8.

229. Myler RK, Shaw RE, Stertzer SH, Clark DA, Fishman J, Murphy MC. Recurrence after coronary angioplasty. Cathet Cardiovasc Diag 1987; 13:77–86.

230. Hirshfeld JW Jr, Goldberg S, MacDonald R, et al. Lesion and procedure-related variables predictive of restenosis after PTCA—A report from the M-HEART Study. Circulation 1987; 76(Suppl):IV215.

231. Stone GW, Rutherford BD, McConahay DR, et al. A randomized trial of corticosteroids for the prevention of restenosis in 102 patients undergoing repeat coronary angioplasty. Cathet Cardiovasc Diag 1989; 18:227–31.

232. Gruentzig AR, Schlumpf M, Siegenthaler W. Long-term results after coronary angioplasty. Circulation 1984; 70(Suppl):II–323.

233. Kouz S, David PR, Bourassa MG. Clinical and angiographic follow-up between 18 months and 3 to 4 years after transluminal coronary angioplasty (PTCA). Circulation 1985; 72(Suppl):III-370.

234. Gruentzig AR, King SB III, Schlumpf M, Siegenthaler W. Long-term follow-up

after percutaneous transluminal coronary angioplasty: The early Zurich experience. N Engl J Med 1987; 316:1127–32.

235. Rupperecht HJ, Brennecke R, Bernhard G, Erbel R, Pop T, Meyer J. Analysis of risk factors of restenosis after PTCA. Cathet Cardiovasc Diag 1990; 19:151–9.

236. Arora RR, Konrad K, Badwar K, Hollman J. Restenosis after transluminal coronary angioplasty: A risk factor analysis. Cathet Cardiovasc Diag 1990; 19:17–22.

237. Lembo NJ, Black AJ, Roubin GS, et al. Effects of pretreatment with aspirin plus dipyridamole on frequency and type of acute complications of percutaneous transluminal coronary angioplasty. Am J Cardiol 1990; 65:422–6.

238. Beatt KJ, Serruys PW, Hugenholtz PG. Restenosis after coronary angioplasty: new standards for clinical studies. J Am Coll Cardiol 1990; 15:491–8.

239. Botman CJ, el Gamal M, el Deeb F, et al. Percutaneous transluminal coronary angioplasty more than twice for the same coronary lesion. Eur Heart J 1989; 10(Suppl H):112–6.

240. Bourassa MG, Fisher LD, Campeau L, Gillespie MJ, McConney M, Lesperance J. Long-term fate of bypass grafts: The Coronary Artery Surgery Study (CASS) and Montreal Heart Institute experience. Circulation 1985; 72:V71–8.

241. Sharma GV, Khuri SF, Josa M, Folland ED, Parisi AF. The effect of antiplatelet therapy on saphenous vein coronary artery bypass graft patency. Circulation 1983; 68(Suppl):II218–21.

242. Campeau L, Lesperance J, Bourassa MG. Natural history of saphenous vein aortocoronary bypass grafts. Mod Concepts Cardiovasc Diag 1984; 53:59–63.

243. Palac RT, Meadows WR, Hwang MH, Loeb HS, Pifarre R, Gunmar RM. Risk factors related to progressive narrowing in aorto coronary vein grafts studies 1 and 5 years after surgery. Circulation 1982; 66(Suppl):140–4.

244. Brower RWm Laird Meeter K, Serruys PW, Meester GT, Hugenholtz PG. Long-term follow-up after coronary artery bypass graft surgery: progression and regression of disease in native coronary circulation and bypass grafts. Br Heart J 1983; 50:42–7.

245. Lylte BW, Loop FD, Cosgrove DM, Ratliff NB, Easley K, Taylor PC. Long-term (5–12 years) serial studies of internal mammary artery and saphenous vein coronary bypass grafts. J Thorac Cardiovasc Surg 1985; 89:248–58.

246. FitzGibbon GM, Leach AJ, Keon WJ, Burton JR, Kafka HP. Coronary bypass graft fate: angiographic study of 1,179 vein grafts early, one, and five years after operation. J Thorac Cardiovasc Surg 1986; 91:773–8.

247. Bjork VO, Ekestrom S, Henze A, Ivert T, Landou C. Early and late patency of aortocoronary vein grafts. Scand J Thorac Cardiovasc Surg 1981; 15:11–21.

248. Chesebro JH, Clements IP, Fuster V, et al. A platelet-inhibitor drug trial in coronary artery bypass operations: Benefit of perioperative dipyridamole and aspirin therapy on early postoperative vein graft patency. N Engl J Med 1982; 307:73–8.

249. Chesebro JH, Fuster V, Elveback LR, et al. Effect of dipyridamole and aspirin on late vein-graft patency after coronary bypass operations. N Engl J Med 1984; 210:209-14.

250. Brooks N., Wright J, Sturridge M, et al. Randomized placebo controlled trial of

aspirin and dipyridamole in the prevention of coronary vein graft occlusions. Br Heart J 1985; 53:201–7.

251. Pantely GA, Goodnight SH Jr, Rahimtoola SH, et al. Failure of antiplatelet and anticoagulant therapy to improve patency of grafts after coronary artery bypass: A controlled, randomized study. N Engl J Med 1979; 301:962–6.

252. Grondin CM, Campeau L, Lesperance J, Enjalbert M, Bourassa MG. Comparison of late changes in internal mammary artery and saphenous vein grafts in two consecutive series of patients 10 years after operation. Circulation 1984; 70(Suppl):208–12.

253. Cosgrove DM, Loop FD, Lytle BW, et al. Does mammary artery grafting increase surgical risk? Circulation 1985; 72(Suppl):170–4.

254. Jones JW, Ochsner JL, Mills NL, Hughes L. Clinical comparison between patients with saphenous vein and internal mammary artery as a coronary graft. J Thorac Cardiovasc Surg 1980; 80:334–41.

255. Spencer FC. The internal mammary artery: The ideal coronary bypass graft? N Engl J Med 1986; 314:50–1.

256. Loop FD, Lytle BW, Cosgrove DM, et al. Influence of the internal-mammary-artery graft on 10-year survival and other cardiac events. N Engl J Med 1986; 314:1–6.

257. Bourassa MG, Wilson JW, Detre KM, Kelsey SF, Robertson T, Passamani ER. Long-term follow-up of coronary angioplasty: The 1977–1981 National Heart, Lung, and Blood Institute registry. Eur Heart J 1989; 10(Suppl G):36–41.

258. Faxon DP, Ruocco N, Jacobs AK. Long-term outcome of patients after percutaneous transluminal coronary angioplasty. Circulation 1990; 81:IV9–13.

259. Cowley MJ, DiSciascio G, Kelly K, et al. Long term efficacy of multiple vessel coronary angioplasty. Circulation 1987; 76(Suppl):IV466.

260. Roubin G, Weintraub WS, Sutor C, et al. Event free survival after successful angioplasty in multivessel coronary artery disease. J Am Coll Cardiol 1987; 9:15A (Abstract).

261. The NHLBI PTCA Registry Investigators. One-year follow-up of 1985–86 NHLBI PTCA Registry. Circulation 1987; 76(Suppl):IV466.

262. Califf RM, Harrell FE Jr, Lee KL, et al. The evolution of medical and surgical therapy for coronary artery disease: A 15-year perspective. JAMA 1989; 261:2077–86.

263. Kelly ME, Taylor GJ, Moses HW, et al. Comparative cost of myocardial revascularization: Percutaneous transluminal angioplasty and coronary artery bypass surgery. J Am Coll Cardiol 1985; 5:16–20.

264. Black AJ, Roubin GS, Sutor C, et al. Comparative costs of percutaneous transluminal coronary angioplasty and coronary artery bypass grafting in multivessel coronary artery disease. Am J Cardiol 1988; 62:809–11.

265. Jang GC, Block PC, Cowley MJ, et al. Comparative cost analysis of coronary angioplasty and coronary bypass surgery: Results from a national cooperative study. Circulation 1982; 66(Suppl):II124.

266. Wittels E, Hay JW, Gotto AM. Medical costs of coronary artery disease in the United States. Am J Cardiol 1990; 65:432–40.

267. Wilson JM, Dunn EJ, Wright CB, et al. The cost of simultaneous surgical

standby for percutaneous transluminal coronary angioplasty. J Thorac Cardiovasc Surg 1986; 91:362–70.

268. Holmes DR Jr, Vliestra RE, Fisher LD, et al. Follow-up of patients from the Coronary Artery Surgery Study (CASS) potentially suitable for percutaneous transluminal coronary angioplasty. Am Heart J 1983; 106:981–8.

269. Knudtson ML, Hansen JL, Manyari DE, Roth DL, Flintoft VF. The role of incomplete revascularization by PTCA in patients with multivessel coronary artery disease. Circulation 1984; 70(Suppl):II–108.

270. Schaff HV, Gersch BJ, Fisher LD, et al. Detrimental effect of peri-operative myocardial infarction on late survival after coronary artery bypass. Report from the Coronary Artery Surgery Study—CASS. J Thorac Cardiovasc Surg 1984; 88:972–81.

271. Cameron A, Kemp HG Jr, Shimomura S, et al. Aortocoronary bypass surgery: A 7-year follow-up. Circulation 1978; 60(Suppl):I9–13.

272. Buda AJ, Macdonald IL, Anderson MJ, Strauss HD, David TE, Berman ND. Long-term results following coronary bypass operation: importance of preoperative factors and complete revascularization. J Thorac Cardiovasc Surg 1981; 82:383–90.

273. Jones EL, Craver JM, King SB III, et al. Clinical, anatomic, and functional descriptors influencing morbidity, survival, and adequacy of revascularization following coronary bypass. Ann Surg 1980; 192:390–402.

274. Jones EL, Craver JM, Guyton RA, Bone DK, Hatcher CR Jr, Riechwald N. Importance of complete revascularization in performance of the coronary artery bypass operation. Am J Cardiol 1983; 51:7–12.

275. Foster ED, Fisher LD, Kaiser GC, Myers WO. Comparison of operative mortality and morbidity for initial and repeat coronary artery bypass grafting: The Coronary Artery Surgery Study (CASS) registry experience. Ann Thorac Surg 1984; 38:563–70.

276. Weintraub WS, Jones EL, King SB III, et al. Changing use of coronary angioplasty and coronary bypass surgery in the treatment of chronic coronary artery disease. Am J Cardiol 1985; 56:712–7.

Index

Acute occlusive syndrome
 with PTCA, 319, 362–363
Age
 risk factor for CABG, 162, 164,
  171, 172, 174, 195, 389,
  390
 risk factor for PTCA, 221, 318,
  377
Angina
 changing pattern (crescendo), 4,
  63, 81, 238
 equivalent, 3, 63
 exertional, 4
 new onset, 5, 63, 81, 238
 postmyocardial infarction, 4–9,
  63, 269, 274
 progressive, 4, 63, 81, 238
 type I unstable, 122, 238
 type II unstable, 123, 238
 unstable, 3, 41, 63, 81, 121,
  183, 238, 430–431

Angiography
 coronary, 11, 43, 48, 50, 60,
  70–71, 105, 123, 127, 273
 ventriculography, 11, 123
Angioplasty (see also Percutaneous
  transluminal coronary
  angioplasty)
 "culprit lesion," 223, 240, 256
 morbidity, 216, 217, 240–243,
  247, 254, 281
 mortality, 216, 217, 240–243,
  247, 254, 281, 318,
  328–331, 390–394
 multivessel disease, 223, 240,
  256
 for rest angina, 224, 390–394
 single vessel disease, 222
 success rates, 241–243, 247,
  255, 295
  anatomic factors, 295, 298
  technical factors, 294, 299

Angioplasty (*cont.*)
  support, mechanical
    coronary sinus retroperfusion,
      269–292, 293–314, 317–336
  support, pharmacologic
    anticoagulation, 339–342
    antiplatelet therapy, 342–345
    beta blockers, 351
    calcium blockers, 347–349
    fibrinolytic therapy, 345–347
    nitrates, 349–350
    oxygen carriers (perfluoro
      chemicals), 320–321,
      351–354, 368–369
  treatment of unstable angina,
    106, 215–236, 237–252,
    253–267
    patients with prior CABG,
      293–314
    patients with reduced LVEF,
      253–267
    patients with recent MI,
      269–292
    patients requiring IABP
    patients requiring IV
      nitroglycerin
Angioscopy, 49, 51, 71
Anticoagulation
  heparin, 87–91, 101, 107–109,
    112
  coumadin (warfarin), 84, 88
Antiplatelet agents
  aspirin, 85–90, 101, 107–109,
    112
  dipyridamole, 88
  suffinpyrazone, 87
  ticlopidine, 89, 101
Aspirin, 85–90, 101, 107–109,
  112
Atenolol, 90–91, 107–109
Autoperfusion catheter, 320–322,
  365–368

BARI (Bypass Angioplasty
  Revascularization
  Investigation), 36, 106,
  230, 433
Beta blocker
  atenolol, 90–91, 107–109
  metoprolol, 96, 97, 107–109
  propranolol, 90–97, 107–109
BHAT (Beta-blocker Heart Attack
  Trial), 278
Bias, selection, 35, 82, 154, 190,
  232, 431
Bifurcation lesions, PTCA,
  318–319

CABG (coronary artery bypass
  grafting)
  for failed angioplasty, 177
  on incidence of myocardial
    infarction, 192
  on quality of life, 138
  on rehospitalization, 138
  for relief of angina, 139, 191
  on return to work, 141
  on treadmill exercise, 141, 191
  on ventricular fraction, 192
CABRI (Coronary Angioplasty
  Bypass Revascularization
  Investigation), 106
Calcified lesions, PTCA, 318–319
Calcium channel blocker
  diltiazem, 92–107, 107–109
  nifedipine, 93–98, 107–109
  verapamil, 93, 107–109
Canadian multicenter aspirin study,
  87
CASS (Coronary Artery Surgery
  Study), 16, 35, 50, 174,
  175, 192, 193, 227
Chest pain, 186
  ischemic versus non-ischemic,
    187

Clinical trials
BARI, 106
CABRI, 106
CASS, 16, 35, 50, 174, 175,
192, 193, 227
concurrent control, 84, 91
Diltiazem Reinfarction Study,
65, 273
DUAST (Dutch Angioplasty
Surgery Trials), 106
EAST (Emory Angioplasty
Surgery Trials), 106
European Coronary Surgery
Study, 192
GABI (German Angioplasty
Bypass Investigation), 106
HINT (Holland Interuniversity
Nifedipine Metoprolol
Trial), 96
ISIS (International Study
of Infarct Survival), 16
National Cooperative Medical
versus Surgical Unstable
Angina, 14, 145–155, 190
Netherlands Sixty Plus
Reinfarction Study, 84
randomized control, 14, 83,
85–89, 91, 122, 145–155,
190–194, 227, 405–417,
431–434
VA Cooperative Aspirin Study,
14, 35, 61, 85–87, 110
VA Cooperative Medical versus
Surgical Unstable Angina,
14, 110, 121–143, 148, 190
Collateral vessel, 257, 276, 278
Comorbidity, 165, 172, 201,
393–394
Complex lesions, 43, 45, 50, 60,
70–71, 218, 237, 278
concentric, 45
eccentric, 45, 278

Complications
of intraaortic balloon pump, 323,
371–372
of percutaneous bypass,
326–331, 373
(COPD) Chronic obstructive
pulmonary disease
risk for CABG, 168, 171, 172,
201–202
Coronary artery
digital angiography, 420–422
Doppler flow velocity, 422
thrombosis, 42, 48, 50, 51, 54,
60, 69–76, 82, 218, 275,
337–338
ultrasound, 423
Videodensitometry, 423
Coronary sinus retroperfusion, 258,
322
Crossover
angioplasty to surgery, 434
medical to angioplasty, 432
medical to surgery, 128, 148,
190, 432
surgery to angioplasty, 434

Definitions
"clinical," 15
"investigational," 153–154,
430–431
"medically refractory," 99,
105–112
"unstable angina," 99, 105–112
Digital angiography, 420–422
Diltiazem, 92–97, 107–109
Diltiazem Reinfarction Study, 65,
273, 278
Dipyridamole, 88
DUAST (Dutch Angioplasty
Surgery Trial), 106
Dyspnea, angina equivalent, 3,
63

EAST (Emory Angioplasty Surgery
    Trial), 106
Ejection fraction (left ventricular),
    133, 148, 174
  risk factor for CABG, 163, 167,
    172, 179, 193, 388
  risk factor for PTCA, 391, 392
Electrocardiographic changes
    with rest angina, 10, 63,
    81, 112, 149–150, 186–189,
    238, 239
Emergency CABG for failed
    angioplasty, 218, 240, 281,
    295, 361–384
Endothelial injury, 59, 61, 62, 65,
    66, 72, 275, 338
End points
  "hard," 105, 124, 148–151,
    230, 433
  "soft," 105, 230, 433
Esophageal pain, 189
Estimated mortality, 159, 195
European Coronary Surgery Study,
    192
Exclusions from clinical studies,
    12–13, 16–17, 35–36, 124,
    127, 147, 190, 230

Fibrinopeptide A, 71

GABI (German Angioplasty Bypass
    Investigation), 106
General medical condition, risk
    for CABG, 169, 393–394

Hemopump for PTCA, 332
Heparin, 87–90, 91, 101, 107–109,
    112
  after angioplasty, 341–342
  before angioplasty, 339–341
  during angioplasty, 341

High risk
  for CABG, 151–152, 162–181,
    184, 194, 207, 386–390,
    393–394
  for PTCA, 218, 240, 246, 253,
    254, 318–339, 362, 363,
    390–394
Hypothesis, 34, 53, 145, 193, 230,
    405–407

Identifying viable myocardium,
    261, 274, 282
  dobutamine echo, 282
  thallium scan, 261, 274, 282
  PET scan, 262, 274, 282
Inclusion criteria, 4–9, 190, 230
  National Cooperative unstable
    angina trial, 146
  VA Cooperative Aspirin Study,
    86
  VA Cooperative Medical versus
    Surgical Unstable Angina
    Trial, 122–127
Infarction, myocardial (*see also*
    Myocardial infarction), 9,
    48, 54, 59, 63, 81, 123,
    133, 269–292
Infarct-related artery, 275
Intention to treat, 36, 133, 154,
    431
Internal mammary artery, 128,
    153, 293, 405–417
Intraaortic balloon counterpulsation,
    386–389
  risk for CABG, 165, 168, 171,
    172, 179
  risk for PTCA, 390–394
  support for PTCA, 322–323,
    369–372
Intravascular ultrasound, 51
Intravenous balloon pumping,
    support for CABG, 376

Intravenous Nitroglycerin
  risk for CABG, 165, 168, 171,
    172, 179, 386–389
  risk for PTCA, 390–394
Ischemia, myocardial
  at a distance, 270, 274
  of the infarct zone, 270, 274
  silent, 3, 63, 74
  symptomatic, 3, 4, 59
ISIS (International Study of Infarct
    Survival), 16

Late vessel closure after PTCA,
    329–330
Left anterior descending artery,
    150–151, 412
Left main stenosis
  risk for CABG, 122, 147, 163,
    169, 174, 204, 387
  risk for PTCA, 329, 377, 393

Medically refractory angina,
    105–112, 128, 152
  risk factor for CABG, 171, 172,
    175, 179, 195, 386–389
  risk factor for PTCA, 390–394
Medical treatment of unstable
    angina, 74, 81–102,
    105–112, 245
Metanalysis, 97, 101
Metoprolol, 96, 97, 107, 109
Multivariate analysis, 161
Myocardial infarction, 9, 48, 54,
    59, 63, 81, 123, 133,
    269–292
  Q-wave, 41, 64, 124, 269
  non-Q-wave, 41, 64, 124, 269

National Cooperative Medical
    versus Surgical Trial
    (unstable angina), 14, 35,
    110, 145–155, 190, 193

National Registry of Supported
    Angioplasty, 328–331,
    376–379
New York State Surgical
    Surveillance, 178
Nifedipine, 93–98, 107–109
Nitroglycerin, intravenous, 98–100,
    107–109, 112
Norwegian Timolol Trial, 278

Observed mortality, 159, 195
Observer bias, 190
Only patent vessel, 330, 377
"Open artery hypothesis" (late
    reperfusion), 265, 275
Operative morbidity, 124, 149
Operative mortality, 124, 149, 157,
    183, 244, 386–390
Operative survival, 128, 148
Oxygen-carrying solution (Fluosol),
    PTCA support, 320–321,
    351–354, 368–369

Pathology
  coronary artery, 69
  saphenous vein grafts, 299–309
Pathophysiology of unstable
    angina, 5, 274–476
  progression of atherosclerosis,
    43, 70
  thrombosis, 42, 48, 51, 69–71,
    82
  unstable plaque, 42, 43, 69–71,
    82
  vasospasm, 61, 73, 92
Percutaneous cardiopulmonary
    bypass, 258, 322–331,
    372–374
Perioperative infarction, 191, 244
Pharmacologically assisted PTCA,
    319–322, 337–360

Placebo effect, 190
Plaque disruption, 41, 54, 69–71,
    82, 237, 275, 338
Platelet aggregation, 71, 82, 237,
    275, 338
Postmyocardial infarction
  angina, 269, 274–278
  prognosis, 272
    age, 274
    coronary anatomy, 273, 274,
      276–278
    ejection fraction, 273, 274,
      276–278
    thrombolytic therapy, 275
Preangioplasty heparin, 218,
    339–341
Pressure gradient, angioplasty
    (PTCA) results, 302, 420
Prinzmetal's angina, 41, 73, 93
Prior CABG
  risk factor for CABG, 165, 168,
    171, 172, 179, 201, 390
  risk factor for PTCA, 221,
    295–296, 391
Propranolol, 90–91, 92–97,
    107–109
Prospective versus retrospective,
    34, 122, 405–406, 431
Prostacyclin, 62, 71, 100
Percutaneous transluminal coronary
    angioplasty (PTCA)
  event-free survival, 227
  myocardial infarction, 220, 231
  on quality of life, 231
  registry (NHLBI), 34, 222, 227
  relief of angina, 216, 220, 231
  on survival, 231
  on treadmill exercise, 219
  on ventricular function, 219,
    224, 231, 259
Pump perfusion for angioplasty,
    320–322

Quality of care, 159, 195
Quality of life, CABG, 138

RITA (randomized interventional
    treatment of angina), 106
Recent myocardial infarction (30
    days)
  risk factor for CABG, 168, 171,
    172, 279, 280, 387–390
  risk factor for PTCA, 221, 269,
    281, 391–394
Restenosis, 62, 65, 219, 239,
    295–296
Risks of emergent CABG
    for failed PTCA
Risk factors
  for CABG
    age, 162, 164, 171, 172, 174,
      195, 389, 390
    ejection fraction, 163, 167,
      172, 179, 193, 388
    general medical condition,
      169, 393–394
    IABP, 165, 168, 171, 172,
      179
    intravenous nitroglycerin, 165,
      168, 171, 172, 179,
      386–389
    left main stenosis, 122, 147,
      163, 169, 174, 204, 387
    medically refractory angina,
      171, 172, 175, 179, 195,
      386–389
    prior CABG, 165, 168, 171,
      172, 179, 201, 390
    recent myocardial infarct, 168,
      171, 172, 279, 280,
      387–390
  for PTCA
    age, 221, 318, 377
    anatomy, 245, 298
    ejection fraction, 391, 392

Risk factors (*cont.*)
  IABP, 390–394
  intravenous nitroglycerin,
    390–394
  left main stenosis, 329, 377,
    393
  medically refractory angina,
    390–394
  prior CABG, 221, 295–296,
    391
  recent myocardial infarction,
    221, 269, 281, 391–394
  technical factors, 294, 299

Sample size, 35, 36, 82, 125, 154,
    405–417, 431
Saphenous vein graft, 128, 185,
    293, 298–312
Skeletal muscle pain, 189
Staged angioplasty, 257, 331
ST segment on surface ECG
  depression, 149–150, 238, 273
  elevation, 149–150, 273
Stroma-free hemoglobin, 368–369
Stunned or hibernating
    myocardium, 257, 261
Sulfinpyrazone, 87
Supply versus demand,
    pathophysiology of
    ischemia, 41, 73, 82, 92,
    110
Surgical treatment (CABG)
    of unstable angina, 106,
    121–143, 145–155,
    157–181, 183–212, 244,
    386–390, 394

Tandem lesions, PTCA, 319
Ticlopidine (antiplatelet agent), 89,
    101
Total occlusions, PTCA, 223

Transseptal-supported PTCA,
    331–332
Treatment of unstable angina
  algorithms for unstable angina,
    245, 246, 282–284
  angioplasty (PTCA), 215–236,
    237–252, 253–267,
    269–292, 293–314
  medical
    anticoagulants, 42, 50, 71,
    83–85
    antiplatelet agent, 71, 85–90
  beta blockers, 90–98
  calcium blockers, 90–98
  nitrates, 98–100
  surgical (CABG) 121–143,
    145–155, 157–181, 183–212
  thrombolytics, 48, 71

Unfavorable anatomy for PTCA,
    229, 318, 377, 393
Univariate analysis, 161
Unstable angina, 3, 41, 59, 63,
    81, 183, 238–239, 430–434

VA Cooperative Aspirin Study, 14,
    35, 61, 85–87, 434
VA Cooperative Medical vs
    Surgical Trial (stable
    angina), 192
VA Cooperative Medical vs
    Surgical Trial (unstable
    angina), 14, 35, 110,
    121–143, 148, 190, 193,
    434
VA Surgical Registry, 18,
    157–181, 184, 194–195,
    386–390
Vasospasm, 61, 62, 73, 92, 338
Ventricular assist devices, 153,
    374–376

Ventricular function
  risk for CABG
  risk for PTCA, 246, 253, 318,
    377, 391, 392
Verapamil, 93, 107–109

Viable muscle, risk for PTCA,
  318–319, 377, 392–394

Warfarin (coumadin), 84, 88

About the Editors

DOUGLASS ANDREW MORRISON is Director, Cardiac Catheterization Laboratory, Veterans Affairs Medical Center, and Associate Professor of Cardiology, Department of Medicine, the University of Colorado, Denver. The author or coauthor of over 60 journal articles, book chapters, and abstracts, he is a Fellow of the American College of Physicians, American College of Chest Physicians, American College of Cardiology, Clinical Council of the American Heart Association, and Society for Cardiac Angiography and Interventions. Dr. Morrison received the B.A. degree (1969) in biochemistry from Harvard University, Cambridge, Massachusetts, and M.D. degree (1973) from the University of Pittsburgh, Pennsylvania.

PATRICK W. SERRUYS is Professor of Interventional Cardiology, Interuniversity Cardiological Institute of the Netherlands, and Director of the Clinical Research Program of the Catheterization Laboratory, Thoraxcenter, Erasmus University, Rotterdam, The Netherlands. The author or coauthor of over 650 scientific papers and editor or coeditor of five books, he is a Fellow of the American College of Cardiology and scientific council of the International College of Angiology. Dr. Serruys received the M.D. degree (1972) from the Catholic University of Louvain, Louvain, Belgium.